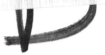

VOX

Super-Mini

MEDICAL

SPANISH
and
ENGLISH
Dictionary

VOX

Super-Mini

MEDICAL

SPANISH
and
ENGLISH
Dictionary

The McGraw·Hill Companies

1 2 3 4 5 6 7 8 9 10 11 12   QLM/QLM   1 9 8 7 6 5 4 3 2

ISBN 978-0-07-178863-2
MHID 0-07-178863-8

e-ISBN 978-0-07-178864-9
e-MHID 0-07-178864-6

Dirección editorial: Jordi Induráin Pons
Coordinación editorial: María José Simón Aragón
Informática editorial: Marc Escarmís Arasa
Realización: Marc Escarmís Arasa

De la parte English-Spanish:
    Responsable: Emilio Ortega Arjonilla
    Redacción: Ana Belén Martínez López y Félix Martínez López
    Revisión: Andrew Hastings y Mercè Piera Fernández

De la parte Español-Inglés:
    Responsable: Andrew Hastings
    Revisión: Mercè Piera Fernández

McGraw-Hill products are available at special quantity discounts to use as premiums and sales promotions or for use in corporate training programs. To contact a representative, please e-mail us at bulksales@ mcgraw-hill.com.

This book is printed on acid-free paper.

Foreword

This *Vox Super-Mini Medical Spanish and English Dictionary* is aimed at professionals in the field of healthcare who in the course of their work come into contact with speakers of Spanish, but it will also prove enormously useful to those users who, having Spanish as their native tongue, need to obtain an accurate English translation for terms from the fields of medicine and health in general.

This Dictionary, with a detailed English-Spanish / Spanish-English bilingual glossary, aims to fill a long-felt gap in Spanish-language medical lexicography: an area where mere approximation or similarity is insufficient, where scientific and terminological precision are de rigueur. The Dictionary was compiled by a wide-ranging team of medical professionals so that not only all specialist fields might be adequately covered, but also nursing, diagnosis and therapeutics.

In the first section of the dictionary, the English-Spanish glossary, there are 6,522 headwords and 5,042 sub-headwords, while in the second part,

Prólogo

El *Vox Super-Mini Medical Spanish and English Dictionary* está destinado a profesionales del ámbito de la salud que por su trabajo tienen relación con personas de origen y habla hispana. Del mismo modo, su contenido puede ser de gran utilidad para todos aquellos usuarios que poseyendo el español como lengua materna, tienen la necesidad de obtener una traducción precisa y rigurosa al inglés de los términos del entorno médico y de la salud.

Es pues este Diccionario un detallado glosario bilingüe inglés-español / español-inglés que pretende cubrir una importante laguna en el ámbito léxico-médico en lengua española, un área donde no cabe una aproximación por similitud o semejanza, sino que requiere del máximo rigor científico y terminológico. En la elaboración del contenido que aquí se presenta ha trabajado un extenso equipo de profesionales en activo de la medicina para poder abarcar todas las diferentes especialidades, además de la terminología propia del ámbito de la enfermería, auxiliaría de clínica, diagnosis y terapéutica.

the Spanish-English glossary, there are 6,204 headwords and 5,092 sub-headwords. All of which adds up to a total of 22,860 references and makes this Dictionary a complete yet portable resource for health care professionals.

In both the subheadwords and in the translations in both languages, we have chosen neither to abbreviate the headword nor substitute it with any special symbol. We have done this in the interests of clarity and to help the user to find the answer to his queries as rapidly as possible. To distinguish them from main headwords, subheadwords appear in italics and in a smaller typeface; this will help the user to orient himself more easily. In this way, the often extensive blocks of subheadwords may be readily identified.

This *Vox Super-Mini Medical Spanish and English Dictionary* also contains a Medical Spanish Phrasebook that will prove invaluable for the production of both written and spoken messages in Spanish.

THE PUBLISHERS

En la primera parte del diccionario, inglés-español, se presentan 6,522 entradas principales y 5,042 suben-tradas; mientras que en la segunda parte, español-inglés, hay 6,204 en-tradas y 5,092 subentradas. Todo ello suma un total de 22,860 regis-tros, lo que hace de este diccionario una herramienta completa y mane-jable para los profesionales de la salud.

En la correlación alfabética de las voces que conforman el diccionario se ha optado por la presentación por extenso de las entradas, evitando en ambos idiomas el uso de elementos de abreviación o sustitución, todo ello con la idea de facilitar al máx-imo la consulta del diccionario y la rápida localización de las dudas del usuario. Para marcar las subentra-das se ha empleado la tipografía cur-siva, además de un cuerpo de letra menor, lo que facilita saber si esta-mos ante una voz principal o ante su conjunto, a veces extenso, de suben-tradas o acepciones.

El *Vox Super-Mini Medical Spanish and English Dictionary* se completa con una **Fraseología médica espa-ñola** muy útil para elaborar men-sajes hablados o escritos en español.

LOS EDITORES

Contents   Índice

Abbreviations used in this dictionary

Abreviaturas usadas en este diccionario

adjective	*adj.*	adjetivo
adverb	*adv.*	adverbio
feminine noun	*f.*	nombre femenino
masculine noun	*m.*	nombre masculino
noun	*n.*	nombre
verb	*v.*	verbo

English - Spanish
Inglés - Español

A

abacterial *adj.* abacteriano, -na.

abalienation *n.* enajenación.
 mental abalienation enajenación mental.

abandonment *n.* abandono.

abasia *n.* abasia.

abbau *n.* descomposición.

abdomen *n.* abdomen.
 acute abdomen abdomen agudo.
 surgical abdomen abdomen quirúrgico.

abdominal *adj.* abdominal.

abdominalgia *n.* abdominalgia.

abduction *n.* abducción.

abductor *adj.* abductor.

aberrant *adj.* aberrante.

aberratio *n.* aberración, aberratio.

aberration *n.* aberración.
 chromosomal aberration aberración cromosómica.
 chromosome aberration aberración cromosómica.

abetalipoproteinemia *n.* abetalipoproteinemia.

ability *n.* habilidad.

ablatio *n.* ablación, ablatio.
 ablatio placentae ablación placentaria, ablatio placentae.
 ablatio retinae ablación retiniana, ablatio retinae.

ablephary *n.* ablefaria.

abnormal *adj.* anormal.

abnormality *n.* anormalidad.

abort *v.* abortar.

abortient *adj.* abortante.

abortigenic *adj.* abortante, abortifaciente.

abortion *n.* aborto.
 abortion in progress aborto en curso.
 accidental abortion aborto accidental.
 elective abortion aborto electivo.
 illegal abortion aborto ilegal.
 induced abortion aborto provocado.
 inevitable abortion aborto inevitable.
 missed abortion aborto diferido, aborto retenido.
 spontaneous abortion aborto espontáneo.
 therapeutic abortion aborto terapéutico.

abortive *adj.* abortivo, -va.

abortus *n.* aborto, abortus.

abrasio *n.* abrasio, abrasión.
 abrasio dentium abrasio dentium, abrasion of the teeth, tooth abrasion.

abrasion *n.* abrasio, abrasión.
 abrasion of the teeth abrasio dentium, abrasión dental, abrasión dentaria.
 corneal abrasion abrasio corneae, abrasión corneal.
 tooth abrasion abrasio dentium, abrasión dental, abrasión dentaria.

abscess *n.* absceso.
 abdominal abscess absceso abdominal.
 acute abscess absceso agudo.
 alveolar abscess absceso alveolar.
 anorectal abscess absceso anorrectal.

biliary abscess absceso biliar.

brain abscess absceso cerebral.

cerebral abscess absceso cerebral.

dental abscess absceso dental, absceso dentoalveolar.

dentoalveolar abscess absceso dental, absceso dentoalveolar.

orbital abscess absceso orbitario.

peridental abscess absceso periodóntico, absceso peridental, absceso periodontal.

periodontal abscess absceso periodóntico, absceso peridental, absceso periodontal.

pulmonary abscess absceso pulmonar.

renal abscess absceso renal.

tonsillar abscess absceso amigdalino.

absence *n.* ausencia.

epileptic absence ausencia epiléptica.

absorption *n.* absorción.

cutaneous absorption absorción cutánea.

drug absorption absorción de fármaco.

intestinal absorption absorción intestinal.

parenteral absorption absorción parenteral.

pathologic absorption absorción patológica.

pathological absorption absorción patológica.

percutaneous absorption absorción percutánea.

abstinence *n.* abstinencia.

alimentary abstinence abstinencia alimentaria.

abstract *n.* abstracto.

abulia *n.* abulia.

abulic *adj.* abúlico, -ca.

abuse *n.* abuso, malos tratos.

abuse of the elderly abuso de ancianos, malos tratos al anciano.

child abuse abuso del niño, malos tratos a menores.

drug abuse abuso de medicamentos.

elder abuse abuso de ancianos, malos tratos al anciano.

emotional abuse malos tratos emocionales.

physical abuse malos tratos físicos.

sexual abuse malos tratos sexuales.

sexual abuse of an adult abuso sexual del adulto.

sexual child abuse abuso sexual del niño.

abutment *n.* contrafuerte, lindero.

acanthosis *n.* acantosis.

acariasis *n.* acariasis.

acaudate *adj.* acaudado, -da, acáudeo, -a.

accelerator *n.* acelerador.

acceptance *n.* aceptación.

access *n.* acceso.

accessorius *n.* accesorio.

accessory *adj.* accesorio, -ria.

accident *n.* accidente.

cerebrovascular accident (CVA) accidente cerebrovascular (ACV).

occupational accident accidente laboral.

professional accident accidente laboral.

accidental *adj.* accidental.

accommodation *n.* acomodación.

accommodation of the eye acomodación del ojo.
accouchement *n.* alumbramiento.
accuracy *n.* exactitud, precisión.
acellular *adj.* acelular.
acephalia *n.* acefalia.
acephalus *n.* acéfalo, acephalus.
acephaly *n.* acefalia.
acetabulum *n.* acetábulo, acetabulum.
acetic *adj.* acético, -ca.
acetone *n.* acetona.
acetonemia *n.* acetonemia.
acetonuria *n.* acetonuria.
ache *n.* dolencia, dolorimiento.
achlorhydria *n.* aclorhidria.
acholia *n.* acolia.
acholuria *n.* acoluria.
acholuric *adj.* acolúrico, -ca.
achondroplasia *n.* acondroplasia.
achondroplasty *n.* acondroplasia.
acid *n.* ácido.
acidic *adj.* acídico, -ca.
acidification *n.* acidificación.
acidify *v.* acidificar.
acidity *n.* acidez.
acidity of the stomach acidez del estómago.
acidosis *n.* acidosis.
compensated acidosis acidosis compensada.
diabetic acidosis acidosis diabética.
lactic acidosis acidosis láctica.
metabolic acidosis acidosis metabólica.
renal acidosis acidosis renal.
respiratory acidosis acidosis respiratoria.
uncompensated acidosis acidosis descompensada.

acidum *n.* ácido, acidum.
aciduria *n.* aciduria.
Acinetobacter *n.* Acinetobacter.
acinic *adj.* acínico, -ca.
acinus *n.* ácino, acinus.
acne *n.* acne, acné.
acne conglobata acné conglobata.
acne rosacea acné rosácea.
acne sebacea acné sebácea.
acne vulgaris acné vulgar.
common acne acné común.
conglobate acne acné conglobata.
infantile acne acné infantil.
acquired *adj.* adquirido, -da.
acrocyanosis *n.* acrocianosis.
acromegalia *n.* acromegalia.
acromegalic *adj.* acromegálico, -ca.
acromegaly *n.* acromegalia.
acromion *n.* acromion.
act *n.* acto.
compulsive act acto compulsivo.
impulsive act acto impulsivo.
reflex act acto reflejo.
voluntary act acto voluntario.
Actinobacillus *n.* Actinobacillus.
Actinomyces *n.* Actinomyces.
actinomycosis *n.* actinomicosis.
action *n.* acción.
drug action acción farmacológica.
reflex action acción refleja.
active *adj.* activo, -va.
activity *n.* actividad.
biological activity actividad biológica.
cholinergic activity actividad colinérgica.
enzyme activity actividad enzimática.
acuity *n.* acuidad, agudeza.

visual acuity agudeza visual.

acupuncture *n.* acupuntura.

acupuncturist *n.* acupuntor, -ra.

acusis *n.* acusia.

adaptation *n.* adaptación.

dark adaptation adaptación a la oscuridad.

adapter *n.* adaptador.

adaptive *adj.* adaptable.

adaptor *n.* adaptador.

addict *n.* adicto, -ta.

drug addict drogadicto, -ta.

addiction *n.* adicción.

Addisonian *adj.* addisoniano, -na, adisoniano, -na.

additive *adj.* aditivo, -va.

food additive aditivo alimentario.

adduct *v.* aducir.

adduction *n.* adducción, aducción.

adductor *adj.* adductor, -ra, aductor, -ra.

adenitis *n.* adenitis.

adenocarcinoma *n.* adenocarcinoma.

adenohypophysis *n.* adenohipófisis.

adenoidectomy *n.* adenoidectomía.

adenoiditis *n.* adenoiditis.

adenoids *n.* adenoides.

adenoma *n.* adenoma.

adenoma of the kidney adenoma renal.

adrenal adenoma adenoma adrenal.

bronchial adenoma adenoma bronquial.

toxic adenoma adenoma tóxico.

adenosis *n.* adenosis.

adenotonsillectomy *n.* adenoamigdalectomía.

adhere *v.* adherir.

adherence *n.* adherencia.

adherent *adj.* adherente.

adhesio *n.* adhesio, adhesión.

adhesion *n.* adherencia, adhesio, adhesión.

abdominal adhesion adherencia abdominal, adhesión abdominal.

amniotic adhesion adherencia amniótica, adhesión amniótica.

traumatic uterine adhesion adherencia traumática uterina.

adhesive *adj.* adhesivo, -va.

adipocyte *n.* adipocito.

adipogenesis *n.* adipogénesis, adipogenia.

adipositas *n.* adiposidad, adipositas.

adiposity *n.* adiposidad.

adjacent *adj.* adyacente.

adjustment *n.* ajuste.

adjuvant *adj.* adyuvante, coadyuvante.

administration *n.* administración.

administration of parenteral fluids administración de líquidos parenterales.

buccal administration of medication administración bucal de la medicación.

drug administration administración de fármacos.

inhalation administration of medication administración de medicación mediante inhalación.

ophthalmic administration of medication administración oftálmica de medicamentos.

adnexa *n.* adnexa, anejos, anexos.

adnexectomy *n.* anexectomía.

adnexitis *n.* anexitis.

adolescence *n.* adolescencia.

adolescent *n.* adolescente.

adrenal *adj.* adrenal, suprarrenal.

adrenalectomy *n.* adrenalectomía.

adrenaline *n.* adrenalina.

adrenergic *adj.* adrenérgico, -ca.

adult *adj., n.* adulto, -ta.

adulteration *n.* adulteración.

adulthood *n.* adultez, edad adulta.

aerate *v.* airear.

aerial *adj.* aéreo, -a.

aerobe *adj.* aerobio, -bia.

aerobic *adj.* aeróbico, -ca.

aerodynamics *n.* aerodinámica.

aerophagia *n.* aerofagia.

aerophagy *n.* aerofagia.

aerosol *n.* aerosol.

aerotherapeutics *n.* aeroterapia.

aerotherapy *n.* aeroterapia.

afebrile *adj.* afebril.

affected *adj.* afectado, -da, afecto, -ta.

affection *n.* afección.

affectivity *n.* afectividad.

affirmation *n.* afirmación.

afterpains *n.* entuertos.

agalactia *n.* agalactia, agalaxia.

agalactorrhea *n.* agalactorrea.

agammaglobulinemia *n.* agammaglobulinemia.

age *n.* edad.
   bone age edad ósea.
   childbearing age edad fértil.
   fetal age edad fetal.
   gestational age edad gestacional.
   menarcheal age edad de la menarquia.

   menarchial age edad de la menarquia.
   mental age edad mental.

agenesia *n.* agenesia.
   agenesia corticalis agenesia cortical.
   agenesia of the corpus callosum agenesia del cuerpo calloso.
   gonadal agenesia agenesia gonadal.
   ovarian agenesia agenesia ovárica.
   renal agenesia agenesia renal.
   thymic agenesia agenesia tímica.
   vaginal agenesia agenesia vaginal.

agenesis *n.* agenesia, agénesis.

agent *n.* agente.
   activating agent agente activador.
   alkylating agent agente alquilante.
   antianxiety agent agente ansiolítico, agente antiansiedad.
   antipsychotic agent agente antipsicótico.
   beta-adrenergic receptor blocking agent agente bloqueador de los receptores beta-adrenérgicos.
   blocking agent agente bloqueador, agente bloqueante.
   calcium channel blocking agent agente bloqueador de los canales del calcio.
   change agent agente de cambio.
   chelating agent agente quelante, quelante.
   chemical agent agente químico.
   chemotherapeutic agent agente quimioterápico.
   diluting agent agente diluyente.
   dispersing agent agente dispersante.

embolization agent agente embolizador.

fixing agent agente fijadores.

masking agent agente enmascarador.

mydriatic and cyclopegic agent agente midriático y ciclopéjico.

neuromuscular blocking agent agente bloqueador neuromuscular.

oxidizing agent agente oxidante.

pharmacological agent agente farmacológico.

progestational agent agente progestacional.

reducing agent agente reductor.

surfactant agent agente tensioactivo.

synergistic agent agente sinérgico.

teratogenic agent agente teratógeno.

agglutinable *adj.* aglutinable.

agglutinant *adj.* aglutinante.

agglutination *n.* aglutinación.

platelet agglutination aglutinación plaquetaria.

agglutinin *n.* aglutinina.

anti-RH agglutinin aglutinina anti-RH.

immune agglutinin aglutinina inmune.

aggregated *adj.* agregado, -da.

aggregation *n.* agregación.

aggregation of platelets agregación plaquetaria.

familial aggregation agregación familiar.

platelet aggregation agregación plaquetaria.

red cell aggregation agregación de hematíes.

aggression *n.* agresión.

destructive aggression agresión destructiva.

inward aggression agresión autodestructiva, agresión interna.

aggressive *adj.* agresivo, -va.

aging *n.* envejecimiento.

agitated *adj.* agitado, -da.

agitation *n.* agitación.

pyschomotor agitation agitación psicomotriz.

aglossia *n.* aglosia.

agnosia *n.* agnosia.

acoustic agnosia agnosia auditiva.

auditory agnosia agnosia auditiva.

body-image agnosia agnosia de la imagen corporal.

optic agnosia agnosia óptica.

tactile agnosia agnosia táctil.

visual agnosia agnosia visual.

visual-spatial agnosia agnosia visuoespacial.

visuospatial agnosia agnosia visuoespacial.

agonadal *adj.* agonadal.

agonal *adj.* agónico, -ca.

agonist *adj.* agonista.

agony *n.* agonía.

agranulocytosis *n.* agranulocitosis.

agraphia *n.* agrafia.

literal agraphia agrafia literal.

mental agraphia agrafia mental.

verbal agraphia agrafia verbal.

agraphic *adj.* agráfico, -ca.

air *n.* aire.

alveolar air aire alveolar.

reserve air aire de reserva.

akinesia *n.* acinesia, acinesis, aquinesia.

alalia *n.* alalia.

alanine *n.* alanina.

albinism *n.* albinismo.

  oculocutaneous albinism albinismo oculocutáneo.

albino *adj.* albino, -na.

albuginea *n.* albugínea.

albuginitis *n.* albuginitis.

albumin *n.* albúmina.

  circulating albumin albúmina circulante.

  normal human serum albumin albúmina normal del suero humano, albúmina sérica humana normal.

  serum albumin albúmina sérica.

albuminemia *n.* albuminemia.

albuminuria *n.* albuminuria.

  cardiac albuminuria albuminuria cardíaca.

  false albuminuria albuminuria falsa.

  physiologic albuminuria albuminuria fisiológica.

  physiological albuminuria albuminuria fisiológica.

  serous albuminuria albuminuria sérica.

  transient albuminuria albuminuria transitoria.

  true albuminuria albuminuria verdadera.

alcohol *n.* alcohol.

alcoholemia *n.* alcoholemia.

alcoholic *adj.* alcohólico, -ca.

alcoholism *n.* alcoholismo.

  acute alcoholism alcoholismo agudo.

alcoholization *n.* alcoholización.

aldosterone *n.* aldosterona.

aldosteronism *n.* aldosteronismo.

  primary aldosteronism aldosteronismo primario.

  secondary aldosteronism aldosteronismo secundario.

alexia *n.* alexia.

  motor alexia alexia motora.

  musical alexia alexia musical.

algid *adj.* álgido, -da.

alignment *n.* alineación, alineamiento.

alimentary *adj.* alimentario, -ria.

alimentation *n.* alimentación.

  artificial alimentation alimentación artificial.

  forced alimentation alimentación forzada.

  parenteral alimentation alimentación parenteral.

  total parenteral alimentation alimentación parenteral total.

alive *adj.* vivo, -va.

alkalinity *n.* alcalinidad.

alkalosis *n.* alcalosis.

  compensated alkalosis alcalosis compensada.

  decompensated alkalosis alcalosis descompensada.

  metabolic alkalosis alcalosis metabólica.

  respiratory alkalosis alcalosis por acapnia, alcalosis respiratoria.

alkaptonuria *n.* alcaptonuria.

allantoid *adj.* alantoide.

allantois *n.* alantoides.

allele *n.* alelo.

  codominant allele alelo codominante, alelo isomorfo.

  dominant allele alelo dominante.

  multiple allele alelo múltiple.

recessive allele alelo recesivo.

silent allele alelo amorfo, alelo silencioso.

allelic *adj.* alélico, -ca.

allergen *n.* alergeno.

allergenic *adj.* alergénico, -ca.

allergic *adj.* alérgico, -ca.

allergology *n.* alergología.

allergy *n.* alergia.

cold allergy alergia al frío.

delayed allergy alergia retardada, alergia tardía.

drug allergy alergia a fármacos, alergia medicamentosa.

food allergy alergia alimentaria.

induced allergy alergia fisiológica, alergia normal, alergia provocada.

pollen allergy alergia al polen.

alliance *n.* alianza.

therapeutic alliance alianza terapéutica.

alloantibody *n.* aloanticuerpo.

alloantigen *n.* aloantígeno.

allodynia *n.* alodinia.

allograft *n.* aloinjerto.

allogroup *n.* alogrupo.

alloimmune *adj.* aloinmune.

allosensitization *n.* alosensibilización.

allotype *n.* alotipo.

allotypy *n.* alotipia.

alopecia *n.* alopecia.

alopecia androgenetica alopecia androgénica.

alopecia areata alopecia areata.

alopecia circumscripta alopecia circunscrita.

alopecia congenitalis alopecia congénita.

alopecia generalisata alopecia generalizada.

alopecia hereditaria alopecia hereditaria.

alopecia orbicularis alopecia orbicular.

alopecia prematura alopecia prematura.

alopecia seborrheica alopecia seborreica.

alopecia senilis alopecia senil.

alopecia totalis alopecia total.

alopecia toxica alopecia tóxica.

alopecia universalis alopecia universal.

androgenetic alopecia alopecia androgénica.

androgenic alopecia alopecia androgénica.

cicatricial alopecia alopecia cicatricial, alopecia cicatrisata.

congenital alopecia alopecia congénita.

male pattern alopecia alopecia de distribución masculina, alopecia de patrón masculino, alopecia de tipo masculino.

postpartum alopecia alopecia posparto.

premature alopecia alopecia prematura.

pressure alopecia alopecia por compresión, alopecia por presión.

psychogenic alopecia alopecia psicógena.

radiation alopecia alopecia por radiación.

senile alopecia alopecia senil.

stress alopecia alopecia de estrés.

X-ray alopecia alopecia por rayos X.

alopecic *adj.* alopécico, -ca.

alpha1-antitrypsin *n.* alfa1-antitripsina.

alpha2-macroblogulin *n.* alfa2-macroglobulina.

alpha-beta-blocker *n.* alfa-beta-bloqueante.

alpha-fetoprotein (AFP) *n.* alfa-fetoproteína (AFP).

alpha-globulin *n.* alfa-globulina.

alpha-lipoprotein *n.* alfa-lipoproteína.

alteration *n.* alteración.

  qualitative alteration alteración cualitativa.

  quantitative alteration alteración cuantitativa.

alternans *n.* alternancia.

alternation *n.* alternación.

altruism *n.* altruismo.

aluminosis *n.* aluminosis.

alveobronchiolitis *n.* alveobronquiolitis.

alveolitis *n.* alveolitis.

  allergic alveolitis alveolitis alérgica, alveolitis alérgica extrínseca.

  extrinsic allergic alveolitis alveolitis alérgica, alveolitis alérgica extrínseca.

alveolus *n.* alveolo, alvéolo.

amalgam *n.* amalgama.

  dental amalgam amalgama dental, amalgama dentaria.

amaurosis *n.* amaurosis.

  amaurosis congenita amaurosis congénita.

  amaurosis fugax amaurosis fugaz.

  congenital amaurosis amaurosis congénita.

  diabetic amaurosis amaurosis diabética.

ambidexter *adj.* ambidextro, -tra.

ambisexual *adj.* ambisexual.

ambivalence *n.* ambivalencia.

Amblyomma *n.* Amblyomma.

amblyopia *n.* ambliopía.

  strabismic amblyopia ambliopía estrábismica.

amblyopiatrics *n.* ambliopiatría.

amblyopic *n.* ambiópico, -ca.

amblyoscope *n.* ambliocospio.

ambo *n.* ambo, ambón.

ambomalleal *adj.* ambomaleal.

ambulance *n.* ambulancia.

ambulant *adj.* ambulatorio, -a.

ambulatory *adj.* ambulatorio, -a.

amebiasis *n.* amebiasis.

  hepatic amebiasis amebiasis hepática.

  intestinal amebiasis amebiasis intestinal.

amebicidal *adj.* amebicida.

amelioration *n.* mejoría.

amenorrhea *n.* amenorrea.

  amenorrhea postpartum amenorrea posparto.

  emotional amenorrhea amenorrea emocional.

  hypophyseal amenorrhea amenorrea hipofisaria.

  hypothalamic amenorrhea amenorrea hipotalámica.

  nutritional amenorrhea amenorrea nutricional.

  ovarian amenorrhea amenorrea ovárica.

  pathologic amenorrhea amenorrea patológica.

physiologic amenorrhea amenorrea fisiológica.

postpill amenorrhea amenorrea pospíldora.

premenopausal amenorrhea ameno-rrea premenopáusica.

secondary amenorrhea amenorrea secundaria.

stress amenorrhea amenorrea por estrés.

traumatic amenorrhea amenorrea traumática.

amenorrheal *adj.* amenorreico, -ca.

amenorrheic *adj.* amenorreico, -ca.

ametropia *n.* ametropía, ecmetropía.

aminoacid *n.* aminoácido.

essential aminoacid aminoácido esencial.

non-essential aminoacid aminoácido no esencial.

aminoacidopathy *n.* aminoacidopatía.

aminoaciduria *n.* aminoaciduria.

ammonia *n.* amoniaco, amoníaco.

ammoniemia *n.* amoniemia.

ammoniuria *n.* amoniuria.

amnesia *n.* amnesia.

anterograde amnesia amnesia anterógrada.

auditory amnesia amnesia auditiva.

continuous amnesia amnesia continua.

dissociative amnesia amnesia disociativa.

emotional amnesia amnesia emocional.

episodic amnesia amnesia episódica.

generalized amnesia amnesia generalizada.

infantile amnesia amnesia infantil.

lacunar amnesia amnesia lacunar, amnesia lagunar.

organic amnesia amnesia orgánica.

postcontussional amnesia amnesia poscontusional.

posthypnotic amnesia amnesia posthipnótica.

retroanterograde amnesia amnesia retroanterógrada.

retrograde amnesia amnesia retrógada.

selective amnesia amnesia selectiva.

tactile amnesia amnesia táctil.

traumatic amnesia amnesia traumática.

verbal amnesia amnesia verbal.

visual amnesia amnesia visual.

amniocentesis *n.* amniocentesis.

amniochorial *adj.* amniocorial, amniocoriónico, -ca.

amnion *n.* amnios.

amnionitis *n.* amnionitis.

amniorrhexis *n.* amniorrexis.

amnioscope *n.* amnioscopio.

amnioscopia *n.* amnioscopia.

amniotic *adj.* amniótico, -ca.

amniotitis *n.* amnionitis.

amorpha *n.* amorfa.

amorphous *adj.* amorfo, -fa.

amorphus *n.* amorfo.

amplification *n.* amplificación.

amplitude *n.* amplitud.

amplitude of convergence amplitud de convergencia.

ampoule *n.* ampolla, ámpula.

ampular *adj.* ampollar.

ampule *n.* ampolla, ámpula.

ampulla *n.* ampolla.

ampullary *adj.* ampollar.

amputation *n.* amputación.

  amniotic amputation amputación amniótica.

  aperiosteal amputation amputación aperióstica.

  below-knee (B-K) amputation amputación por debajo de la rodilla (B-K).

  birth amputation amputación natural.

  cervical amputation amputación cervical.

  circus amputation amputación circular.

  cirular amputation amputación circular.

  closed amputation amputación cerrada.

  complete amputation amputación completa.

  eccentric amputation amputación excéntrica.

  flap amputation amputación con colgajos, amputación de colgajo.

  flapless amputation amputación sin colgajos, amputación sin colgajos.

  immediate amputation amputación inmediata.

  intrauterine amputation amputación intrauterina.

  minor amputation amputación menor.

  musculocutaneous amputation amputación musculocutánea.

  natural amputation amputación natural.

  oblique amputation amputación oblicua.

  open amputation amputación abierta.

  operative amputation amputación operatoria.

  oval amputation amputación oval.

  partial amputation amputación parcial.

  pathologic amputation amputación patológica.

  quadruple amputation amputación cuádruple.

  spontaneous amputation amputación espontánea.

amputee *n.* amputado, -da.

amyelinic *adj.* amielínico, -ca.

amygdala *n.* amígdala.

amygdalectomy *n.* amigdalectomía.

amyloid *n.* amiloide.

amyloidosis *n.* amiloidosis.

  amyloidosis cutis amiloidosis cutánea, amiloidosis cutis.

  cutaneous amyloidosis amiloidosis cutánea, amiloidosis cutis.

  familial amyloidosis amiloidosis familiar.

  hereditary amyloidosis amiloidosis hereditaria, amiloidosis heredofamiliar.

  heredofamilial amyloidosis amiloidosis hereditaria, amiloidosis heredofamiliar.

  idiopathic amyloidosis amiloidosis idiopática.

  nodular amyloidosis amiloidosis nodular.

  primary amyloidosis amiloidosis primaria.

secondary amyloidosis amiloidosis secundaria.

senile amyloidosis amiloidosis senil.

amyotrophy *n.* amiotrofia.

anabolism *n.* anabolismo.

anabolite *n.* anabolito.

anaerobe *adj.* anaerobio, -a.

anaerobiotic *adj.* anaerobiótico, -ca.

anagen *n.* anagen, anágeno.

anal *adj.* anal.

analgesia *n.* analgesia.

analgesia dolorosa analgesia dolorosa.

audio analgesia analgesia auditiva.

infiltration analgesia analgesia por infiltración.

inhalation analgesia analgesia por inhalación.

surface analgesia analgesia superficial.

analgesic *adj.* analgésico, -ca.

analog *adj.* análogo, -ga.

analogy *n.* analogía.

analysis *n.* análisis, valoración.

analysis of variance análisis de la varianza (ANOVA).

bioelectrical impedance analysis (BIA) análisis de impedancia bioeléctrica (AIB).

volumetric analysis análisis volumétrico.

analyzer *n.* analizador.

anamnesis *n.* anamnesis.

anaphase *n.* anafase.

anaphylactic *adj.* anafiláctico, -ca.

anaphylaxis *n.* anafilaxia, anafilaxis.

acquired anaphylaxis anafilaxia adquirida.

antiserum anaphylaxis anafilaxia de antisuero.

generalized anaphylaxis anafilaxia generalizada.

indirect anaphylaxis anafilaxia indirecta.

passive anaphylaxis anafilaxia pasiva.

systemic anaphylaxis anafilaxia sistémica.

anaplasia *n.* anaplasia.

anaplastic *adj.* anaplásico, -ca.

anasarca *n.* anasarca.

anastomose *v.* anastomosar.

anastomosis *n.* anastomosis.

arteriovenous anastomosis anastomosis arteriovenosa.

iliorectal anastomosis anastomosis iliorrectal.

microvascular anastomosis anastomosis microvascular.

termino-terminal anastomosis anastomosis terminoterminal.

transureteroureteral anastomosis anastomosis transureteroureteral.

ureteroureteral anastomosis anastomosis ureteroureteral.

anastomotic *adj.* anastomótico, -ca.

anatomic *adj.* anatómico, -ca.

anatomical *adj.* anatómico, -ca.

anatomicopathological *adj.* anatomopatológico, -ca.

anatomy *n.* anatomía.

applied anatomy anatomía aplicada.

clinical anatomy anatomía clínica.

comparative anatomy anatomía comparada.

dental anatomy anatomía dental.

descriptive anatomy anatomía descriptiva.

functional anatomy anatomía funcional.

general anatomy anatomía general.

gross anatomy anatomía macroscópica.

histological anatomy anatomía histológica.

macroscopic anatomy anatomía macroscópica.

microscopic anatomy anatomía microscópica.

minute anatomy anatomía microscópica.

pathological anatomy anatomía patológica.

physiological anatomy anatomía fisiológica.

surgical anatomy anatomía quirúrgica.

anchorage *n.* anclaje.

androgen *n.* andrógeno.

androgenesis *n.* androgénesis.

androgenization *n.* androgenización.

androsterone *n.* androsterona.

anemia *n.* anemia.

acute anemia anemia aguda.

acute hemolytic anemia anemia hemolítica aguda.

anemia lymphatica anemia linfática.

anemia neonatorum anemia neonatal.

anemia splenica anemia esplénica.

aregenerative anemia anemia arregenerativa.

autoimmune hemolytic anemia (AIHS) anemia hemolítica autoinmune.

congenital hemolytic anemia anemia hemolítica congénita.

deficiency anemia anemia carencial, anemia deficitaria.

drug-induced immune hemolytic anemia anemia hemolítica inmune inducida por fármacos.

erythroblastic anemia of childhood anemia eritroblástica de la infancia.

familial erythroblastic anemia anemia eritroblástica familiar.

folic acid deficiency anemia anemia por deficiencia de ácido fólico.

hemolytic anemia anemia hemolítica.

hemorrhagic anemia anemia hemorrágica.

hypoferric anemia anemia hipoférrica.

immune hemolytic anemia anemia hemolítica inmune.

immunohemolytic anemia anemia hemolítica inmune.

infectious hemolytic anemia anemia hemolítica infecciosa.

iron deficiency anemia anemia ferropénica, anemia por deficiencia de hierro.

juvenile pernicious anemia anemia perniciosa juvenil.

local anemia anemia local.

macrocytic anemia anemia macrocítica.

macrocytic anemia of pregnancy anemia macrocítica del embarazo.

malignant anemia anemia maligna.

megaloblastic anemia anemia megaloblástica.

megalocytic anemia anemia megalocítica.

metaplastic anemia anemia metaplásica.

miners' anemia anemia de los mineros.

mountain anemia anemia de las montañas.

normochromic anemia anemia normocrómica.

normocytic anemia anemia normocítica.

nutritional anemia anemia nutricional.

nutritional macrocytic anemia anemia macrocítica nutricional.

pernicious anemia anemia perniciosa.

physiologic anemia anemia fisiológica.

posthemorrhagic anemia anemia poshemorrágica.

posthemorrhagic anemia of the newborn anemia poshemorrágica neonatal.

pure red cell anemia anemia de glóbulos rojos puros, anemia eritrocítica pura.

refractory anemia anemia rebelde, anemia refractaria.

scorbutic anemia anemia escorbútica.

sickle cell anemia anemia de células falciformes, anemia drepanocítica.

sideroachrestic anemia anemia sideroacréstica.

sideroblastic anemia anemia sideroblástica.

sideropenic anemia anemia sideropénica.

spherocytic anemia anemia esferocítica.

splenic anemia anemia esplénica.

traumatic anemia anemia traumática.

anemic *adj.* anémico, -ca.

anencephalia *n.* anencefalia.

anencephalic *adj.* anencefálico, -ca.

anencephalous *adj.* anencefálico, -ca.

anencephalus *n.* anencéfalo.

anephric *adj.* anéfrico, -ca.

anergic *adj.* anérgico, -ca.

anergy *n.* anergia.

negative anergy anergia negativa.

non-specific anergy anergia inespecífica.

positive anergy anergia positiva.

specific anergy anergia específica.

anesthesia *n.* anestesia.

anesthesia dolorosa anestesia dolorosa.

block anesthesia anestesia bloqueante, anestesia bloqueo.

bulbar anesthesia anestesia bulbar.

caudal anesthesia anestesia caudal.

central anesthesia anestesia central.

closed anesthesia anestesia cerrada.

compression anesthesia anestesia por compresión.

conduction anesthesia anestesia por conducción.

crossed anesthesia anestesia cruzada.

dissociated anesthesia anestesia disociada.

electric anesthesia anestesia eléctrica.

epidural anesthesia anestesia epidural.

facial anesthesia anestesia facial.

frost anesthesia anestesia por congelación.

general anesthesia anestesia general.

hypothermic anesthesia anestesia hipotérmica.

hysterical anesthesia anestesia histérica.

infiltration anesthesia anestesia por infiltración.

inhalation anesthesia anestesia por inhalación.

intercostal anesthesia anestesia intercostal.

intranasal anesthesia anestesia intranasal.

intraoral anesthesia anestesia intrabucal.

intraosseous anesthesia anestesia intraósea.

intravenous anesthesia anestesia intravenosa.

local anesthesia anestesia local.

lumbar epidural anesthesia anestesia epidural lumbar.

muscular anesthesia anestesia muscular.

olfactory anesthesia anestesia olfatoria.

paraneural anesthesia anestesia paraneural.

paravertebral anesthesia anestesia paravertebral.

peridural anesthesia anestesia peridural.

perineural anesthesia anestesia perineural.

peripheral anesthesia anestesia periférica.

pharyngeal anesthesia anestesia faríngea.

pressure anesthesia anestesia por presión.

rectal anesthesia anestesia rectal.

refrigeration anesthesia anestesia por refrigeración.

regional anesthesia anestesia regional.

sacral anesthesia anestesia sacra.

saddle block anesthesia anestesia en silla de montar.

segmental anesthesia anestesia segmentaria.

spinal anesthesia anestesia espinal, anestesia raquídea, raquianestesia.

surface anesthesia anestesia de superficie.

surgical anesthesia anestesia quirúrgica.

tactile anesthesia anestesia táctil.

thermal anesthesia anestesia térmica.

thermic anesthesia anestesia térmica.

topical anesthesia anestesia tópica.

total anesthesia anestesia completa.

unilateral anesthesia anestesia unilateral.

visceral anesthesia anestesia visceral.

anesthesiology *n.* anestesiología.

anesthetic *n.* anestésico, -ca.

general anesthetic anestésico general.

intravenous anesthetic anestésico endovenoso.

local anesthetic anestésico local.

spinal anesthetic anestésico raquídeo.

topical anesthetic anestésico tópico.

anesthetist *n.* anestesista.

aneuploid *adj.* aneuploide.

aneuploidy *n.* aneuploidía.

aneurysm *n.* aneurisma.

abdominal aneurysm aneurisma abdominal.

aneurysm by anastomosis aneurisma anastomático, aneurisma por anastomosis.

aortic aneurysm aneurisma aórtico.

arteriovenous aneurysm aneurisma arteriovenoso.

atherosclerotic aneurysm aneurisma arterioesclerótico.

bacterial aneurysm aneurisma bacteriano.

cardiac aneurysm aneurisma cardíaco.

cerebral aneurysm aneurisma cerebral.

compound aneurysm aneurisma compuesto.

congenital cerebral aneurysm aneurisma cerebral congénito.

dissecting aneurysm aneurisma disecante.

embolic aneurysm aneurisma embólico.

false aneurysm aneurisma falso.

infected aneurysm aneurisma infectado.

intracranial aneurysm aneurisma intracraneal.

lateral aneurysm aneurisma lateral.

mycotic aneurysm aneurisma micótico.

orbital aneurysm aneurisma orbitario.

pelvic aneurysm aneurisma pélvico.

renal aneurysm aneurisma renal.

syphilitic aneurysm aneurisma sifilítico.

thoracic aneurysm aneurisma torácico.

traumatic aneurysm aneurisma traumático.

true aneurysm aneurisma verdadero.

varicose aneurysm aneurisma varicoso.

ventricular aneurysm aneurisma ventricular.

anger *n.* ira.

angiectasia *n.* angiectasia, angiectasis.

angiectasis *n.* angiectasia, angiectasis.

angiitis *n.* angeítis, angiítis.

allergic cutaneous angiitis angiítis alérgica cutánea.

necrotizing angiitis angiítis necrosante.

angina *n.* angina.

angina acuta angina aguda.

angina catarrhalis angina catarral.

angina diphtheritica angina diftérica.

angina dyspeptica angina dispéptica.

angina pectoris angina de pecho.

angina rheumatica angina reumática.

angina trachealis angina traqueal.

exudative angina angina exudativa.

false angina angina falsa.

intestinal angina angina intestinal.

neutropenic angina angina neutropénica.

angioblastoma *n.* angioblastoma.

angiocardiogram *n.* angiocardiograma.

angiocardiopathy *n.* angiocardiopatía.

angioedema *n.* angioedema.

angiogenesis *n.* angiogénesis.

angiogenic *adj.* angiogénico, -ca.

angiography *n.* angiografía.

radioisotope angiography gamma-angiografía.

angioma *n.* angioma.

angioma cavernosum angioma cavernoso.

angioma cutis angioma del cutis.

angioma lymphaticum angioma linfático.

angioma senile angioma senil.

arteriovenous angioma of the brain angioma arteriovenoso del cerebro.

capillary angioma angioma capilar.

cavernous angioma angioma cavernoso.

cherry angioma angioma en cereza.

strawberry angioma angioma en fresa.

telangiectatic angioma angioma telangiectásico.

angiomatosis *n.* angiomatosis.

angiopathic *adj.* angiopático, -ca.

angiopathy *n.* angiopatía.

angioplasty *n.* angioplastia.

percutaneous transluminal coronary angioplasty (PTCA) angioplastia coronaria transluminal percutánea (ACTP).

angioscope *n.* angioscopio.

angioscopy *n.* angioscopia.

angitis *n.* angiítis, angitis.

angle *n.* ángulo.

angle of aberration ángulo de aberración.

angle of aperture ángulo de abertura, ángulo de abertura, ángulo de apertura.

angor *n.* angor.

angular *adj.* angular.

angulus *n.* ángulo.

anhidrosis *n.* anhidrosis.

anhydride *n.* anhídrido.

anima *n.* ánima.

anion *n.* anión.

anionic *adj.* aniónico, -ca.

ankle *n.* tobillo.

ankylopoietic *adj.* anquilopoyético, -ca.

ankylosed *adj.* anquilosado, -da.

ankylosis *n.* anquilosis.

artificial ankylosis anquilosis artificial.

bony ankylosis anquilosis ósea.

dental ankylosis anquilosis dental.

extracapsular ankylosis anquilosis extracapsular.

false ankylosis anquilosis falsa.

fibrous ankylosis anquilosis fibrosa.

intracapsular ankylosis anquilosis intracapsular.

spurious ankylosis anquilosis espuria.

stapedial ankylosis anquilosis del estribo.

true ankylosis anquilosis verdadera.

anmiotitis *n.* amniotitis.

annular *adj.* anular.

annulus *n.* anillo, annulus.

annulus umbilicalis anillo umbilical.

anococcygeal *adj.* anococcígeo, -a, anocoxígeo, -a.

anode *n.* ánodo.

anodyne *adj.* anodino, -na.

anodynia *n.* anodinia.

anomaly *n.* anomalía.

chromosomal anomaly anomalía cromosómica.

chromosome anomaly anomalía cromosómica.

congenital cardiac anomaly anomalía cardíaca congénita.

developmental anomaly anomalía de desarrollo.

gestant anomaly anomalía gestante.

anophthalmia *n.* anoftalmía.

anorchia *n.* anorquia, anorquidia.

anorchid *adj.* anórquido, -da.

anorchidic *adj.* anórquidico, -ca.

anorchidism *n.* anorquia, anorquidia.

anorchism *n.* anorquismo.

anorectal *adj.* anorrectal.

anoretic *adj.* anoréxico, -ca.

anorexia *n.* anorexia.

anorexia nervosa anorexia nerviosa.

anorexiant *n.* anorexígeno.

anorexic *adj.* anoréxico, -ca.

anorgasmia *n.* anorgasmia.

anorgasmy *n.* anorgasmia.

anoscope *n.* anoscopio.

anoscopy *n.* anoscopia.

anosigmoidoscopy *n.* anosigmoidoscopia.

anosmia *n.* anosmia.

anosmia gustatoria anosmia gustatoria.

anosmia respiratoria anosmia respiratoria.

preferential anosmia anosmia preferencial.

anosmic *adj.* anósmico, -ca.

anovulation *n.* anovulación.

anovulatory *adj.* anovulatorio, -a.

anoxia *n.* anoxia.

anoxia neonatorum anoxia del neonato.

anoxic *adj.* anóxico, -ca.

antacid *n.* antiácido, -da.

antagonism *n.* antagonismo.

antagonist *adj.* antagonista, antistático, -ca.

aldosterone antagonist antagonista aldosterona.

associated antagonist antagonista asociado.

calcium antagonist antagonista del calcio.

competitive antagonist antagonista competitivo.

direct antagonist antagonista directo.

enzyme antagonist antagonista enzimático.

folic acid antagonist antagonista del ácido fólico.

narcotic antagonist antagonista de los narcóticos, antagonista narcótico.

antalgesic *adj.* antálgico, -ca, antiálgico, -ca.

antalgic *adj.* antálgico, -ca, antiálgico, -ca.

antarthritic *adj.* antiartrítico, -ca.

antasthmatic *adj.* antiasmático, -ca.

antebrachial *adj.* antebraquial.

antebrachium *n.* antebrachium, antebrazo.

anteflexio *n.* anteflexio, anteflexión.

anteflexion *n.* anteflexio, anteflexión.

anteflexion of the iris anteflexión del iris.

uterine anteflexion anteflexio uteri, anteflexión uterina.

antenatal *adj.* antenatal.

anterior *adj.* anterior.

anteroexternal *adj.* anteroexterno, -na.

anterograde *adj.* anterógrado, -ra.

anteroinferior *adj.* anteroinferior.

anterointernal *adj.* anterointerno, -na.

anterolateral *adj.* anterolateral.

anteromedial *adj.* anteromedio, -dia.

anteromedian *adj.* anteromediano, -na.

anteroposterior *adj.* anteroposterior.

anteroseptal *adj.* anteroseptal.

anterosuperior *adj.* anterosuperior.

anteroventral *adj.* anteroventral.

anteversion *n.* anteversión.

anthemorrhagic *adj.* antihemorrágico, -ca.

antherpetic *adj.* antiherpético, -ca.

anthocyanidin *n.* antocianidina.

anthracosis *n.* antracosis.

anthrax *n.* carbunco.

cerebral anthrax carbunco cerebral.

cutaneous anthrax carbunco cutáneo.

gastrointestinal anthrax carbunco gastrointestinal.

inhalational anthrax carbunco por inhalación.

intestinal anthrax carbunco intestinal.

meningeal anthrax carbunco meníngeo.

pulmonary anthrax carbunco pulmonar.

anthropology *n.* antropología.

antiabortifacient *n.* antiabortivo.

antiacid *n.* antiácido, -da.

antiadrenergic *n.* antiadrenérgico, -ca.

antiandrogenic *adj.* antiandrógeno, -na.

antiantibody *n.* antianticuerpo.

antiantidote *n.* antiantídoto.

antiarrhythmic *adj.* antiarrítmico, -ca.

antiarthritic *adj.* antiartrítico, -ca.

antiasthmatic *adj.* antiasmático, -ca.

antibacterial *adj.* antibacteriano, -na, antibactérico, -ca.

antibiogram *n.* antibiograma, antibioticograma.

antibiotic *adj.* antibiótico, -ca.

antibiotic-resistant *adj.* antibioticorresistente.

antibody *n.* anticuerpo.

agglutinating antibody anticuerpo aglutinante.

anaphylactic antibody anticuerpo anafiláctico.

anti-basement membrane antibody anticuerpo antimembrana basal.

anti-D antibody anticuerpo anti-D.

anti-DNA antibody anticuerpo anti-ADN.

anti-glomerular basement membrane antibody anticuerpo antimembrana basal glomerular (anti-MBG).

antimicrosomal antibody anticuerpo antimicrosomal.

antimitochondrial antibody anticuerpo antimitocondrial, anticuerpo antimitocóndrico.

antinuclear antibody (ANA) anticuerpo antinuclear (ANA).

antireceptor antibody anticuerpo antirreceptor.

antithyroglobulin antibody anticuerpo antitiroglobulina.

antithyroid antibody anticuerpo antitiroideo.

antologous antibody anticuerpo autólogo.

bispecific antibody anticuerpo biespecífico.

bivalent antibody anticuerpo bivalente.

blocking antibody anticuerpo bloqueante.

cell-bound antibody anticuerpo fijo a célula, anticuerpo ligado a la célula.

cell-fixed antibody anticuerpo fijo a célula, anticuerpo ligado a la célula.

cold antibody anticuerpo frío, anticuerpo frío-reactivo.

cold-reactive antibody anticuerpo frío, anticuerpo frío-reactivo.

complement-fixing antibody anticuerpo fijador del complemento.

complete antibody anticuerpo completo.

cross-reacting antibody anticuerpo de reacción cruzada.

cytotoxic antibody anticuerpo citotóxico.

detectable circulating antibody anticuerpo circulante.

fluorescent antibody anticuerpo fluorescente.

heteroclitic antibody anticuerpo heteroclítico.

heterocytotropic antibody anticuerpo heterocitotrópico.

heterogenetic antibody anticuerpo heterogenético.

heterophil antibody anticuerpo heterófilo.

heterophile antibody anticuerpo heterófilo.

horse-type antibody anticuerpo de tipo equino.

hybrid antibody anticuerpo híbrido.

idiotype antibody anticuerpo idiotipo.

immune antibody anticuerpo inmunitario.

incomplete antibody anticuerpo incompleto.

inhibiting antibody anticuerpo inhibidor.

lymphocytotoxic antibody anticuerpo linfocitotóxico.

mitochondrial antibody anticuerpo mitocondrial.

monoclonal antibody anticuerpo monoclonal.

natural antibody anticuerpo natural.

neutralizing antibody anticuerpo neutralizante.

normal antibody anticuerpo normal.

polyclonal antibody anticuerpo policlonal.

protective antibody anticuerpo protector.

reaginic antibody anticuerpo reagínico.

Rh antibody anticuerpo Rh.

saline antibody anticuerpo salino.

sensitizing antibody anticuerpo sensibilizante.

treponema-immobilizing antibody anticuerpo antitreponema.

treponemal antibody anticuerpo treponémico.

univalent antibody anticuerpo univalente.

warm antibody anticuerpo caliente, anticuerpo caliente-reactivo.

warm-reactive antibody anticuerpo caliente, anticuerpo caliente-reactivo.

anticalculous *adj.* anticalculoso, -sa.

anticancer *adj.* anticanceroso, -sa.

anticarcinogen *adj.* anticarcinógeno, -na.

anticarcinogenic *adj.* anticarcinogénico, -ca.

anticariogenic *adj.* anticariogénico, -ca.

anticatalyzer *adj.* anticatalizador, -ra.

anticatarrhal *adj.* anticatarral.

anticholinergic *adj.* anticolinérgico, -ca.

anticholinesterase *n.* anticolinesterasa.

anticoagulant *adj.* anticoagulante.

anticoagulation *n.* anticoagulación.

anticomplement *n.* anticomplemento.

anticonvulsive *adj.* anticonvulsivo, -va.

antidepressant *adj.* antidepresivo, -va.

antidiabetic *adj.* antidiabético, -ca.

antidiarrheal *adj.* antidiarreico, -ca.

antidiarrheic *adj.* antidiarreico, -ca.

antidiuretic *adj.* antidiurético, -ca.

antidote *n.* antídoto.

chemical antidote antídoto químico.

mechanical antidote antídoto mecánico.

physiologic antidote antídoto fisiológico.

universal antidote antídoto universal.

antiemetic *adj.* antemético, -ca, antiemético, -ca.

antiepileptic *adj.* antiepiléptico, -ca.

antistreptokinase *n.* antiestreptoquinasa.

antiestrogen *n.* antiestrógeno.

antifebrile *adj.* antifebril.

antiflatulent *adj.* antiflatulento, -ta.

antifungal *adj.* antifúngico, -ca.

antigen *n.* antígeno.

allogenic antigen antígeno alogénico.

Australia antigen antígeno Australia.

blood group antigen antígeno de grupo sanguíneo.

carbohydrate antigen antígeno hidrocarbonado.

carcinoembryonic antigen antígeno carcinoembrionario (CEA).

class I antigen antígeno clase I.

class II antigen antígeno clase II.

class III antigen antígeno clase III.

common antigen antígeno común.

common leukocyte antigen antígeno leucocitario común.

complete antigen antígeno completo.

conjugated antigen antígeno conjugado.

cross-reacting antigen antígeno de reacción cruzada.

delta antigen antígeno delta.

envelope antigen antígeno de cubierta.

extractable nuclear antigen (ena) antígeno nuclear extraíble (ena).

F antigen antígeno F.

febrile antigen antígeno febril.

group antigen antígeno de grupo.

hepatitis associated antigen (HAA) antígeno asociado a hepatitis.

hepatitis b surface antigen (hb-sag) antígeno de superficie del virus de la hepatitis b.

heterogenetic antigen antígeno heterogénico, antígeno heterógeno.

heterologous antigen antígeno heterólogo.

histocompatibility antigen antígeno de histocompatibilidad.

histocompatibility major antigen antígeno de histocompatibilidad mayor.

histocompatibility minor antigen antígeno de histocompatibilidad menor.

homologous antigen antígeno homólogo.

human leukemia-associated antigen antígeno asociado a las leucemias humanas.

human lymphocyte antigen (HLA) antígeno de los linfocitos humanos (hla), antígeno leucocitario humano.

nuclear antigen antígeno nuclear.

o antigen antígeno o.

oncofetal antigen antígeno oncofetal.

organ-specific antigen antígeno específico de órgano.

partial antigen antígeno parcial.

pollen antigen antígeno del polen.

private antigen antígeno privado.

prostate specific antigen antígeno prostático específico (psa).

public antigen antígeno público.

recall antigen antígeno de recuerdo.

self-antigen antígeno propio.

sensitized antigen antígeno sensibilizado.

sequestered antigen antígeno secuestrado.

sero-defined antigen antígeno serodefinido (sd).

serologically defined antigen antígeno serodefinido (sd).

shock antigen antígeno de shock.

soluble antigen antígeno soluble.

somatic antigen antígeno somático.

species-specific antigen antígeno específico de especie.

specific antigen antígeno específico.

SS-a antigen antígeno SS-a.

SS-b antigen antígeno SS-b.

Tac antigen antígeno Tac.

theta antigen antígeno theta, antígeno Thy.

Thy antigen antígeno theta, antígeno Thy.

tissue-specific antigen antígeno específico de tejido.

transplantation antigen antígeno de trasplante.

tumor antigen antígeno tumoral.

tumor associated antigen antígeno asociado a tumor.

tumor-specific antigen (TSA) antígeno específico de tumor.

tumor-specific transplantation antigen (ttet) antígeno de trasplante específico del tumor.

antigenic *adj.* antigénico, -ca.

antiglobulin *n.* antiglobulina.

antihemolytic *adj.* antihemolítico, -ca.

antihemorrhagic *adj.* antihemorrágico, -ca.

antiherpetic *adj.* antiherpético, -ca.

antihistaminic *adj.* antihistamínico, -ca.

antihypercholesteronemic *adj.* antihipercolesterolémico, -ca.

antihyperglycemic *adj.* antihiperglucémico, -ca.

antihyperlipoproteinemic *adj.* antihiperlipoproteico, -ca.

antihypertensive *adj.* antihipertensivo, -va.

anti-infectious *adj.* antiinfeccioso, -sa.

anti-inflammatory *adj.* antiinflamatorio, -ria.

antiketogenetic *adj.* anticetogénico, -ca.

antiketogenic *adj.* anticetógeno, -na, antiquetógeno, -na.

antimicrobial *adj.* antimicrobiano, -na.

antimicrobic *adj.* antimicrobiano, -na.

antimycotic *adj.* antimicótico, -ca.

antineoplastic *adj.* antineoplásico, -ca.

antioncogene *n.* antioncogen.

antioxidant *n.* antioxidante.

antipaludial *adj.* antipalúdico, -ca.

antiparalytic *adj.* antiparalítico, -ca.

antiparasitic *adj.* antiparasitario, -ria.

antiparkinsonian *adj.* antiparkinsoniano, -na.

antipedicular *adj.* antipedicular, antipediculoso, -sa.

antiperistaltic *adj.* antiperistáltico, -ca.

antiperspirant *adj.* antiperspirante, antisudoríparo, -ra.

antiplatelet *adj.* antiplaquetario, -ria.

antipruritical *adj.* antipruriginoso, -sa, antiprurítico, -ca, antipruritoso, -sa.

antipsychotic *adj.* antipsicótico, -ca.

antipyretic *adj.* antipirético, -ca.

antiscabietic *adj.* antiescabiético, -ca, antiescabioso, -sa.

antiscarlatinal *adj.* antiescarlatinoso, -sa.

antiscorbutic *adj.* antiescorbútico, -ca.

antiseptic *adj.* antiséptico, -ca.

antiserum *n.* antisuero.
  blood group antiserum antisuero de grupos sanguíneos.
  heterologous antiserum antisuero heterólogo.
  homologous antiserum antisuero homólogo.
  monovalent antiserum antisuero monovalente.
  polyvalent antiserum antisuero polivalente.
  Rh antiserum antisuero Rh.
  specific antiserum antisuero específico.

antisocial *adj.* antisocial.

antispasmodic *n.* antiespasmódico, antispasmódico.
  billiary antispasmodic antiespasmódico biliar.
  bronchial antispasmodic antiespasmódico bronquial.

antispastic *adj.* antiespástico, -ca.

antitetanic *adj.* antitetánico, -ca.

antithermic *adj.* antitérmico, -ca.

antithrombin *n.* antitrombina.

antithromboplastin *n.* antitromboplastina.

antithrombotic *adj.* antitrombótico, -ca.

antitoxin *n.* antitoxina.
  botulinum antitoxin antitoxina botulínica.
  botulism antitoxin antitoxina botulínica.
  diphtheria antitoxin antitoxina diftérica.

antitrypsin *n.* antitripsina.

antitubercular *adj.* antituberculoso, -sa.

antituberculous *adj.* antituberculoso, -sa.

antitussive *adj.* antitusígeno, -na, antitusivo, -va.

antiulcerative *adj.* antiulceroso, -sa.

antivenereal *adj.* antivenéreo, -a.

antivenin *n.* antiponzoñoso, -sa, antitoxina, antiveneno.

antivenomous *adj.* antivenenoso, -sa.

antiviral *adj.* antiviral, antivírico, -ca.

antrum *n.* antro, antrum.

anuclear *adj.* anuclear.

anuria *n.* anuria.
  calculus anuria anuria calculosa.
  obstructive anuria anuria obstructiva.
  postrenal anuria anuria posrenal.
  prerenal anuria anuria prerrenal.
  renal anuria anuria renal.
  suppressive anuria anuria por supresión.

anus *n.* ano, anus.
  anus vesicalis ano vesical.
  artificial anus ano artificial, ano contra natura.
  ectopic anus ano ectópico.
  imperforate anus ano imperforado.
  vestibular anus ano vestibular, ano vulvovaginal.
  vulvovaginal anus ano vestibular, ano vulvovaginal.

anvil *n.* yunque.

anxiety *n.* angustia, ansiedad.
  anticipatory anxiety ansiedad anticipatoria, ansiedad de señal.

basic anxiety ansiedad básica.

separation anxiety ansiedad de separación.

situation anxiety ansiedad de situación.

stranger anxiety ansiedad ante los extraños.

traumatic anxiety ansiedad traumática.

anxiolytic *adj.* ansiolítico, -ca.

aorta *n.* aorta.

aortic *adj.* aórtico, -ca.

aortitis *n.* aortitis.

aortography *n.* aortografía.

apathetic *adj.* apático, -ca.

apathic *adj.* apático, -ca.

apathy *n.* apatía.

aphagia *n.* afagia.

aphasia *n.* afasia.

anosmic aphasia afasia anósmica.

auditory aphasia afasia auditiva.

Broca's aphasia afasia de Broca.

central aphasia afasia central.

childhood aphasia afasia infantil.

complete aphasia afasia completa.

global aphasia afasia global.

graphic aphasia afasia gráfica, afasia grafomotora.

graphomotor aphasia afasia gráfica, afasia grafomotora.

motor aphasia afasia motora.

optic aphasia afasia óptica.

verbal aphasia afasia verbal.

visual aphasia afasia visual.

Wernicke's aphasia afasia de Wernicke.

aphasiac *n.* afásico, -ca.

aphonia *n.* afonía.

aphonic *adj.* afónico, -ca.

aphrodisiac *adj.* afrodisíaco, -ca.

aphtha *n.* afta.

aphthoid *adj.* aftoide.

aplasia *n.* aplasia.

aplasia of the ovary aplasia ovárica.

aplasia pilorum propia aplasia pilorum propia.

ovarian aplasia aplasia ovárica.

thymic aplasia aplasia tímica.

aplastic *adj.* aplásico, -ca.

apnea *n.* apnea, apneustia.

apnea neonatorum apnea neonatal.

apnea vera apnea vera, apnea verdadera.

cardiac apnea apnea cardíaca.

central apnea apnea central.

central sleep apnea apnea central del sueño.

deglutition apnea apnea de deglución.

induced apnea apnea inducida.

late apnea apnea tardía.

mixed sleep apnea apnea del sueño mixta.

obstructive apnea apnea obstructiva.

obstructive sleep apnea apnea obstructiva del sueño (SAOS).

periodic apnea of the newborn apnea periódica del recién nacido.

peripheral apnea apnea periférica.

primary apnea apnea primaria.

reflex apnea apnea refleja.

secondary apnea apnea secundaria.

sleep apnea apnea del sueño.

sleep-induced apnea apnea inducida por el sueño.

true apnea apnea vera, apnea verdadera.

apneic *adj.* apneico, -ca.

apocrine *adj.* apocrino, -na.

apolipoprotein *n.* apolipoproteína.

aponeurosis *n.* aponeurosis.

apophysis *n.* apófisis.

apophysitis *n.* apofisitis.

apoplexia *n.* apoplejía.

apoplexia uterina apoplejía uterina.

apoplexy *n.* apoplejía.

abdominal apoplexy apoplejía abdominal.

bulbar apoplexy apoplejía bulbar.

cerebellar apoplexy apoplejía cerebelar, apoplejía cerebelosa.

cutaneous apoplexy apoplejía cutánea.

embolic apoplexy apoplejía embólica.

functional apoplexy apoplejía funcional.

heat apoplexy apoplejía por calor.

intestinal apoplexy apoplejía intestinal.

neonatal apoplexy apoplejía neonatorum.

pancreatic apoplexy apoplejía pancreática.

pituitary apoplexy apoplejía hipofisaria, apoplejía pituitaria.

placental apoplexy apoplejía placentaria.

pontil apoplexy apoplejía pontina.

pontile apoplexy apoplejía pontina.

renal apoplexy apoplejía renal.

spasmodic apoplexy apoplejía espasmódica.

spinal apoplexy apoplejía medular.

thrombotic apoplexy apoplejía trombótica.

uteroplacental apoplexy apoplejía uteroplacentaria.

apoptosis *n.* apoptosis.

apparatus *n.* aparato.

apparatus digestorius aparato digestivo.

digestive apparatus aparato digestivo.

respiratory apparatus aparato respiratorio.

urinary apparatus aparato urinario.

appendage *n.* apéndice.

appendicectomy *n.* apendicectomía, apendicotomía.

appendicitis *n.* apendicitis.

acute appendicitis apendicitis aguda.

appendicitis by contiguity apendicitis por contigüedad.

chronic appendicitis apendicitis crónica.

focal appendicitis apendicitis focal.

foreign-body appendicitis apendicitis por cuerpo extraño.

fulminating appendicitis apendicitis fulminante.

gangrenous appendicitis apendicitis gangrenosa.

left-sided appendicitis apendicitis izquierda.

lumbar appendicitis apendicitis lumbar.

obstructive appendicitis apendicitis obstructiva.

perforating appendicitis apendicitis destructiva, apendicitis perforante, apendicitis perforativa.

purulent appendicitis apendicitis purulenta.

recurrent appendicitis apendicitis recurrente.

segmental appendicitis apendicitis segmentaria.

suppurative appendicitis apendicitis supurada, apendicitis supurativa.

traumatic appendicitis apendicitis traumática.

verminous appendicitis apendicitis verminosa.

appendix *n.* apéndice.

appetite *n.* apetito.

appetition *n.* apetencia.

appliance *n.* aparato, dispositivo.

orthodontic appliance aparato ortodóncico, dispositivo ortodóncico.

approach *n.* abordaje.

apraxia *n.* apraxia.

akinetic apraxia apraxia acinética.

amnestic apraxia apraxia amnésica.

constructional apraxia apraxia constructiva, apraxia de construcción.

developmental apraxia apraxia del desarrollo.

gait apraxia apraxia de la marcha.

ideational apraxia apraxia ideomotriz, apraxia de ideación, apraxia ideatoria.

ideomotor apraxia apraxia ideomotora.

kinetic apraxia apraxia cinética.

sensory apraxia apraxia sensitiva.

apraxic *adj.* apráxico, -ca.

arachnoid *adj.* aracnoide.

arachnoidal *adj.* aracnoidal.

arachnoidea *n.* aracnoides.

arcade *n.* arcada.

dental arcade arcada Alveolar, arcada dentaria.

arch *n.* arco.

pharyngeal arch arco faríngeo.

reflex arch arco reflejo.

arcus *n.* arco, arcus.

arcus senilis arco senil.

ardor *n.* ardor, escozor.

heartburn ardor ardor epigástrico.

area *n.* área, zona.

relief area área de alivio, zona de descarga.

rest area área de descanso, zona de apoyo.

areola *n.* areola, aréola.

areola mammae areola de la mama, areola del pezón.

areola of mammary gland areola de la mama, areola del pezón.

areola of the nipple areola de la mama, areola del pezón.

areola papillaris areola papilar.

areola umbilicus areola umbilical.

second areola areola secundaria.

umbilical areola areola umbilical.

argyria *n.* argiria.

arm *n.* brazo.

armless *adj.* manco, -ca.

armpit *n.* axila.

arousal *n.* despertar.

arrhythmia *n.* arritmia.

cardiac arrhythmia arritmia cardíaca.

continuous arrhythmia arritmia continua.

juvenile arrhythmia arritmia juvenil.

perpetual arrhythmia arritmia perpetua.

phasic arrhythmia arritmia fásica.

respiratory arrhythmia arritmia respiratoria.

sinus arrhythmia arritmia de seno, arritmia sinusal.

arrhythmic *adj.* arrítmico, -ca.

artefact *n.* artefacto.

arteria *n.* arteria.

arterial *adj.* arterial.

arterialization *n.* arterialización, arterización.

arteriocapillary *adj.* arteriocapilar.

arteriodilating *n.* arteriodilatación.

arteriogenesis *n.* arteriogénesis.

arteriogram *n.* arteriograma.

arteriography *n.* arteriografía.

catheter arteriography arteriografía por sonda.

cerebral arteriography arteriografía cerebral.

selective coronary arteriography arteriografía selectiva coronaria.

spinal arteriography arteriografía espinal.

arteriola *n.* arteriola.

arteriolar *adj.* arteriolar.

arteriole *n.* arteriola.

arteriolitis *n.* arteriolitis.

necrotizing arteriolitis arteriolitis necrosante.

arteriopathy *n.* arteriopatía.

arteriosclerosis *n.* arterioesclerosis, arteriosclerosis.

cerebral arteriosclerosis arterioesclerosis cerebral.

coronary arteriosclerosis arterioesclerosis coronaria.

hypertensive arteriosclerosis arterioesclerosis hipertensiva.

peripheral arteriosclerosis arterioesclerosis periférica.

presenile arteriosclerosis arterioesclerosis presenil.

senile arteriosclerosis arterioesclerosis senil.

arteriosclerotic *adj.* arterioesclerótico, arteriosclerótico, -ca.

arteriospasm *n.* arterioespasmo, arteriospasmo.

arteriostenosis *n.* arterioestenosis, arteriostenosis.

arteriovenosus *adj.* arteriovenoso, -sa.

arteriovenous *adj.* arteriovenoso, -sa.

arteritis *n.* arteritis.

coronary arteritis arteritis coronaria.

cranial arteritis arteritis craneal.

rheumatic arteritis arteritis reumática.

arterocapillary *adj.* arteriocapilar.

artery *n.* arteria.

arthralgia *n.* artralgia, artronalgia.

arthritis *n.* artritis.

acute arthritis artritis aguda.

acute gouty arthritis artritis gotosa aguda.

acute rheumatic arthritis artritis reumática aguda.

arthritis deformans artritis deformante.

arthritis fungosa artritis fúngica, artritis fungosa.

arthritis mutilans artritis mutilante.

arthritis nodosa artritis nudosa.

arthritis sicca artritis seca.

chronic inflammatory arthritis artritis inflamatoria crónica.

climactic arthritis artritis climatérica.

degenerative arthritis artritis degenerativa.

exudative arthritis artritis exudativa.

fungal arthritis artritis fúngica, artritis fungosa.

gonoccocal arthritis artritis blenorrágica, artritis gonocócica, artritis gonorreica.

gouty arthritis artritis gotosa.

infectious arthritis artritis infecciosa.

juvenile arthritis artritis juvenil, artritis juvenil crónica.

juvenile chronic arthritis artritis juvenil, artritis juvenil crónica.

juvenile rheumatoid arthritis artritis reumatoide juvenil.

lyme arthritis artritis de lyme.

menopausal arthritis artritis menopáusica.

mycotic arthritis artritis micótica.

neuropathic arthritis artritis neuropática.

rheumatoid arthritis artritis reumatoide.

septic arthritis artritis séptica.

suppurative arthritis artritis supurada.

syphilitic arthritis artritis sifilítica.

tuberculous arthritis artritis tuberculosa.

viral arthritis artritis vírica.

arthropathia *n.* artropatía.

arthropathy *n.* artropatía.

Charcot's arthropathy artropatía de Charcot.

diabetic arthropathy artropatía diabética.

inflammatory arthropathy artropatía inflamatoria.

neurogenic arthropathy artropatía neurógena.

osteopulmonary arthropathy artropatía osteopulmonar.

syphilitic arthropathy artropatía sifilítica.

tabetic arthropathy artropatía tabética.

arthropod *n.* artrópodo.

arthroscope *n.* artroscopio.

arthroscopy *n.* artroscopia.

arthrosis *n.* artrosis.

arthrosis deformans artrosis deformans, artrosis deformante.

temporomandibular arthrosis artrosis temporomandibular.

articulate *adj.* articular.

articulated *adj.* articulado, -da.

articulatio *n.* articulación, articulatio.

articulation *n.* articulación.

articulator *n.* articulador.

artificial *adj.* artificial.

asbestosis *n.* asbestosis.

ascertainment *n.* comprobación, determinación, indagación.

complete ascertainment comprobación completa, determinación completa, indagación completa.

incomplete ascertainment comprobación incompleta, determinación incompleta.

multiple ascertainment comprobación múltiple.

single ascertainment comprobación única, determinación aislada, indagación única.

truncate ascertainment comprobación truncada, determinación trunca, indagación truncada.

ascites *n.* ascitis.

ascites adiposus ascitis adiposa.

ascites chylosus ascitis quilosa.

ascites praecox ascitis precoz.

bloody ascites ascitis sanguinolenta.

chyliform ascites ascitis quiliforme.

chylous ascites ascitis quilosa.

exudative ascites ascitis exudativa.

fatty ascites ascitis grasa.

hemorrhagic ascites ascitis hemorrágica.

milky ascites ascitis lechosa.

ascitic *adj.* ascítico, -ca.

asemia *n.* asemia.

asepsis *n.* asepsia, asepsis.

aseptic *adj.* aséptico, -ca.

aspect *n.* aspecto.

aspergilloma *n.* aspergiloma.

aspergillosis *n.* aspergilosis.

asphyxia *n.* asfixia.

asphyxia carbonica asfixia carbónica.

asphyxia livida asfixia lívida.

asphyxia neonatorum asfixia neonatal, asfixia neonatorum.

asphyxia pallida asfixia pálida.

asphyxia reticularis asfixia reticular.

blue asphyxia asfixia azul.

cyanotic asphyxia asfixia cianótica.

fetal asphyxia asfixia fetal.

local asphyxia asfixia local.

secondary asphyxia asfixia secundaria.

traumatic asphyxia asfixia traumática.

white asphyxia asfixia blanca.

asphyxiant *adj.* asfixiante.

asphyxiate *v.* asfixiar.

aspirate *adj.* aspirado, -da, aspirar.

aspiration *n.* aspiración.

bronchoscopic aspiration aspiración broncoscópica.

meconium aspiration aspiración de meconio, aspiración meconial.

post-tussive aspiration aspiración postusiva.

vacuum aspiration aspiración al vacío.

aspirator *n.* aspirador.

assay *n.* ensayo, valoración.

enzyme-linked immunosorbent assay ensayo de inmunoadsorción ligado a enzimas, ensayo enzimoinmunoensayo.

assessment *n.* valoración.

gestational assessment valoración gestacional.

neurologic assessment valoración neurológica.

pain assessment valoración del dolor.

physical assessment valoración física.

assistant *n.* soporte.

associated *adj.* asociado, -da.

association *n.* asociación.

association of ideas asociación de ideas.

controlled association asociación controlada, asociación dirigida.

dream association asociación de sueño, asociación onírica.

free association asociación libre.

genetic association asociación genética.

assonance *n.* asonancia.

assortment *n.* agrupación.

asthenia *n.* astenia, languidez.

myalgic asthenia astenia miálgica.

asthenopia *n.* astenopía.

asthma *n.* asma.

abdominal asthma asma abdominal.

allergic asthma asma alérgica.

alveolar asthma asma alveolar.

asthma convulsivum asma convulsiva.

atopic asthma asma atópica.

bacterial asthma asma bacteriana.

bronchial asthma asma bronquial.

bronchitic asthma asma bronquítica.

cardiac asthma asma cardíaca.

cat asthma asma de los gatos.

catarrhal asthma asma catarral.

dust asthma asma por polvo.

essential asthma asma esencial.

extrinsic asthma asma extrínseca.

food asthma asma alimentaria.

hay asthma asma del heno.

Heberden's asthma asma de Heberden, asma enfisematosa.

horse asthma asma caballar, asma equina.

humid asthma asma húmeda.

infective asthma asma infecciosa.

intrinsic asthma asma intrínseca.

miner's asthma asma de los mineros.

nervous asthma asma nerviosa.

pollen asthma asma por polen.

potter's asthma asma de los alfareros.

reflex asthma asma refleja.

renal asthma asma renal.

sexual asthma asma sexual.

spasmodic asthma asma espasmódica.

summer asthma asma de verano.

thymic asthma asma tímica.

true asthma asma verdadera.

asthmatic *adj.* asmático, -ca.

astigmatism *n.* astigmatismo.

acquired astigmatism astigmatismo adquirido.

astigmatism against the rule astigmatismo anormal.

compound astigmatism astigmatismo compuesto.

congenital astigmatism astigmatismo congénito.

corneal astigmatism astigmatismo corneal.

direct astigmatism astigmatismo directo.

hypermetropic astigmatism astigmatismo hipermetrópico, astigmatismo hiperópico.

hyperopic astigmatism astigmatismo hipermetrópico, astigmatismo hiperópico.

inverse astigmatism astigmatismo inverso.

irregular astigmatism astigmatismo irregular.

lenticular astigmatism astigmatismo lenticular.

mixed astigmatism astigmatismo mixto.

physiological astigmatism astigmatismo fisiológico.
astragalus *n.* astrágalo.
astringent *n.* astringente.
astrocyte *n.* astrocito.
astrocytoma *n.* astrocitoma.
astroglia *n.* astroglia.
asymmetric *adj.* asimétrico, -ca.
asymmetrical *adj.* asimétrico, -ca.
asymmetry *n.* asimetría.
asymptomatic *adj.* asintomático, -ca.
asystole *n.* asistolia.
asystolia *n.* asistolia.
asystolic *adj.* asistólico, -ca.
ataxia *n.* ataxia.
acute ataxia ataxia aguda.
alcoholic ataxia ataxia alcohólica.
ataxia cordis ataxia cardíaca, ataxia cordis.
autonomic ataxia ataxia autónoma.
central ataxia ataxia central.
cerebellar ataxia ataxia cerebelosa.
cerebral ataxia ataxia cerebral.
frontal ataxia ataxia frontal.
hereditary ataxia ataxia hereditaria.
hysterical ataxia ataxia histérica.
kinetic ataxia ataxia cinética, ataxia dinámica.
labyrinthic ataxia ataxia laberíntica.
locomotor ataxia ataxia locomotora, ataxia locomotriz.
ocular ataxia ataxia ocular.
optic ataxia ataxia óptica.
sensory ataxia ataxia sensitiva.
spinal ataxia ataxia espinal.
static ataxia ataxia estática.

atelectasis *n.* atelectasia.
compression atelectasis atelectasia compresiva.
congenital atelectasis atelectasia congénita.
lobular atelectasis atelectasia lobular.
obstructive atelectasis atelectasia obstructiva.
segmental atelectasis atelectasia segmentaria.
atheroembolism *n.* ateroembolia, ateroembolismo.
atheroembolus *n.* ateroémbolo.
atherogenesis *n.* aterogénesis.
atherogenic *adj.* aterogenético, -ca, aterogénico, -ca.
atheroma *n.* ateroma.
atheromatosis *n.* ateromatosis.
athetosis *n.* atesia, atetosis.
atlas *n.* atlas.
atom *n.* átomo.
atonic *adj.* atónico, -ca.
atony *n.* atonía.
atopia *n.* atopia.
atopic *adj.* atópico, -ca.
atresia *n.* atresia.
anal atresia atresia del ano.
aortic atresia atresia aórtica.
atresia iridis atresia del iris, atresia irídica.
biliary atresia atresia biliar.
choanal atresia atresia de las coanas.
duodenal atresia atresia duodenal.
esophageal atresia atresia esofágica.
intestinal atresia atresia intestinal.
mitral atresia atresia mitral.

pulmonary atresia atresia pulmonar.

tricuspid atresia atresia tricúspide, atresia tricuspídea.

vaginal atresia atresia vaginal.

atresic *adj.* atrésico, -ca, atrético, -ca.

atrial *adj.* atrial.

atrium *n.* atrio, atrium, aurícula.

atrophia *n.* atrofia.

atrophic *adj.* atrófico, -ca.

atrophy *n.* aridura, atrofia.

atrophy cutis atrofia cutis.

atrophy of disuse atrofia por desuso, atrofia por inacción.

atrophy unguium atrofia ungueal.

bone atrophy atrofia ósea.

cerebellar atrophy atrofia cerebelosa.

degenerative atrophy atrofia degenerativa.

exhaustion atrophy atrofia por agotamiento.

gastric atrophy atrofia gástrica, gastratrofia.

gingival atrophy atrofia gingival.

hemifacial atrophy atrofia hemifacial.

hemilingual atrophy atrofia hemilingual.

infantile atrophy atrofia infantil.

inflammatory atrophy atrofia inflamatoria.

muscular atrophy atrofia muscular.

myopathic muscular atrophy atrofia miopática.

pathologic atrophy atrofia patológica.

periodontal atrophy atrofia periodontal.

spinal atrophy atrofia espinal.

atropinism *n.* atropinismo, atropismo.

attachment *n.* inserción, unión.

attack *n.* acceso, ataque.

heart attack ataque cardíaco.

panic attack ataque de pánico.

sleep attack ataque de sueño.

transient ischemic attack ataque isquémico transitorio.

vagal attack ataque vagal.

vasovagal attack ataque vasovagal.

attention *n.* atención.

attenuate *v.* atenuar.

attenuation *n.* atenuación.

attitude *n.* actitud.

attraction *n.* atracción.

atypia *n.* atipia.

atypical *adj.* atípico, -ca.

audiogram *n.* audiograma.

audiometry *n.* audiometría.

audition *n.* audición.

auditive *adj.* auditivo, -va.

auditory *adj.* auditivo, -va.

aura *n.* aura.

auditory aura aura auditiva.

aura asthmatica aura asmática.

aura hysterica aura histérica.

electric aura aura eléctrica.

epigastric aura aura epigástrica.

epileptic aura aura epiléptica.

intellectual aura aura intelectual.

kinesthetic aura aura cinestésica.

reminescent aura aura reminiscente.

vertiginous aura aura vertiginosa.

auricular *adj.* auricular.

auris *n.* oído.

auris externa auris externa, oído externo.

auris interna auris interna, oído interno.

auris media auris media, oído medio.

auscult *v.* auscultar.

auscultate *v.* auscultar.

auscultation *n.* auscultación.

direct auscultation auscultación directa.

immediate auscultation auscultación inmediata.

obstetric auscultation auscultación obstétrica.

autism *n.* autismo.

autistic *adj.* autista.

autoagglutination *n.* autoaglutinación.

autoagglutinin *n.* autoaglutinina.

autoantibody *n.* autoanticuerpo.

autoclave *n.* autoclave.

autoimmune *adj.* autoinmune, autoinmunitario, -ria.

autoimmunity *n.* autoinmunidad.

autoimmunization *n.* autoinmunización.

autoinoculation *n.* autoinoculación.

autolesion *n.* autolesión, automutilación.

automatism *n.* automatismo.

ambulatory automatism automatismo ambulatorio, automatismo deambulante.

command automatism automatismo de orden.

autonomic *adj.* autonómico, -ca.

autonomy *n.* autonomía.

autopsia *n.* autopsia.

autopsy *n.* autopsia.

autoregulation *n.* autorregulación.

autotransfusion *n.* autotransfusión.

autotransplantation *n.* autotrasplante.

avascular *adj.* avascular.

average *n.* medio, medium.

axilla *n.* axila.

axillary *adj.* axilar.

axis *n.* axis, eje.

axon *n.* axón.

axonal *adj.* axonal, axónico, -ca.

azoospermatism *n.* azoospermia.

azoospermia *n.* azoospermia.

azotemia *n.* azoemia, hiperazoemia.

azotemic *adj.* azoémico, -ca.

B

baby *n.* bebé, neonato.

blue baby bebé azul, neonato azul.

immature baby bebé inmaduro.

test-tube baby bebé probeta.

babyhood *n.* infancia.

bacillar *adj.* bacilar.

bacillary *adj.* bacilar.

bacilleferous *adj.* bacilífero, -ra.

bacillemia *n.* bacilemia.

bacilliform *adj.* baciliforme.

bacillus *n.* bacilo.

back *n.* dorso, espalda.

backache *n.* dorsalgia.

background *n.* antecedentes.

bacterial *adj.* bacteriano, -na.

bactericide *n.* bactericida.

bacteriemia *n.* bacteriemia.

bacteriocide *n.* bactericida.

bacteriologic *adj.* bacteriológico, -ca.
bacteriological *adj.* bacteriológico, -ca.
bacteriologist *n.* bacteriólogo, -ga.
bacteriology *n.* bacteriología.
 clinical diagnostic bacteriology
bacteriología clínica.
 medical bacteriology bacteriología médica.
 public health bacteriology bacteriología higiénica.
 sanitary bacteriology bacteriología sanitaria.
 systematic bacteriology bacteriología sistemática.
bacteriophage *n.* bacteriófago, mi-
crobívoro.
bacteriosis *n.* bacteriosis.
bacterium *n.* bacteria.
bacteriuria *n.* bacteriuria.
 asymptomatic bacteriuria bacteriuria asintomática.
 pregnancy bacteriuria bacteriuria
gravídica.
 significant bacteriuria bacteriuria
significativa.
bacteriuric *adj.* bacteriúrico, -ca.
bacteruria *n.* bacteriuria.
bag *n.* bolsa.
 bag of waters bolsa de aguas.
 colostomy bag bolsa de colostomía.
 forewaters bag bolsa de aguas.
 ileostomy bag bolsa de ileostomía.
 micturition bag bolsa para micción.
 testicular bag bolsa testicular.
balance *n.* balance, balanza, equilibrio.

 acid-base balance balance acidobásico, equilibrio ácido-base, equilibrio acidobásico.
 calcium balance balance cálcico.
 electrolyte balance balance electrolítico, equilibrio electrolítico.
 energy balance balance calórico,
balance energético.
 enzyme balance balance enzimático.
 fluid balance balance líquido.
 genic balance balance genético.
 glomerulotubular balance balance glomérulo-tubular.
 inhibition-action balance balance
de inhibición y acción.
 nitrogen balance balance de nitrógeno, balance nitrogenado, equilibrio
nitrogenado, equilibrio nitrógeno.
 occlusal balance balance oclusal,
equilibrio oclusal.
 water balance balance hídrico.
balanitis *n.* balanitis.
bald *adj.* calvo, -va.
baldness *n.* calvicie.
 common male baldness calvicie
masculina común.
 congenital baldness calvicie congénita.
 male pattern baldness calvicie de
distribución masculina.
 pubic baldness calvicie del pubis.
ball *n.* bola, pelota.
 fatty ball of Bichat bola adiposa de
Bichat, bola grasa de Bichat.
 food ball bola alimentaria, bola de
alimento, pelota de comida.
 fungus ball bola fúngica, bola micótica.

balloon *n.* balón, balonizar.
  balloon angioplasty angioplastia con balón.
balm *n.* bálsamo.
balneotherapeutics *n.* balneoterapia.
balneotherapy *n.* balneoterapia.
balsamic *adj.* balsámico, -ca.
band *n.* banda, bandaleta, bandeleta, cintilla.
  amniotic band banda amniótica.
  belly band banda abdominal.
  clamp band banda abrazadera, banda clamp.
bandage *n.* venda, vendaje.
  adhesive bandage vendaje adhesivo.
  elastic bandage venda elástica, vendaje elástico.
  immobilizing bandage vendaje de inmovilización.
banding *n.* bandaje, bandeo, banding.
bank *n.* banco.
  blood bank banco de sangre.
  embryo bank banco de embriones.
  eye bank banco de ojos.
  gene bank banco de genes.
  semen bank banco de semen.
  serum bank banco de suero.
  sperm bank banco de esperma.
bar *n.* barra.
barba *n.* barba.
barbiturate *n.* barbitúrico.
bariatric *adj.* bariátrico, -ca.
bariatrics *n.* bariatría.
barium *n.* bario.
baroceptor *n.* baroceptor.
baroreceptor *n.* barorreceptor.

barotrauma *n.* barotrauma, barotraumatismo.
barrier *n.* barrera.
  blood-brain barrier (BBB) barrera hematocerebral, barrera hematoencefálica (BHE).
  blood-cerebral barrier barrera hematocerebral, barrera hematoencefálica (BHE).
  blood-cerebrospinal fluid barrier barrera hematocerebroespinal.
  gastric mucosal barrier barrera de la mucosa gástrica, barrera mucosa.
  placental barrier barrera placentaria.
  protective barrier barrera protectora.
  skin barrier barrera cutánea.
bartholinitis *n.* bartholinitis, bartolinitis.
basal *adj.* basal.
base *n.* base.
  nitrogenous base base nitrogenada.
basic *adj.* básico, -ca.
basilar *adj.* basilar.
basilaris *adj.* basilar, basilaris.
basophil *n.* basófilo, -la.
basophilia *n.* basofilia.
bath *n.* baño.
  antipyretic bath baño antipirético.
  antiseptic bath baño antiséptico.
  astringent bath baño astringente.
  hip bath baño de asiento.
  lukewarm bath baño templado.
  mood bath baño de barro, baño de fango, baño de limo, baño de lodo.
  mud bath baño de barro.
  seawater bath baño de agua de mar.

sitz bath baño de asiento.

water bath baño de agua, baño de María.

battery *n.* batería.

beam *n.* balancín, haz, traviesa.

X-ray beam haz de rayos X.

beard *n.* barba.

beat *n.* latido, latir.

ectopic beat latido ectópico.

escape beat latido de escape.

escaped beat latido de escape.

heart beat latido cardíaco.

bed *n.* lecho.

capillary bed lecho capilar.

nail bed lecho ungueal.

behavior *n.* comportamiento, conducta.

sexual behavior comportamiento sexual.

behaviorism *n.* behaviorismo, conductismo.

behaviorist *adj.* conductista.

belch *n.* eructar, eructo.

belly *n.* vientre.

wooden belly vientre de madera, vientre en tabla.

benign *adj.* benigno, -na.

bereavement *n.* aflicción, duelo.

beriberi *n.* beriberi.

beta *n.* beta.

beta fetoprotein beta fetoproteína.

beta-blocker *n.* betabloqueante.

beta-carotene *n.* betacaroteno.

beta-lipoprotein *n.* beta-lipoproteína.

bevel *n.* bisel, biselar.

bezoar *n.* bezoar.

biarticular *adj.* biarticular.

biarticulate *adj.* biarticulado, -da.

bias *n.* desviación, sesgo.

detection bias sesgo de detección.

bicarbonate *n.* bicarbonato.

blood bicarbonate bicarbonato sanguíneo.

plasma bicarbonate bicarbonato del plasma.

sodium bicarbonate bicarbonato de sodio, bicarbonato sódico.

standard bicarbonate bicarbonato estándar.

biceps *n.* bíceps.

bicipital *adj.* bicipital.

biclonal *adj.* biclonal.

biconcave *adj.* bicóncavo, -va.

biconvex *adj.* biconvexo, -xa.

bicornate *adj.* bicorne.

bicornous *adj.* bicorne.

bicornuate *adj.* bicorne.

bicuspid *n.* bicúspide.

bidet *n.* bidé, bidet.

bidimensional *adj.* bidimensional.

bifidobacterium *n.* bifidobacteria.

bifocal *adj.* bifocal.

bifurcate *adj.* bifurcado, -da.

bifurcated *adj.* bifurcado, -da.

bifurcatio *n.* bifurcación, bifurcatio.

bifurcatio aortae bifurcatio aortae.

bifurcatio aortica bifurcatio aortae.

bifurcatio carotidis bifurcatio carotidis.

bifurcatio trunci pulmonalis bifurcatio trunci pulmonalis.

bifurcation *n.* bifurcación, bifurcatio.

bifurcation of the aorta bifurcación aórtica, bifurcación de la aorta, bifurcatio aortae.

bifurcation of the pulmonary

trunk bifurcación del tronco pulmonar, bifurcatio trunci pulmonalis.

carotid bifurcation bifurcación de la carótida, bifurcato carotidis.

bigeminal *adj.* bigeminado, -da, bigeminal.

bigeminy *n.* bigeminia, bigeminidad, bigeminismo.

bilateral *adj.* bilateral.

bilateralism *n.* bilateralismo.

bile *n.* bilis.

biliary *adj.* biliar.

bilious *adj.* bilioso, -sa.

biliousness *n.* biliosidad.

bilirubin *n.* bilirrubina.

conjugated bilirubin bilirrubina conjugada.

direct bilirubin bilirrubina directa.

direct reacting bilirubin bilirrubina de reacción directa.

free bilirubin bilirrubina libre.

indirect bilirubin bilirrubina indirecta.

indirect reacting bilirubin bilirrubina de reacción indirecta.

total bilirubin bilirrubina total.

unconjugated bilirubin bilirrubina no conjugada.

bilirubinemia *n.* bilirrubinemia.

bilobate *adj.* bilobulado, -da.

bilobed *adj.* bilobulado, -da, bilobular.

binary *adj.* binario, -ria.

bind *v.* unir, vendar.

binder *n.* faja.

abdominal binder faja abdominal.

binuclear *adj.* binuclear.

bioactivity *n.* bioactividad.

bioassay *n.* bioanálisis, bioensayo.

bioavailability *n.* biodisponibilidad.

biochemical *adj.* bioquímico, -ca.

biochemistry *n.* bioquímica.

biocompatibility *n.* biocompatibilidad.

biocompatible *adj.* biocompatible.

biodegradable *adj.* biodegradable.

bioequivalent *adj.* bioequivalente.

bioethics *n.* bioética.

biofeedback *n.* biorretroalimentación.

biogeny *n.* biogenia.

bioimplant *n.* bioimplante.

bioincompatibility *n.* bioincompatibilidad.

biology *n.* biología.

biomarker *n.* biomarcador.

biomechanics *n.* biomecánica.

biomedicine *n.* biomedicina.

biophysics *n.* biofísica.

bioprosthesis *n.* bioprótesis.

biopsy *n.* biopsia.

aspiration biopsy biopsia por aspiración.

bone biopsy biopsia ósea.

cerebral biopsy biopsia cerebral.

cervix uterinic biopsy biopsia del cuello uterino.

chorionic biopsy biopsia coriónica.

chorionic villus biopsy (CVB) biopsia de vellosidad coriónica (BVC).

cone biopsy biopsia cónica, biopsia de cono.

cytological biopsy biopsia citológica.

endometrium biopsy biopsia del endometrio.

endoscopic biopsy biopsia endoscópica.

excision biopsy biopsia escisional, biopsia por escisión.

exploratory biopsy biopsia de exploración.

fine-needle aspiration biopsy biopsia por punción-aspiración con aguja fina.

liver biopsy biopsia hepática.

muscular biopsy biopsia muscular.

needle biopsy biopsia por aguja, biopsia por punción.

negative biopsy biopsia negativa.

percutaneous biopsy biopsia percutánea.

percutaneous renal biopsy biopsia renal percutánea.

positive biopsy biopsia positiva.

punch biopsy biopsia con sacabocados, biopsia de sacabocado.

renal biopsy biopsia renal.

sternal biopsy biopsia esternal.

surface biopsy biopsia de superficie, biopsia exfoliativa, biopsia superficial.

surgical biopsy biopsia quirúrgica.

transvenous renal biopsy biopsia renal transvenosa.

trephine biopsy biopsia por trepanación.

wedge biopsy biopsia en cuña.

biorhythm *n.* biorritmo.

bioscience *n.* biociencia.

biostatistics *n.* bioestadística.

biosynthesis *n.* biosíntesis.

biotechnology *n.* biotecnología.

biotin *n.* biotina.

biotype *n.* biotipo.

biparietal *adj.* biparietal.

biphasic *adj.* bifásico, -ca.

bipolar *adj.* bipolar.

birefringence *n.* birrefringencia.

birth *n.* nacimiento.

complete birth nacimiento completo.

cross birth nacimiento transversal.

dead birth nacimiento con producto muerto.

head birth nacimiento de vértice.

multiple birth nacimiento múltiple.

post-term birth nacimiento tardío.

preterm birth nacimiento prematuro, nacimiento pretérmino.

birthmark *n.* antojo.

bisexual *adj.* bisexual.

bistoury *n.* bisturí.

bite *n.* bocado, dentellada, mordedura, mordida, mordisco.

closed bite mordida cerrada.

cross bite mordida cruzada.

normal bite mordida normal.

open bite mordida abierta.

bitter *adj.* amargo, -ga.

bivalent *adj.* bivalente.

biventricular *adj.* biventricular.

blackout *n.* desmayo.

bladder *n.* vejiga.

urinary bladder vejiga de la orina, vejiga urinaria, vesica urinalis, vesica urinaria.

blanket *n.* manta.

bath blanket manta de baño.

hypothermia blanket manta de hipotermia.

blastemic *adj.* blastémico, -ca.

blastocele *n.* blastocele.

blastocoele *n.* blastocele.

blastocyst *n.* blastocisto.

blastomere *n.* blastómera, blastómero.

blastomycosis *n.* blastomicosis.

blastula *n.* blástula.

bleaching *adj.* blanqueamiento, decolorante, descolorante.

bleb *n.* ampolla.

bleed *v.* sangrar.

bleeding *n.* desangramiento, hemorragia, sangrado, sangramiento.

  dysfunctional uterine bleeding sangrado uterino disfuncional.

  occult bleeding hemorragia oculta.

blennorrhea *n.* blenorrea.

blepharitis *n.* blefaritis.

  blepharitis rosacea blefaritis rosácea.

  blepharitis sicca blefaritis seca.

  blepharitis ulcerosa blefaritis ulcerosa.

  seborrheic blepharitis blefaritis seborreica.

  squamous seborrheic blepharitis blefaritis seborreica escamosa.

  ulcerative blepharitis blefaritis ulcerosa.

blepharospasm *n.* blefaroespasmo, blefarospasmo.

blepharospasmus *n.* blefaroespasmo.

blind *adj.* ciego, -ga.

blindness *n.* ceguera.

  color blindness ceguera para los colores.

  mind blindness ceguera mental.

  music blindness ceguera musical.

  night blindness ceguera nocturna.

  psychic blindness ceguera psíquica.

  smell blindness ceguera para el olfato.

blister *n.* ampolla, blíster, vesícula.

block *n.* bloque, bloquear, bloqueo.

  air block bloqueo de aire.

  atrioventricular block bloqueo auriculoventricular bloqueo A-V).

  A-V block bloqueo auriculoventricular bloqueo A-V).

  bundle-branch block (BBB) bloqueo de rama (BR).

  congenital complete heart block bloqueo cardíaco congénito.

  congenital heart block bloqueo cardíaco congénito.

  ear block bloqueo auditivo.

  epidural block bloqueo epidural.

  heart block bloqueo cardíaco, bloqueo del corazón.

  intercostal block bloqueo intercostal.

  interventricular block bloqueo de rama (BR).

  intra-atrial block bloqueo intraauricular.

  intraspinal block bloqueo intraespinal.

  nerve block bloqueo nervioso.

  neuromuscular block bloqueo neuromuscular.

  non-depolarizing block bloqueo no despolarizante.

  paracervical block bloqueo paracervical.

  perineural block bloqueo perineural.

  presacral block bloqueo presacro.

  protective block bloqueo protector.

  spinal block bloqueo espinal.

blockade *n.* bloqueo.
  renal blockade bloqueo renal.
  vagal blockade bloqueo vagal.
  vagus nerve blockade bloqueo vagal.
blocker *n.* bloqueador, -ra, bloqueante.
  alpha-blocker bloqueante alfa-adrenérgico.
  beta-blocker bloqueante beta-adrenérgico.
  calcium channel blocker bloqueante de la vía del calcio, bloqueante de los canales de calcio.
blocking *n.* bloqueo.
  affective blocking bloqueo afectivo, bloqueo emocional.
  mental blocking bloqueo mental.
  thought blocking bloqueo del pensamiento.
blood *n.* sangre.
  arterial blood sangre arterial.
  central blood sangre central.
  cord blood sangre del cordón.
  mixed venous blood sangre venosa mixta.
  occult blood sangre oculta.
  peripheral blood sangre periférica.
  sludged blood sangre estancada, sangre lodosa.
  venous blood sangre venosa.
  whole blood sangre entera, sangre total.
bloodletting *n.* sangradura, sangría.
blurring *n.* borrosidad.
body *n.* cuerpo.
  vitreous body cuerpo vítreo, cuerpo vítreo.
boil *n.* botón, divieso, furúnculo.

bolus *n.* bolo.
  alimentary bolus bolo alimentario, bolo alimenticio.
  intravenous bolus bolo endovenoso, bolo intravenoso.
bonding *n.* vinculación, vinculación afectiva.
  maternal-infant bonding vinculación maternoinfantil.
bone *n.* hueso.
bonelet *n.* huesecillo.
bony *adj.* óseo, -a.
boot *n.* bota.
border *n.* borde.
  striated border borde estriado.
borderline *adj.* borderline, limítrofe.
bottle *n.* botella, frasco.
  nursing bottle biberón.
botulin *n.* botulina.
botulinal *adj.* botulínico, -ca.
botulism *n.* botulismo.
  wound botulism botulismo en heridas, botulismo por herida.
bougie *n.* bujía.
  ear bougie bujía auditiva.
bouillon *n.* caldo.
bourdonnement *n.* zumbido.
bout *n.* brote.
bouton *n.* botón.
  bouton terminale botón terminal, bouton terminale.
  synaptic bouton botón sináptico.
  terminal bouton botón terminal, bouton terminale.
brace *n.* abrazadera, braguero, corsé.
bracelet *n.* brazalete.
brachial *adj.* braquial.
brachialgia *n.* braquialgia.

brachialgia statica paresthestica braquialgia estática parestésica.

bradycardia *n.* bradicardia.

cardiomuscular bradycardia bradicardia cardiomuscular.

central bradycardia bradicardia central.

essential bradycardia bradicardia esencial.

fetal bradycardia bradicardia fetal.

idiopathic bradycardia bradicardia idiopática.

nodal bradycardia bradicardia nodal.

postinfectious bradycardia bradicardia posinfecciosa, bradicardia postinfecciosa.

postinfective bradycardia bradicardia posinfecciosa, bradicardia postinfecciosa.

sinoatrial bradycardia bradicardia sinoauricular.

sinus bradycardia bradicardia sinusal.

vagal bradycardia bradicardia vagal.

ventricular bradycardia bradicardia ventricular.

bradycardiac *adj.* bradicárdico.

bradycardic *adj.* bradicárdico.

bradykinesia *n.* bradicinesia, bradiquinesia.

bradypnea *n.* bradipnea.

bradypsychia *n.* bradipsiquia.

braille *n.* braille.

brain *n.* cerebro, encéfalo.

branch *n.* rama, ramo.

branching *adj.* ramificado, -da.

break *n.* ruptura.

breast *n.* mama.

breast-feeding *n.* lactancia materna.

breath *n.* aliento.

bad breath mal aliento.

liver breath aliento hepático.

uremic breath aliento urémico.

breathing *n.* respiración.

shallow breathing respiración superficial.

bridge *n.* puente.

bromatologist *n.* bromatólogo, -ga.

bromatology *n.* bromatología.

bronchial *adj.* bronquial.

bronchiectasia *n.* bronquiectasis.

bronchiectasic *adj.* bronquiectásico.

bronchiectasis *n.* bronquiectasis.

bronchiectatic *adj.* bronquiectático.

bronchiole *n.* bronquiolo, bronquíolo.

lobular bronchiole bronquiolo lobulillar.

terminal bronchiole bronquiolo terminal.

bronchiolitis *n.* bronquiolitis.

acute obliterating bronchiolitis bronquiolitis aguda obliterante.

bronchiolitis obliterans bronquiolitis obliterante.

bronchiolus *n.* bronquiolo, bronquíolo.

bronchismus *n.* broncoespasmo.

bronchitis *n.* bronquitis.

acute bronchitis bronquitis aguda.

bronchitis obliterans bronquitis obliterante.

catarrhal bronchitis bronquitis catarral.

chronic bronchitis bronquitis crónica.

croupous bronchitis bronquitis crupal.

dry bronchitis bronquitis seca.

epidemic bronchitis bronquitis epidémica.

exudative bronchitis bronquitis exudativa.

infectious asthmatic bronchitis bronquitis asmática infecciosa.

membranous bronchitis bronquitis membranosa.

obliterative bronchitis bronquitis obliterante.

productive bronchitis bronquitis productiva.

putrid bronchitis bronquitis fétida, bronquitis pútrida.

staphylococcus bronchitis bronquitis estafilocócica.

streptococcal bronchitis bronquitis estreptocócica.

bronchoalveolitis *n.* broncoalveolitis.

bronchoaspiration *n.* broncoaspiración.

bronchoconstriction *n.* broncoconstricción.

bronchoconstrictor *n.* broncoconstrictor.

bronchodilatation *n.* broncodilatación.

bronchodilator *n.* broncodilatador.

bronchofiberscope *n.* broncofibroscopio.

bronchofiberscopy *n.* broncofibroscopia.

bronchofibroscope *n.* broncofibroscopio.

bronchofibroscopy *n.* broncofibroscopia.

bronchopathy *n.* broncopatía.

bronchopneumonia *n.* bronconeumonía.

postoperative bronchopneumonia bronconeumonía postoperatoria.

tuberculous bronchopneumonia bronconeumonía tuberculosa.

virus bronchopneumonia bronconeumonía por virus.

bronchopneumonic *adj.* bronconeumónico, -ca.

bronchopneumonitis *n.* bronconeumonitis.

bronchorrhea *n.* broncorrea.

bronchoscopy *n.* broncoscopia.

fiberoptic bronchoscopy broncoscopia de fibra óptica, broncoscopia fibroóptica.

laser bronchoscopy broncoscopia láser.

bronchospasm *n.* broncoespasmo, broncospasmo.

bronchus *n.* bronchus, bronquio.

stem bronchus bronquio de sostén, bronquio fuente.

tracheal bronchus bronquio traqueal.

broth *n.* caldo.

brucellosis *n.* brucelosis.

bruit *n.* ruido.

brush *n.* cepillo.

denture brush cepillo dental.

bruxism *n.* bruxismo.

buba *n.* buba, bubas.

bubas *n.* buba, bubas.

bubo *n.* bubón.

buccal *adj.* bucal.

bud *n.* brote, yema.

bronchial bud brote bronquial, yema bronquial.

lung bud brote pulmonar, yema pulmonar.

tail bud brote caudal.

vascular bud brote vascular, yema vascular.

buffer *n.* amortiguador, buffer, tampón.

buffering *n.* amortiguamiento.

bulb *n.* bulbo, bulbus.

bulbar *adj.* bulbar.

bulbitis *n.* bulbitis.

bulbus *n.* bulbo, bulbus.

bulimia *n.* bulimia.

bulimia nervosa bulimia nerviosa.

bulimic *adj.* bulímico, -ca.

bulla *n.* bulla.

bulla ethmoidalis bulla etmoidal.

bulla ossea bulla ossea.

emphysematous bulla bulla enfisematosa.

ethmoid bulla bulla etmoidal.

ethmoidal bulla bulla etmoidal.

pulmonary bulla bulla pulmonar.

bullosis *n.* bullosis.

bullous *adj.* bulloso, -sa.

bundle *n.* banda, fascículo.

bunion *n.* bunio, juanete.

burden *n.* carga.

body burden carga corporal.

tumor burden carga tumoral.

burn *n.* quemadura.

chemical burn quemadura química.

electric burn quemadura eléctrica.

electrical burn quemadura eléctrica.

radiation burn quemadura por radiación.

second degree burn quemadura de segundo grado.

solar burn quemadura solar.

sun burn quemadura solar.

superficial burn quemadura superficial.

thermal burn quemadura por agentes térmicos, quemadura térmica.

third degree burn quemadura de tercer grado.

X-ray burn quemadura por rayos X.

burning *n.* quemazón.

bursa *n.* bolsa, bursa.

bursitis *n.* bursitis.

Achilles bursitis bursitis aquilea, bursitis aquiliana.

olecranal bursitis bursitis del olécranon, bursitis oleocraniana.

popliteal bursitis bursitis poplítea.

prepatellar bursitis bursitis prerrotuliana.

radiohumeral bursitis bursitis radiohumeral.

retrocalcaneal bursitis bursitis retrocalcánea.

button *n.* botón.

Oriental button botón de Oriente, botón oriental.

by pass *n.* derivación.

C

cabinet *n.* gabinete.

cachectic *adj.* caquéctico, -ca.

cachexia *n.* caquexia.

cachexia suprarrenalis caquexia suprarrenal.

cachexia thyroidea caquexia tiroidea.

malarial cachexia caquexia palúdica.

cadaver *n.* cadáver.

cadaveric *adj.* cadavérico, -ca.

cadaverous *adj.* cadavérico, -ca.

caduca *n.* caduca.

caecum *n.* caecum, ciego.

calcaneus *n.* calcáneo.

calcemia *n.* calcemia.

calcification *n.* calcificación.

   pathologic calcification calcificación patológica.

   pulp calcification calcificación de la pulpa.

calcinosis *n.* calcinosis.

calcium *n.* calcio.

calciuria *n.* calciuria.

calculus *n.* cálculo, calculus.

   arthritic calculus cálculo artrítico.

   articular calculus cálculo articular.

   biliary calculus cálculo biliar.

   bladder calculus cálculo de la vejiga.

   bronchial calculus cálculo bronquial.

   cardiac calculus cálculo cardíaco.

   cerebral calculus cálculo cerebral.

   cholesterol calculus cálculo de colesterol.

   cystine calculus cálculo de cistina.

   dental calculus cálculo dental, cálculo dentario.

   encysted calculus cálculo enquistado.

   fibrin calculus cálculo de fibrina.

   gastric calculus cálculo gástrico.

   hepatic calculus cálculo hepático.

   intestinal calculus cálculo intestinal.

   pancreatic calculus cálculo pancreático.

   pharyngeal calculus cálculo faríngeo.

   renal calculus cálculo renal.

   salivary calculus cálculo salival.

   stomachic calculus cálculo gástrico.

   urate calculus cálculo de urato.

   uric acid calculus cálculo de ácido úrico.

   urinary calculus cálculo urinario.

   vesical calculus cálculo vesical.

   xanthic calculus cálculo xantínico.

calentura *n.* calentura.

calenture *n.* calentura.

callosal *adj.* calloso, -sa.

callositas *n.* callosidad.

callosity *n.* callosidad.

callous *adj.* calloso, -sa.

callus *n.* callo.

   hard callus callo duro.

calmative *n.* calmante.

calor *n.* calor.

caloric *adj.* calórico, -ca.

calorie *n.* caloría.

calvaria *n.* calvaria, calvario.

calvities *n.* calvicie.

calyx *n.* cáliz, calyx.

camera *n.* cámara.

   pulp camera cámara pulpar.

canal *n.* canal.

canaliculus *n.* canalículo, canaliculus.

canalis *n.* canal.

canalization *n.* canalización.

cancellated *adj.* canceloso, -sa.

cancellous *adj.* canceloso, -sa.

cancer *n.* cáncer.

   bone cancer cáncer óseo.

   breast cancer cáncer de mama.

   cancer in situ cáncer in situ.

familial cancer cáncer familiar.

latent cancer cáncer latente.

liver cancer cáncer de hígado.

lung cancer cáncer de pulmón.

medullary cancer cáncer medular.

occult cancer cáncer oculto.

pipe-smoker's cancer cáncer de los fumadores de pipa.

stump cancer cáncer del muñón.

cancerigenic *adj.* cancerígeno, -na.

cancerogenic *adj.* cancerígeno, -na.

cancerous *adj.* canceroso, -sa, carcinoso, -sa.

Candida *n.* Candida.

candidemia *n.* candidemia.

candidiasis *n.* candidiasis, candidiosis.

cutaneous candidiasis candidiasis cutánea.

endocardial candidiasis candidiasis endocárdica.

candidosis *n.* candidosis.

cane *n.* bastón.

canine *n.* canino.

cannabis *n.* cannabis.

cannula *n.* cánula.

tracheostomy cannula cánula de traqueostomía.

cannulization *n.* canulización.

cap *n.* capuchón.

capacitation *n.* capacitación.

capacity *n.* capacidad.

buffer capacity capacidad buffer.

forced vital capacity (FVC) capacidad vital (CV), capacidad vital forzada (CVF).

heat capacity capacidad térmica.

hypnotic capacity capacidad hipnótica.

inspiratory capacity capacidad inspiratoria.

iron-binding capacity (IBC) capacidad de fijación de hierro (CFH).

oxygen capacity capacidad de oxígeno.

residual capacity capacidad residual.

respiratory capacity capacidad respiratoria.

thermal capacity capacidad térmica.

total lung capacity (TLC) capacidad pulmonar total (CPT).

vital capacity (VC) capacidad vital (CV), capacidad vital forzada (CVF).

capillarity *n.* capilaridad.

capillary *n.* capilar.

capillus *n.* cabello, capillus.

capsid *n.* cápsida, cápside.

capsula *n.* capsula, cápsula.

capsule *n.* capsula, cápsula.

nasal capsule cápsula nasal.

optic capsule cápsula óptica.

otic capsule cápsula ótica.

capsulitis *n.* capsulitis.

adhesive capsulitis capsulitis adhesiva.

hepatic capsulitis capsulitis hepática.

capture *n.* captura.

caput *n.* cabeza, caput.

caput medusae cabeza de medusa, caput medusae.

carbon *n.* carbono.

carbuncle *n.* ántrax.

carcinoembryonic *adj.* carcinoembrionario, -ria.

carcinogen *n.* carcinógeno.

carcinogenesis *n.* carcinogénesis, carcinogenia.

carcinogenic *adj.* carcinogénico, -ca.

carcinoid *n.* carcinoide.

carcinoma *n.* carcinoma.

carcinoma in situ carcinoma in situ.

occult carcinoma carcinoma oculto.

preinvasive carcinoma carcinoma preinvasivo.

primary carcinoma carcinoma primario.

cardia *n.* cardias.

cardiac *adj.* cardíaco, -ca.

cardinal *adj.* cardinal.

cardioesophageal *adj.* cardioesofágico, -ca.

cardiogram *n.* cardiograma.

cardiograph *n.* cardiógrafo.

cardiologist *n.* cardiólogo, -ga.

cardiology *n.* cardiología.

cardiomegaly *n.* cardiomegalia.

cardiomyopathy *n.* cardiomiopatía.

alcoholic cardiomyopathy cardiomiopatía alcohólica.

congestive cardiomyopathy cardiomiopatía congestiva.

dilated cardiomyopathy cardiomiopatía de dilatación.

hypertrophic cardiomyopathy cardiomiopatía hipertrófica.

idiopathic cardiomyopathy cardiomiopatía idiopática.

postpartum cardiomyopathy cardiomiopatía posparto, cardiomiopatía postpartum.

restrictive cardiomyopathy cardiomiopatía restrictiva.

cardiopath *n.* cardiópata.

cardiopathia *n.* cardiopatía.

cardiopathy *n.* cardiopatía.

cardiopulmonary *adj.* cardiopulmonar.

cardiospasm *n.* cardioespasmo, cardiospasmo.

cardiotonic *adj.* cardiotónico, -ca.

cardiotoxic *adj.* cardiotóxico, -ca.

cardiovascular *adj.* cardiovascular.

cardiovasculorenal *adj.* cardiovasculorrenal.

cardioversion *n.* cardioversión.

cardioverter *n.* cardioversor.

carditis *n.* carditis.

care *n.* cuidado.

intensive care cuidado intensivo.

palliative care cuidado paliativo.

postoperative care cuidado posoperatorio.

postpartal care cuidado posparto.

caries *n.* caries.

buccal caries caries bucal.

incipient caries caries incipiente.

occlusal caries caries oclusal.

recurrent caries caries recurrente.

carina *n.* carina.

carotene *n.* caroteno.

carotid *n.* carótida, carotídeo, -a.

carpal *adj.* carpiano, -na.

carpocarpal *adj.* carpocarpiano, -na.

carpometacarpal *adj.* carpometacarpiano, -na.

carpophalangeal *adj.* carpofalángico, -ca.

carpus *n.* carpo.

carrier *n.* portador, - ra.

cartilage *n.* cartílago.

calcified cartilage cartílago calcificado.

metaphyseal cartilage cartílago de crecimiento, cartílago metafisario.

cartilaginous *n.* cartilaginoso.

cartilago *n.* cartílago.

case *n.* caso.

caseous *adj.* caseoso, -sa.

cast *n.* cilindro, enyesado, escayola, modelo, molde, moldear, yeso.

diagnostic cast cilindro modelo diagnóstico, modelo de diagnóstico, molde diagnóstico.

master cast cilindro modelo patrón, modelo patrón, molde maestro.

plaster cast escayola de yeso.

preoperative cast modelo preoperatorio.

renal cast cilindro renal.

study cast modelo de estudio.

casting *n.* colado, escayolar, moldeado, vaciado.

castrate *v.* castrar.

castration *n.* castración.

catabolic *adj.* catabólico, -ca.

catabolism *n.* catabolismo.

catabolite *n.* catabolito.

catalepsy *n.* catalepsia.

cataleptic *adj.* cataléptico, -ca.

catalysis *n.* catálisis.

catalyst *n.* catalizador.

catalyzer *n.* catalizador.

cataplasm *n.* cataplasma.

cataract *n.* catarata.

capsular cataract catarata capsular.

complete cataract catarata completa, catarata general.

complicated cataract catarata complicada.

crystalline cataract catarata cristalina.

diabetic cataract catarata diabética.

glaucomatous cataract catarata glaucomatosa.

hard cataract catarata dura.

immature cataract catarata inmadura.

incipient cataract catarata incipiente.

infantile cataract catarata infantil.

juvenile cataract catarata juvenil.

mature cataract catarata madura.

membranous cataract catarata membranosa.

overripe cataract catarata supermadura.

perinuclear cataract catarata perinuclear.

peripheral cataract catarata periférica.

progresssive cataract catarata progresiva.

ripe cataract catarata madura.

rubella cataract catarata por rubéola.

secondary cataract catarata secundaria.

senile cataract catarata senil.

soft cataract catarata blanda.

traumatic cataract catarata traumática.

vascular cataract catarata vascular.

cataracta *n.* catarata.

catarrh *n.* catarro.

catatonia *n.* catatonía.

catatonic *adj.* catatónico, -ca.

catechin *n.* catequina.

catecholamine *n.* catecolaminas.

catgut *n.* catgut.

catharsis *n.* catarsis.

cathartic *adj.* catártico, -ca.

catheter *n.* catéter.

  central venous catheter catéter venoso central.

catheterization *n.* cateterismo, cateterización.

  female catheterization sondaje femenino.

  male catheterization sondaje masculino.

cathode *n.* cátodo.

cation *n.* catión.

caudal *adj.* caudal.

caudate *adj.* caudado, -da.

cause *n.* causa.

  local cause causa local.

  necessary cause causa necesaria.

  predisposing cause causa predisponente.

  primary cause causa primaria.

  secondary cause causa secundaria.

  specific cause causa específica.

  sufficient cause causa suficiente.

  ultimate cause causa última.

caustic *adj.* cáustico, -ca.

cauterization *n.* cauterización.

cavern *n.* caverna.

cavernous *adj.* cavernoso, -sa.

cavitas *n.* cavidad.

cavitation *n.* cavitación.

cavity *n.* cavidad.

  amniotic cavity cavidad amniótica.

  tooth-decay cavity cavidad cariosa, cavidad de caries.

cell *n.* célula.

  adipose cell célula adiposa.

  B-cell célula B.

  bone cell célula ósea.

  bronchic cell célula bronquial.

  brood cell célula madre.

  cardiac muscle cell célula muscular estriada cardíaca.

  cardiac muscle cell of the myocardium célula miocárdica.

  egg cell célula cigoto, célula huevo.

  endothelial cell célula endotelial.

  epithelial cell célula epitelial.

  killer cell célula asesina.

  mother cell célula madre.

  necrotic cell célula necrótica.

  nerve cell célula nerviosa.

  osseous cell célula ósea.

  pigment cell célula pigmentaria.

  red blood cell célula roja de la sangre.

  skeletal muscle cell célula muscular estriada esquelética.

  smooth muscle cell célula muscular lisa.

  striated muscle cell célula muscular estriada.

  T cell célula T.

  T cytotoxic cell célula T citotóxica, célula TC.

  target cell célula diana, célula en diana.

  TC cell célula T citotóxica, célula TC.

  TH cell célula T colaboradora, célula TH.

  T-helper cell célula T colaboradora, célula TH.

  TS cell célula T supresora, célula TS.

  T-suppressor cell célula T supresora, célula TS.

cellularity *n.* celularidad.

cellulitis *n.* celulitis.

  gangrenous cellulitis celulitis gangrenosa.

necrotizing cellulitis celulitis necrotizante.

orbital cellulitis celulitis orbitaria.

pelvic cellulitis celulitis pélvica.

center *n.* centro.

active center centro activo.

center of ossification centro de osificación.

expiratory center centro espiratorio.

feeding center centro de la alimentación.

inspiratory center centro inspiratorio.

ossific center centro de osificación.

satiety center centro de la saciedad.

secondary center of ossification centro secundario de osificación.

vasomotor center centro vasomotor.

vital center centro vitales.

central *adj.* central.

centric *adj.* céntrico, -ca.

centrum *n.* centro, centrum.

cenuriasis *n.* cenuriasis, cenurosis.

cephalalgia *n.* cefalalgia.

cephalic *adj.* cefálico, -ca.

ceramide *n.* ceramida.

ceratin *n.* queratina.

cerclage *n.* cerclaje.

cerebellitis *n.* cerebelitis.

cerebellum *n.* cerebelo.

cerebral *adj.* cerebral.

cerebritis *n.* cerebritis.

cerebrovascular *adj.* cerebrovascular.

cerebrum *n.* cerebro, cerebrum.

cerumen *n.* cerumen.

cervical *adj.* cervical.

cervicitis *n.* cervicitis.

cervix *n.* cérvix, cuello.

cesarean *n.* cesárea.

cestoid *adj.* cestoideo, -a.

chain *n.* cadena.

chair *n.* silla.

birthing chair silla de parto.

chalasia *n.* calasia.

chalasis *n.* calasia, calasis.

chalazion *n.* calacio, chalazión.

chamber *n.* cámara.

pulp chamber cámara pulpar.

chancre *n.* chancro.

hard chancre chancro duro, chancro sifilítico.

change *n.* cambio.

trophic change cambio trófico.

character *n.* carácter.

dominant character carácter dominante.

inherited character carácter hereditario.

Mendelian character carácter mendeliano.

primary sex character carácter sexual primario.

recessive character carácter recesivo.

secondary sex character carácter sexual secundario.

sex-linked character carácter ligado al sexo.

characterization *n.* caracterización.

chart *n.* cuadro, gráfica, gráfico.

cheek *n.* carrillo, mejilla.

cheilitis *n.* queilitis.

cheloid *n.* queloide, queloides.

chemabrasion *n.* quimioabrasión.

chemical *adj.* químico, -ca.

chemist *n.* químico, -ca.

chemistry *n.* química.

chemoprevention *n.* quimioprevención.

chemoprophylaxis *n.* quimioprofilaxis.

chemoreceptor *n.* quimiorreceptor.

chemosis *n.* quemosis.

  conjunctival chemosis quemosis conjuntival.

chemotaxis *n.* quimiotactismo, quimiotaxis.

chemotherapeutic *adj.* quimioterapéutico, -ca, quimioterápico, -ca.

chemotherapy *n.* quimioterapia.

  adjuvant chemotherapy quimioterapia adyuvante.

  chemotherapy (unsealed radioactive) quimioterapia radioactiva.

  combination chemotherapy quimioterapia combinada.

  consolidation chemotherapy quimioterapia de consolidación.

  induction chemotherapy quimioterapia de inducción.

  intensification chemotherapy quimioterapia de intensificación.

  intraarterial chemotherapy quimioterapia I.A., quimioterapia intraarterial.

cherubism *n.* querubismo.

chest *n.* pecho, tórax.

chiasm *n.* quiasma.

  optic chiasm quiasma óptico.

chiasma *n.* quiasma.

  chiasma opticum quiasma óptico.

chiasmatic *adj.* quiasmático, -ca.

chickenpox *n.* varicela.

chilblain *n.* sabañón.

child *n.* niño, -ña.

childhood *n.* infancia, niñez.

chill *n.* escalofrío.

chilosis *n.* quilosis.

chimaera *n.* quimera.

chimera *n.* quimera.

chin *n.* barbilla, mentón.

chiomera *n.* quimera.

chiropractor *n.* quiropráctico$$ca, quiropractor$$ra.

chirurgic *adj.* quirúrgico, -ca.

Chlamydia *n.* Chlamydia, clamidia.

chloasma *n.* cloasma.

chloroform *n.* cloroformo.

chlorosis *n.* clorosis.

choana *n.* coana.

choice *n.* elección.

  free choice of doctor libre elección de médico.

choke *n.* ahogo.

cholangeitis *n.* colangeítis, colangitis.

cholangiocholecystography *n.* colangiocolecistografía.

cholangiogram *n.* colangiograma.

cholangiography *n.* colangiografía.

cholangiohepatitis *n.* colangiohepatitis.

cholangiopancreatography *n.* colangiopancreatografía.

  endoscopic retrograde cholangiopancreatography (ERCP) colangiopancreatografía endoscópica retrógrada, colangiopancreatografía retrógrada endoscópica (CPRE).

cholangioscopy *n.* colangioscopia.

cholangitis *n.* colangitis.

  sclerosing cholangitis colangitis esclerosante.

cholecystectomy *n.* colecistectomía.

cholecystitis *n.* colecistitis.

choledoch *n.* colédoco.

cholera *n.* cólera.

   cholera infantum cólera infantil.

   typhoid cholera cólera tífico, cólera tifoídico.

cholestasis *n.* colestasia, colestasis.

cholestatic *adj.* colestático -ca.

cholesteatoma *n.* colesteatoma.

cholesterol *n.* colesterol.

cholesterolemia *n.* colesterolemia.

cholinephritis *n.* colinefritis.

cholinergic *adj.* colinérgico, -ca.

choluria *n.* coleuria, coluria.

choluric *adj.* colúrico, -ca.

chondritis *n.* condritis.

chondrocyte *n.* condrocito.

chondrodysplasia *n.* condrodisplasia.

   chondrodysplasia punctata condrodisplasia punctata, condrodisplasia punteada, condrodisplasia puntiforme.

chondrogenesis *n.* condrogénesis.

chondroma *n.* condrocele, condroma.

chondromatosise *n.* condromatosis.

chondropathia *n.* condropatía.

chondroskeleton *n.* condroesqueleto, condrosqueleto.

chorda *n.* cuerda.

chorditis *n.* corditis.

   chorditis cantorum corditis de los cantantes.

   chorditis nodosa corditis nudosa.

   chorditis tuberosa corditis tuberosa.

   chorditis vocalis corditis vocal.

   chorditis vocalis inferior corditis vocal inferior.

chorea *n.* corea.

   acute chorea corea aguda.

   chorea festinans corea festinante.

   chorea major corea major, corea mayor.

   chorea minor corea menor, corea minor.

   chronic chorea corea crónica.

   dancing chorea corea danzante.

   degenerative chorea corea degenerativa.

   epidemic chorea corea epidémica.

   Huntington's chorea corea de Huntington.

   hysteric chorea corea histérica.

   hysterical chorea corea histérica.

   juvenile chorea corea juvenil.

   onesided chorea corea unilateral.

   rheumatic chorea corea reumática.

chorion *n.* corion.

   shaggy chorion corion hirsuto, corion velloso.

chorionic *adj.* coriónico, -ca.

choroidea *n.* coroides.

choroiditis *n.* coroiditis.

   anterior choroiditis coroiditis anterior.

   multifocal choroiditis coroiditis multifocal.

   posterior choroiditis coroiditis posterior.

   proliferative choroiditis coroiditis proliferante.

   serous choroiditis coroiditis serosa.

chromatic *adj.* cromático, -ca.

chromatid *n.* cromátida, cromátide.

chromatin *n.* cromatina.

  nucleolar chromatin cromatina nuclear.

  nucleolar-associated chromatin cromatina asociada al núcleo.

  nucleous chromatin cromatina nuclear.

  nucleus-associated chromatin cromatina asociada al núcleo.

  sex chromatin cromatina sexual.

chromatography *n.* cromatografía.

chromosomal *adj.* cromosómico, -ca.

chromosome *n.* cromosoma.

chronic *adj.* crónico, -ca.

chronicity *n.* cronicidad.

chyle *n.* quilo.

chylomicron *n.* quilomicrón.

chylosis *n.* quilosis.

chylous *adj.* quiloso, -sa.

chyluria *n.* quiluria.

chyme *n.* quimo.

cicatrix *n.* cicatriz.

cicatrizant *adj.* cicatrizante.

cicatrization *n.* cicatrización, ulesis.

ciliary *adj.* ciliar.

ciliate *adj.* ciliado, ciliado, -da.

cilium *n.* cilio, cilium.

circle *n.* círculo.

  vicious circle círculo vicioso.

circuit *n.* circuito.

circular *adj.* circular.

circulation *n.* circulación.

  capillary circulation circulación capilar.

  collateral circulation circulación colateral.

  coronary circulation circulación coronaria.

  embryonic circulation circulación embrionaria.

  extracorporeal circulation circulación extracorpórea.

  fetal circulation circulación fetal.

  greater circulation circulación mayor.

  lesser circulation circulación menor.

  lymph circulation circulación linfática.

  placental circulation circulación placentaria.

  portal circulation circulación de la vena porta, circulación portal.

  pulmonary circulation circulación pulmonar.

  systemic circulation circulación general, circulación sistémica.

circulatory *adj.* circulatorio, -ria.

circulus *n.* círculo.

circumcision *n.* circuncisión.

cirrhosis *n.* cirrosis.

  alcoholic cirrhosis cirrosis alcohólica.

  biliary cirrhosis cirrosis biliar.

  fatty cirrhosis cirrosis grasa.

  periportal cirrhosis cirrosis periportal.

  postnecrotic cirrhosis cirrosis posnecrótica.

  primary biliary cirrhosis cirrosis biliar primaria.

clamp *n.* clamp.

  Gaskell's clamp clamp de Gaskell.

classification *n.* clasificación.

claudication *n.* claudicación.

  intermittent claudication claudicación intermitente.

venous claudication claudicación venosa.

claustrophobia *n.* claustrofobia.

claustrophobic *adj.* claustrofóbico, -ca.

clavicle *n.* clavícula.

clavicula *n.* clavícula.

claw *n.* garra.

cleaning *n.* higienización, limpieza.

clearance *n.* aclaramiento, limpieza.

creatinine clearance aclaramiento de creatinina.

drug clearance aclaramiento de fármaco.

cleavage *n.* escisión, segmentación.

climacterium *n.* climaterio.

climate *n.* clima.

climax *n.* clímax.

clinic *n.* clínica.

clinical *adj.* clínico, -ca.

clinician *n.* clínico, -ca.

clinicopathologic *adj.* clinicopatológico, -ca.

clip *n.* grapa.

clitoris *n.* clítoris.

clonal *adj.* clonal.

clone *n.* clon, clonar, clono.

clonic *adj.* clónico, -ca.

cloning *n.* clonación.

clonus *n.* clonus.

clostridium *n.* clostridio.

closure *n.* cierre.

clot *n.* coágulo, grumo.

antemortem clot coágulo ante mortem.

blood clot coágulo sanguíneo.

chicken fat clot coágulo en grasa de pollo.

distal clot coágulo distal.

external clot coágulo externo.

heart clot coágulo cardíaco.

internal clot coágulo interno.

post mortem clot coágulo post mortem.

proximal clot coágulo proximal.

coagulant *adj.* coagulante.

coagulation *n.* coagulación.

diffuse intravascular coagulation coagulación intravascular difusa.

disseminated intravascular coagulation (DIC) coagulación intravascular diseminada (CID).

massive coagulation coagulación masiva.

plasmatic coagulation coagulación plasmática.

coagulopathy *n.* coagulopatía.

coagulum *n.* coágulo.

coaptation *n.* coaptación.

coarctate *adj.* coartado, -da.

coarctation *n.* coartación.

adult type coarctation of the aorta coartación aórtica de tipo adulto.

coarctation of the aorta coartación aórtica, coartación de la aorta.

infantile type coarctation of the aorta coartación aórtica de tipo infantil.

reversed coarctation coartación invertida.

coarticulation *n.* coarticulación.

coat *n.* capa.

cobaltosis *n.* cobaltosis.

cocain *n.* cocaína.

cocaine *n.* cocaína.

cocainist *n.* cocainómano, -na.

coccobacillus *n.* cocobacilo.

coccyx *n.* cóccix, cóxis.

cochlea *n.* caracol, cóclea.

cochlear *adj.* coclear.

cocktail *n.* cocktail, cóctel.

code *n.* código.

  analogical code código analógico.

  digital code código digital.

  genetic code código genético.

codon *n.* codón.

coefficient *n.* coeficiente.

coenurasis *n.* cenuriasis, cenurosis.

coenzyme *n.* coenzima.

cofactor *n.* cofactor.

cognition *n.* cognición.

cognitive *adj.* cognitivo, -va.

cohort *n.* cohorte.

coital *adj.* coital.

coitalgia *n.* coitalgia.

coitus *n.* coito.

cold *n.* enfriamiento, frío, resfriado.

colic *n.* cólico.

  biliary colic cólico biliar, cólico bilioso.

  gallstone colic cólico colelitiásico, cólico por cálculo biliar.

  gastric colic cólico gástrico.

  hepatic colic cólico hepático.

  infantile colic cólico del lactante.

  intestinal colic cólico intestinal.

  menstrual colic cólico menstrual.

  nephritic colic cólico nefrítico.

  pancreatic colic cólico pancreático.

  renal colic cólico renal.

colitis *n.* colicolitis, colitis.

  colitis ulcerativa colitis ulcerosa.

  ulcerative colitis colitis ulcerosa.

collagen *n.* colágena, colágeno.

  type I collagen colágeno tipo I.

  type II collagen colágeno tipo II.

  type III collagen colágeno tipo III.

  type IV collagen colágeno tipo IV.

collagenosis *n.* colagenosis.

collagenous *adj.* colágeno, -na.

collapse *n.* colapso.

  circulatory collapse colapso circulatorio.

  collapse of the lung colapso pulmonar.

  massive collapse colapso masivo.

  pulmonary collapse colapso pulmonar.

collar *n.* collar.

  cervical collar collar ortopédico, collarín cervical.

collateral *adj.* colateral.

collection *n.* toma.

collum *n.* collum, cuello.

collutorium *n.* colutorio.

collutory *n.* colutorio.

colon *n.* colon.

  giant colon colon gigante.

  inactive colon colon inactivo.

  irritable colon colon irritable.

  lazy colon colon perezoso.

colonitis *n.* colonitis.

colonization *n.* colonización.

colonorrhagia *n.* colonorragia.

colonorrhea *n.* colonorrea.

colonoscope *n.* colonoscopio, coloscopio.

colonoscopy *n.* colonoscopia.

colony *n.* colonia.

color *n.* color.

colorectal *adj.* colorrectal.

colorimetry *n.* colorimetría.

colosigmoidoscopy *n.* colosigmoidoscopia.

colostomate *adj.* colostomizado, -da.

colostomy *n.* colostomía.

colostrum *n.* calostro.
  colostrum gravidum calostro gravídico.
  colostrum puerperarum calostro puerperal.
colposcope *n.* colposcopio.
colposcopy *n.* colposcopia.
column *n.* columna.
  vertebral column columna vertebral.
columna *n.* columna.
coma *n.* coma.
  alcoholic coma coma alcohólico.
  barbiturate coma coma por barbitúricos.
  coma hepaticum coma hepático.
  coma hypochloraemicum coma hipoclorémico.
  coma vigil coma vigil.
  diabetic coma coma diabético.
  hepatic coma coma hepático.
  hyperosmolar coma coma hiperosmolar.
  hypoglycemic coma coma hipoglucémico.
  irreversible coma coma irreversible.
  Kussmaul's coma coma de Kussmaul.
  metabolic coma coma metabólico.
  thyrotoxic coma coma tirotóxico.
  trance coma coma de trance.
  uremic coma coma urémico.
comatose *adj.* comatoso, -sa.
combination *n.* combinación.
  new combination combinación nueva.
comedo *n.* comedón.
  closed comedo comedón cerrado.
  open comedo comedón abierto.

  whitehead comedo comedón blanco.
comedogenic *adj.* comedogénico, -ca, comedógeno, -na.
commensal *n.* comensal.
comminuted *adj.* conminuto, -ta.
commissura *n.* comisura.
commisure *n.* comisura.
commitment *n.* internamiento.
commotio *n.* conmoción.
  commotio cerebri conmoción cerebral.
communicans *adj.* comunicante.
communication *n.* comunicación.
  congruent communication comunicación congruente.
  dysfunctional communication comunicación disfuncional.
  impaired verbal communication comunicación verbal alterada.
  incongruent communication comunicación incongruente.
community *n.* comunidad.
  therapeutic community comunidad terapéutica.
comorbidity *n.* comorbilidad.
compact *adj.* compacto, -ta.
compacta *n.* compacta.
comparator *n.* comparador.
compartment *n.* compartimento.
compatibility *n.* compatibilidad.
compatible *adj.* compatible.
compensation *n.* compensación.
  dosage compensation compensación de dosis.
compensatory *adj.* compensador, -ra.
competence *n.* competencia, suficiencia.

cardiac competence competencia cardíaca.

embryonic competence competencia embrionaria, suficiencia embrionaria.

immunological competence competencia inmunológica, suficiencia inmunológica.

competition *n.* competición.

complement *n.* complemento.

complementarity *n.* complementariedad.

complementary *adj.* complementario, - ria.

complementation *n.* complementación.

complex *n.* complejo, -ja.

aberrant complex complejo aberrante.

AIDS dementia complex (ADC) complejo demencia SIDA (CDS).

AIDS related complex (ARC) complejo relacionado con el SIDA (CRS).

anomalous complex complejo anómalo.

antigen-antibody complex complejo antígeno-anticuerpo.

antigenic complex complejo antigénico.

apical complex complejo apical.

atrial complex complejo auricular.

auricular complex complejo auricular.

diphasic complex complejo bifásico.

father complex complejo paterno.

Gohn's complex complejo de Gohn.

Golgi complex complejo de Golgi.

hemoglobin-haptoglobin complex complejo hemoglobina-haptoglobina.

HLA complex complejo HLA.

major histocompatibility complex (MHC) complejo mayor de histocompatibilidad (CMH), complejo principal de histocompatibilidad.

mother complex complejo materno.

Oedipus complex complejo de Edipo.

QRS complex complejo QRS.

QRST complex complejo QRST.

superiority complex complejo de superioridad.

complexion *n.* complexión.

compliance *n.* adaptabilidad, compliance, compliancia, complianza.

brain compliance compliancia cerebral.

compliance of the heart compliancia del corazón.

lung compliance compliancia pulmonar.

specific compliance compliancia específica.

static compliance compliancia estática.

thoracic compliance compliancia torácica.

ventilatory compliance compliancia ventilatoria.

complicated *adj.* complicado, -da.

complication *n.* complicación.

medical complication complicación médica.

surgical complication complicación quirúrgica.

vascular complication complicación vascular.

composition *n.* composición.

compound *adj.* componer, compuesto, -ta.

comprehension *n.* comprensión.

compress *n.* compresa.

cold compress compresa fría.

graduated compress compresa graduada.

gynecologic compress compresa ginegológica.

hot compress compresa caliente.

perinal compress compresa perineal.

wet compress compresa húmeda.

compression *n.* compresión.

cardiac compression compresión cardíaca.

cerebral compression compresión cerebral, compresión del cerebro.

compression of the brain compresión cerebral, compresión del cerebro.

digital compression compresión digital.

instrumental compression compresión instrumental.

medullar compression compresión medular.

nerve compression compresión nerviosa.

spinal compression compresión espinal, compresión raquídea.

spinal cord compression compresión de la médula espinal.

compressor *n.* compresor.

air compressor compresor de aire.

compulsion *n.* compulsión.

compulsive *adj.* compulsivo.

computer *n.* ordenador.

concave *adj.* cóncavo, -va.

concavity *n.* concavidad.

conceive *v.* concebir.

concentrate *v.* concentrado, concentrar.

liver concentrate concentrado de hígado.

packed cell concentrate concentrado celular.

platelet concentrate concentrado de plaquetas.

red blood cell concentrate concentrado de hematíes.

vitamin concentrate concentrado vitamínico.

concentrated *adj.* concentrado, -da.

concentration *n.* concentración.

hemodialysate concentration concentración de hemodiálisis.

maximum cell concentration (MC) concentración celular máxima (CM).

maximum urinary concentration (MUC) concentración urinaria máxima (CUM).

minimal bactericidal concentration concentración bactericida mínima.

minimal lethal concentration (MLC) concentración letal mínima (MCL).

molar concentration concentración molar.

normal concentration concentración normal.

oxygen concentration in blood concentración sérica de oxigeno.

concentric *adj.* concéntrico, -ca.

concept *n.* concepto.

  no-threshold concept concepto de no umbral.

conception *n.* concepción.

  imperative conception concepción imperativa.

conceptive *adj.* conceptivo, -va.

conceptual *adj.* conceptual.

concordance *n.* concordancia.

concordant *adj.* concordante.

concretio *n.* concreción, concretio.

  concretio cordis concreción cardíaca.

concretion *n.* concreción.

  calculous concretion concreción calculosa.

  prostatic concretion concreción prostástica.

  tophic concretion concreción tofácea, concreción tófica.

concussion *n.* concusión.

  abdominal concussion concusión abdominal.

  concussion of the brain concusión cerebral, concusión del cerebro.

  concussion of the labyrinth concusión del laberinto.

  concussion of the retina concusión de la retina.

  concussion of the spinal cord concusión de la médula espinal.

  pulmonary concussion concusión pulmonar.

condensation *n.* condensación.

condenser *n.* condensador.

condition *n.* acondicionar, condición.

  basal condition condición basal.

conditioning *n.* condicionamiento.

  operant conditioning condicionamiento operante, condicionamiento operativo.

  Pavlovian conditioning condicionamiento de Pavlov, condicionamiento pavloviano.

condom *n.* condón, preservativo.

conduction *n.* conducción.

  aberrant ventricular conduction conducción ventricular aberrante.

  accelerated conduction conducción acelerada.

  anomalous conduction conducción anómala.

  anterograde conduction conducción anterógrada.

  atrioventricular conduction (A-V) conducción auriculoventricular (A-V).

  bone conduction conducción ósea.

  conduction of the nervous impulse conducción del impulso nervioso.

  decremental conduction conducción decreciente.

  delayed conduction conducción demorada, conducción retardada.

  forward conduction conducción anterior.

  intraventricular conduction conducción intraventricular.

  nerve conduction conducción nerviosa.

  retrograde conduction conducción retrógrada.

  saltatory conduction conducción saltatoria.

  supranormal conduction conducción supranormal.

synaptic conduction conducción sináptica.

ventricular conduction conducción ventricular.

ventriculoatrial conduction (V-A) conducción ventriculoauricular (V-A).

conductive *adj.* conductor, -ra.

conductor *n.* conductor.

condylar *adj.* condilar, condíleo, -a.

condyle *n.* cóndilo.

condylectomy *n.* condilectomía.

condyloma *n.* condiloma.

cone *n.* cono.

congenital cone cono congénito.

cones *n.* conos.

confidence *n.* confianza.

conflict *n.* conflicto.

approach-approach conflict conflicto de acercamiento-acercamiento, conflicto de enfoque-enfoque.

approach-avoidance conflict conflicto de acercamiento-evitación, conflicto enfoque-evitación.

avoidance-avoidance conflict conflicto de evitación-evitación.

double conflict conflicto doble.

intrapsychic conflict conflicto intrapersonal, conflicto intrapsíquico.

motivational conflict conflicto motivación.

role conflict conflicto de rol.

conformation *n.* conformación.

congelation *n.* congelación.

congenital *adj.* congénito, -ta.

congested *adj.* congestionado, -da.

congestion *n.* congestión.

brain congestion congestión cerebral.

bronchial congestion congestión bronquial.

functional congestion congestión funcional.

hypostatic congestion congestión hipostática.

neurotonic congestion congestión neurotónica.

passive congestion congestión pasiva.

physiologic congestion congestión fisiológica.

pulmonary congestion congestión pulmonar.

rebound congestion congestión de rebote.

congestive *adj.* congestivo, -va.

conic *adj.* cónico, -ca.

conical *adj.* cónico, -ca.

conization *n.* conización.

cautery conization conización por cauterio.

cervical conization conización cervical.

cold conization conización en frío.

conjugation *n.* conjugación.

conjunctiva *n.* conjuntiva.

bulbar conjunctiva conjuntiva bulbar.

palpebral conjunctiva conjuntiva palpebral.

conjunctival *adj.* conjuntival.

conjunctive *adj.* conjuntivo, -va.

conjunctivitis *n.* conjuntivitis.

acute conjunctivitis conjuntivitis aguda.

acute catarrhal conjunctivitis conjuntivitis catarral, conjuntivitis catarral aguda.

acute contagious conjunctivitis conjuntivitis contagiosa aguda.

acute hemorrhagic conjunctivitis conjuntivitis hemorrágica aguda.

allergic conjunctivitis conjuntivitis alérgica, conjuntivitis anafiláctica.

angular conjunctivitis conjuntivitis angular.

atopic conjunctivitis conjuntivitis atópica.

atropine conjunctivitis conjuntivitis atropínica.

bacterial conjunctivitis conjuntivitis bacteriana.

blenorrheal conjunctivitis conjuntivitis blenorrágica.

calcareous conjunctivitis conjuntivitis calcárea.

catarrhal conjunctivitis conjuntivitis catarral.

chemical conjunctivitis conjuntivitis química.

cicatricial conjunctivitis conjuntivitis cicatricial, conjuntivitis cicatrizal.

conjunctivitis medicamentosa conjuntivitis medicamentosa.

conjunctivitis of the newborn conjuntivitis del recién nacido.

conjunctivitis tularensis conjuntivitis tularémica.

diphtheritic conjunctivitis conjuntivitis diftérica.

epidemic conjunctivitis conjuntivitis aguda contagiosa, conjuntivitis epidémica.

gonococcal conjunctivitis conjuntivitis gonocócica.

gonorrheal conjunctivitis conjuntivitis gonorreica.

inclusion conjunctivitis conjuntivitis de inclusión.

infantile purulent conjunctivitis conjuntivitis infantil purulenta, conjuntivitis purulenta infantil.

lacrimal conjunctivitis conjuntivitis lagrimal.

ligneous conjunctivitis conjuntivitis leñosa.

lithiasis conjunctivitis conjuntivitis litiásica.

Meibomian conjunctivitis conjuntivitis de Meibomio.

membranous conjunctivitis conjuntivitis membranosa.

meningococcus conjunctivitis conjuntivitis meningocócica.

neonatal conjunctivitis conjuntivitis neonatal.

phlyctenular conjunctivitis conjuntivitis escrofulosa.

prairie conjunctivitis conjuntivitis de las praderas.

pseudomembranous conjunctivitis conjuntivitis seudomembranosa.

purulent conjunctivitis conjuntivitis purulenta.

simple conjunctivitis conjuntivitis simple.

spring conjunctivitis conjuntivitis primaveral.

swimming pool conjunctivitis conjuntivitis de las piscinas.

toxicogenic conjunctivitis conjuntivitis toxicogénica.

trachomatous conjunctivitis conjuntivitis tracomatosa.

tularemic conjunctivitis conjuntivitis tularémica, conjuntivitis tularensis.

uratic conjunctivitis conjuntivitis urática.

vaccinial conjunctivitis conjuntivitis vacunal.

viral conjunctivitis conjuntivitis vírica.

welder's conjunctivitis conjuntivitis de soldador.

connection *n.* conexión.

connective *adj.* conectivo, -va.

connector *n.* conector.

connexus *n.* conexión.

consanguineous *adj.* consanguíneo, -a.

consanguinity *n.* consanguinidad.

conscience *n.* consciencia.

conscious *adj.* consciente.

consciousness *n.* conciencia.

clouding consciousness conciencia nublada.

double consciousness conciencia doble.

dual consciousness conciencia doble.

moral consciousness conciencia moral.

consecutive *adj.* consecutivo, -va.

consensual *adj.* consensual.

conservation *n.* conservación.

conservation of energy conservación de la energía.

conservation of matter conservación de la materia.

conservative *adj.* conservador, -ra.

consistence *n.* consistencia.

gingival consistence consistencia gingival.

consolidant *adj.* consolidante.

consolidate *adj.* consolidado, -da.

consolidation *n.* consolidación.

constancy *n.* constancia.

constant *n.* constante.

association constant constante de asociación.

binding constant constante de conjugación.

desintegration constant constante de desactivación, constante de desintegración.

diffusion constant constante de difusión.

dissociation constant constante de disociación.

equilibrium constant constante de equilibrio.

velocity constant constante de velocidad.

constipation *n.* estreñimiento.

constituent *n.* componente.

constituent of complement componente del complemento.

constituent of occlusion componente de la oclusión.

metabolic constituent componente metabólico.

respiratory constituent componente respiratorio.

secretory constituent componente secretor.

somatic motor constituent componente somático motor.

somatic sensory constituent componente somático sensitivo.

splanchnic motor constituent componente esplácnico motor, componente visceral motor.

splanchnic sensory constituent componente esplácnico sensitivo, componente visceral sensitivo.

constitution *n.* constitución.

lymphatic constitution constitución linfática.

constitutional *adj.* constitucional.

constriction *n.* constricción.

duodenopyloric constriction constricción duodenopilórica.

primary constriction constricción primaria.

secondary constriction constricción secundaria.

constrictive *adj.* constrictivo, -va.

constrictor *n.* constrictor.

constructive *adj.* constructivo, -va.

consumption *n.* consumo, consunción.

damaging consumption consumo perjudicial.

oxygen consumption consumo de oxígeno.

passive smoking consumption consumo pasivo de tabaco.

systemic oxygen consumption consumo sistémico de oxígeno.

contact *n.* contacto.

complete contact contacto completo.

contact with reality contacto con la realidad.

direct contact contacto directo.

immediate contact contacto inmediato.

initial contact contacto inicial.

mediate contact contacto indirecto.

occlusal contact contacto oclusal.

premature contact contacto prematuro.

proximal contact contacto proximal, contacto próximo.

proximate contact contacto proximal, contacto próximo.

weak contact contacto débil.

working contact contacto de trabajo.

contagion *n.* contagio.

immediate contagion contagio directo, contagio inmediato.

mediate contagion contagio indirecto.

psychic contagion contagio mental, contagio psíquico.

contagious *adj.* contagioso, -sa.

contaminant *adj.* contaminante.

contamination *n.* contaminación.

content *n.* contenido.

continence *n.* continencia.

fecal continence continencia fecal.

urinary continence continencia urinaria.

contraception *n.* anticoncepción, contracepción.

hormonal contraception contracepción hormonal.

intrauterine contraception contracepción intrauterina.

contraceptive *adj.* anticonceptivo, -va, contraceptivo.

barrier contraceptive anticonceptivo de barrera.

combination oral contraceptive anticonceptivo oral combinado.

oral contraceptive anticonceptivo oral.

contractile *adj.* contráctil.

contractility *n.* contractilidad.
  cardiac contractility contractilidad cardíaca.
  idiomuscular contractility contractilidad idiomuscular.
contraction *n.* contracción.
  automatic ventricular contraction contracción ventricular automática.
  Braxton-Hicks contraction contracción Braxton Hicks.
  escaped ventricular contraction contracción ventricular de escape.
  isometric contraction contracción isométrica.
  isotonic contraction contracción isotónica.
  isovolumetric contraction contracción isovolumétrica.
  paradoxical contraction contracción paradójica.
  postural contraction contracción postural.
  premature contraction contracción prematura.
  premature ventricular contraction (PVC) contracción ventricular prematura (CVP).
  tetanic contraction contracción tetánica.
  tonic contraction contracción tónica.
  twich contraction contracción de sacudida.
  twiching contraction contracción espasmódica.
  uterine contraction contracción uterina.
contracture *n.* contractura.

defense contracture contractura de defensa.
  Dupuytren's contracture contractura de Dupuytren.
  functional contracture contractura funcional.
  hypertonic contracture contractura hipertónica.
  hysterical contracture contractura histérica.
  ischemic contracture contractura isquémica.
  ischemic contracture of the left ventricle contractura isquémica del ventrículo izquierdo.
  painful contracture contractura dolorosa.
  physiologic contracture contractura fisiológica.
  Volkmann's contracture contractura de Volkmann.
contraindicated *adj.* contraindicado, -da.
contraindication *n.* contraindicación.
contrast *n.* contraste.
  baric contrast contraste baritado.
  double contrast contraste doble.
  film contrast contraste de la película.
  iodate contrast contraste iodado, contraste yodado.
  liposoluble contrast contraste liposoluble.
  negative contrast contraste negativo.
  radiographic contrast contraste radiográfico.
contrastimulus *n.* contraestímulo.

control *n.* control.
  automatic control control automático.
  biological control control biológico.
  birth control control de la natalidad, control natal.
  control of hemorrhage control de la hemorragia.
  control with placebo in investigation control con placebo en investigación.
  feedback control control por retroalimentación.
  local control control local.
  nudge control control por presion.
  quality control control de calidad.
  reflex control control reflejo.
  respiratory control control respiratorio.
  social control control social.
  synergic control control sinérgico.
  tonic control control tónico.
  vestibulo-equilibratory control control vestibuloequilibratorio.
  volitional control control volitivo, control voluntario.
  voluntary control control volitivo, control voluntario.
contusion *n.* contusión.
  brain contusion contusión cerebral.
  contusion of the spinal cord contusión de la médula espinal.
  countercoup contusion contusión por contragolpe.
  medullar contusion contusión medular.
  renal contusion contusión renal.

  scalp contusion contusión del cuero cabelludo.
  stone contusion contusión por piedra.
  temporal lobe contusion contusión del lóbulo temporal.
conus *n.* cono, conus.
convalescence *n.* convalecencia.
convalescent *adj.* convaleciente.
convergence *n.* convergencia.
  accommodative convergence convergencia acomodativa, convergencia de acomodación.
convulsant *adj.* convulsionante.
convulsion *n.* convulsión.
  clonic convulsion convulsión clónica.
  complex partial convulsion convulsión parcial compleja.
  febrile convulsion convulsión febril.
  generalized tonic-clonic convulsion convulsión tónico-clónica generalizada.
  hysterical convulsion convulsión histérica, convulsión histeroide.
  hysteroid convulsion convulsión histérica, convulsión histeroide.
  infantile convulsion convulsión infantil.
  mimetic convulsion convulsión mímica.
  mimic convulsion convulsión mímica.
  partial convulsion convulsión parcial.
  puerperal convulsion convulsión puerperal.
  salaam convulsion "convulsión en salaam".

static convulsion convulsión estática.

tetanic convulsion convulsión tetánica.

tonic convulsion convulsión tónica.

convulsive *adj.* convulsivo, -va.

convulsotherapy *n.* convulsoterapia.

coordination *n.* coordinación.

motor coordination coordinación motora.

visual-motor coordination coordinación visualmotora.

coproculture *n.* coprocultivo.

cor *n.* cor, corazón.

cor adiposum cor adiposum, corazón adiposo.

cor mobile cor mobile, corazón móvil.

cor pulmonale cor pulmonale, corazón pulmonar.

cor triloculare cor triloculare, corazón de tres cavidades.

cord *n.* cordón, cuerda.

vocal cord cuerda vocal.

corditis *n.* corditis.

corium *n.* corion, corium.

cornea *n.* córnea.

conical cornea córnea cónica.

corneal *adj.* corneal, corneano, -na.

corneitis *n.* corneítis.

cornu *n.* cuerno.

corona *n.* corona.

corona radiata corona radiada, corona radiante.

coronal *adj.* coronal.

coronale *adj.* coronal, coronale.

coronary *adj.* coronario, -ria.

corporeal *adj.* corporal, corpóreo, -a.

corpus *n.* corpus.

corpus albicans cuerpo albicans.

corpus luteum cuerpo lúteo.

corpuscle *n.* corpúsculo.

corpuscular *adj.* corpuscular.

corpusculum *n.* corpúsculo.

correction *n.* corrección.

corrective *adj.* corrector, -ra.

corrector *n.* corrector.

function corrector corrector de función.

correlation *n.* correlación.

correspondence *n.* correspondencia.

anomalous correspondence correspondencia anómala.

dysharmonious correspondence correspondencia inarmónica.

harmonious correspondence correspondencia armoniosa.

retinal correspondence correspondencia retiniana.

corrosion *n.* corrosión.

corrosive *adj.* corrosivo, -va.

corset *n.* corsé.

cortex *n.* corteza.

cortical *adj.* cortical.

corticospinal *adj.* corticoespinal, corticomedular, corticospinal.

corticosteroid *n.* corticoesteroide, corticosteroide.

cortisol *n.* cortisol.

cortisolemia *n.* cortisolemia.

coryza *n.* coriza.

allergic coryza coriza alérgica.

coryza spasmodica coriza espasmódica.

pollen coryza coriza del polen.

costa *n.* costa, costilla.

costiveness *n.* estreñimiento.

costrous *adj.* costroso, -sa.

cotton *n.* algodón.

cotyledon *n.* cotiledón.

cough *n.* tos.

  dry cough tos seca.

  hacking cough tos perruna, tos seca.

  non-productive cough tos no productiva.

  paroxysmal cough tos espasmódica, tos paroxística.

  productive cough tos productiva, tos simpática.

  wet cough tos blanda, tos húmeda.

  whooping cough tos convulsa, tos coqueluchoide, tos ferina, tos quintosa, tosferina.

count *n.* numeración, recuento.

  complete blood count recuento sanguíneo completo.

  differential white blood count recuento sanguíneo diferencial de glóbulos blancos.

counter *n.* contador.

countercurrent *n.* contracorriente.

counting *n.* detección.

coupling *n.* acoplamiento, emparejamiento.

coxa *n.* cadera, coxa.

coxalgia *n.* coxalgia.

crab *n.* ladilla.

crablouse *n.* ladilla.

cramp *n.* calambre.

  heat cramp calambre por calor.

  intermittent cramp calambre intermitente.

  miner's cramp calambre de minero.

  musician's cramp calambre de músico.

  pianist's cramp calambre de pianista.

  recumbency cramp calambre por decúbito.

  stomach cramp retortijón.

  tailor's cramp calambre de los sastres.

  violinist's cramp calambre de violinista.

  watchmaker's cramp calambre de relojero.

  writers' cramp calambre de los escritores.

cranial *adj.* craneal, craneano, -na.

craniotomy *n.* craneotomía.

cranium *n.* cráneo, cranium.

crater *n.* cráter.

  gingival crater cráter gingival.

  interdental crater cráter interdental.

cream *n.* crema.

creatine *n.* creatina.

creatinemia *n.* creatinemia.

creatinin *n.* creatinina.

creatinine *n.* creatinina.

  creatinine height index creatinina de 24 horas.

creatinuria *n.* creatinuria.

crepitant *adj.* crepitante.

crepitation *n.* crepitación.

crepitus *n.* crepitación, crépito, crepitus.

  articular crepitus crepitación articular, crépito articular.

  bony crepitus crepitación ósea, crépito óseo.

  joint crepitus crepitación articular, crépito articular.

  painful tendon crepitus crepitación dolorosa de los tendones.

cretin *n.* cretino, -na.
cretinism *n.* cretinismo.
  familial cretinism cretinismo familiar.
  goitrous cretinism cretinismo bocioso.
  spontaneous cretinism cretinismo espontáneo, cretinismo esporádico.
  sporadic cretinism cretinismo espontáneo, cretinismo esporádico.
  sporadic goitrous cretinism cretinismo esporádico bocioso.
cretinoid *adj.* cretinoide.
cretinous *adj.* cretino, -na.
crib *n.* criba.
cribration *n.* cribado.
crisis *n.* acceso, crisis.
  Addison crisis crisis addisoniana, crisis de Addison.
  Addisonian crisis crisis addisoniana, crisis de Addison.
  adolescent crisis crisis de adolescencia.
  adrenal crisis crisis adrenal, crisis suprarrenal.
  blood crisis crisis sanguínea.
  bronchial crisis crisis bronquial.
  cardiac crisis crisis cardíaca.
  catathymic crisis crisis de catatimia.
  colinergic crisis crisis colinérgica.
  developmental crisis crisis del desarrollo.
  false crisis crisis falsa.
  febrile crisis crisis febril.
  gastric crisis crisis gástrica.
  genital crisis of the newborn crisis genital del neonato.
  hepatic crisis crisis hepática.
  hypertensive crisis crisis hipertensiva.
  identity crisis crisis de identidad.
  intestinal crisis crisis intestinal.
  laryngeal crisis crisis laríngea.
  maturational crisis crisis de maduración.
  ocular crisis crisis ocular.
  pharyngeal crisis crisis faríngea.
  puberal crisis crisis puberal.
  rejection crisis crisis de rechazo.
  renal crisis crisis renal.
  salt-losing crisis crisis con pérdida salina.
  sickle cell crisis crisis drepanocítica.
  situational crisis crisis de situación.
  tabetic crisis crisis tabética.
  therapeutic crisis crisis terapéutica.
  thoracic crisis crisis torácica.
  thyroid crisis crisis tiroidea, crisis tirotóxica.
  thyrotoxic crisis crisis tiroidea, crisis tirotóxica.
  visceral crisis crisis visceral.
criterion *n.* criterio.
  frequency normality criterion criterio de normalidad de frecuencia.
  functional normality criterion criterio de normalidad funcional.
  ideal normality criterion criterio de normalidad ideal.
  normality criterion criterio de normalidad.
  social normality criterion criterio de normalidad social.
critical *adj.* crítico, -ca.
crossed *adj.* cruzado, -da.
cross-eye *n.* estrabismo.
cross-eyed *adj.* bizco, -ca.

crossing-over *n.* crossing-over, entrecruzamiento.

croup *n.* croup, crup.

crown *n.* corona.

  artificial crown corona artificial.

  jacket crown corona funda.

  partial crown corona parcial.

  radiate crown corona radiada, corona radiante.

crust *n.* costra.

  milk crust costra de leche, costra láctea.

crusta *n.* costra, crusta.

  crusta inflammatoria costra inflamatoria.

  crusta lactea costra de leche, costra láctea, crusta lactea.

crustal *adj.* costroso, -sa.

crutch *n.* muleta.

cryoglobulin *n.* crioglobulina.

cryopreservation *n.* crioconservación, criopreservación.

cryptorchidy *n.* criptorquidia.

crystal *n.* cristal.

crystallin *n.* cristalina.

crystallization *n.* cristalización.

cubital *adj.* cubital.

cubitus *n.* cúbito, cubitus.

cue *n.* señal.

cuff *n.* brazal, manguito.

  rotator cuff manguito rotador del hombro.

culture *n.* cultivo.

cuneus *n.* cuña, cuneus.

cup *n.* copa, taza, ventosa.

curative *adj.* curativo, -va.

cure *n.* cura.

curettage *n.* curetaje, legrado, legrado uterino, raspado.

curvated *adj.* curvado, -da.

curvature *n.* curvatura.

cusp *n.* cúspide.

cuspis *n.* cúspide, cuspis, valva.

cut *n.* corte.

cutaneomucosal *adj.* cutaneomucoso, -sa.

cutaneous *n.* cutáneo, -a.

cuticle *n.* cutícula.

cuticula *n.* cutícula.

cutis *n.* cutis.

cyanosis *n.* cianosis.

  compression cyanosis cianosis por compresión.

cyanotic *adj.* cianótico, -ca.

cycle *n.* ciclo.

  anovulatory cycle ciclo anovulatorio.

  cardiac cycle ciclo cardíaco.

  cell cycle ciclo celular.

  hair cycle ciclo del pelo.

  life cycle ciclo vital.

  menstrual cycle ciclo menstrual.

  visual cycle ciclo visual.

cyclic *adj.* cíclico, -ca.

cyclops *adj.* ciclope, cíclope.

cyclothymiac *adj.* ciclotímico, -ca.

cyclotymic *adj.* ciclotímico, -ca.

cylinder *n.* cilindro.

cylindrical *adj.* cilíndrico, -ca.

cyst *n.* quiste.

  Bartholin's cyst quiste de Bartholin, quiste de Bartolino.

  congenital cyst quiste congénito.

  cyst of the liver quiste hepático.

  hepatic cyst quiste hepático.

  hydatid cyst quiste hidatídico.

  intracordal cyst quiste vocal.

  renal cyst quiste renal.

cystadenoma *n.* cistadenoma.
cystectomy *n.* cistectomía, quistectomía.
cystic *adj.* cístico, -ca, quístico, -ca.
cysticercosis *n.* cisticercosis.
cystinuria *n.* cistinuria.
cystitis *n.* cistitis.
　acute catarrhal cystitis cistitis aguda.
　allergic cystitis cistitis alérgica.
　bacterial cystitis cistitis bacteriana.
　cystitis cystica cistitis quística.
　cystitis senilis cistitis senil.
　diphtheritic cystitis cistitis diftérica.
　hemorrhagic cystitis cistitis hemorrágica.
　viral cystitis cistitis vírica.
cystoadenoma *n.* cistadenoma, cistoadenoma.
cystocopy *n.* cistoscopia.
cystogram *n.* cistograma.
cystoma *n.* cistoma.
cystoscope *n.* cistoscopio.
cystose *adj.* quístico, -ca.
cystostomy *n.* cistostomía.
cystous *adj.* cístico, -ca, quístico, -ca.
cytocidal *adj.* citocida.
cytocide *n.* citocida.
cytogenetics *n.* citogenética.
cytokine *n.* citocina.
cytology *n.* citología.
　cervicovaginal cytology citología cervicovaginal.
cytolysis *n.* citólisis.
cytomegalovirus *n.* citomegalovirus.
cytopathology *n.* citopatología.
cytoplasm *n.* citoplasma.
cytoplasmic *adj.* citoplasmático, -ca.

cytosis *n.* citosis.
cytotoxic *adj.* citotóxico, -ca.
cytotoxicity *n.* citotoxicidad.
cytotoxin *n.* citotoxina.

D

dactilar *adj.* dactilar.
dactylitis *n.* dactilitis.
daltonian *adj.* daltónico, -ca.
daltonism *n.* daltonismo.
damping *n.* amortiguación, amortiguamiento.
dance *n.* danza.
　Saint Vitus dance baile de san Vito, danza de san Vito.
dandruff *n.* caspa.
dark *adj.* oscuro, -ra.
database *n.* base de datos.
dead *adj.* muerto, -ta.
deadly *adj.* mortífero, -ra.
deaf *adj.* sordo, -da.
deaf-mute *adj., n.* sordomudo, -da.
deaf-mutism *n.* sordomudez.
deafness *n.* cofosis, sordera.
death *n.* deceso, muerte.
　accidental death muerte accidental.
　apparent death mors putativa, muerte aparente.
　assisted death muerte asistida.
　brain death muerte encefálica.
　cell death muerte celular.
　cerebral death muerte cerebral.
　fetal death muerte fetal.
　infant death muerte infantil.
　maternal death muerte materna.
　natural death muerte natural.

neocortical death muerte neocortical.

neonatal death muerte neonatal.

perinatal death muerte perinatal.

sudden cardiac death muerte cardíaca súbita.

violent death muerte a mano airada, muerte violenta, occisión.

debilitation *n.* debilitación.

debility *n.* debilidad.

mental debility debilidad mental.

débridement *n.* desbridamiento.

surgical débridement desbridamiento quirúrgico.

débris *n.* desecho, detritos.

debt *n.* deuda.

alactic oxygen debt deuda de oxígeno aláctico.

lactacid oxygen debt deuda de oxígeno lactácido.

oxygen debt deuda de oxígeno.

decalcification *n.* decalcificación, descalcificación.

decalcifying *adj.* decalcificante, descalcificante.

decay *n.* decaimiento, descomposición, desintegración.

decease *n.* deceso, óbito.

deceleration *n.* desaceleración.

decenter *v.* descentrar.

decidua *n.* decidua.

decoloration *n.* decoloración, descoloración.

decompensation *n.* descompensación.

decomposition *n.* descomposición.

decompression *n.* descompresión.

decongestant *n.* descongestionante, descongestivo, descongestivo, -va.

nasal decongestant descongestivo nasal.

decortication *n.* decorticación.

decortization *n.* decorticación, decortización.

decrease *n.* disminución.

decubitus *n.* decúbito.

supine decubitus position decúbito supino.

deep *adj.* profundo, -da.

defecation *n.* defecación.

defect *n.* defecto.

acquired defect defecto adquirido.

birth defect defecto congénito, defecto de nacimiento.

filling defect defecto de llenado, defecto de relleno.

genetic defect defecto genético.

neural-tube defect defecto del tubo neural.

visual field defect defecto del campo visual.

defective *adj.* defectuoso, -sa.

defeminization *n.* defeminación, defeminización, desfeminización.

defense *n.* defensa.

muscular defense defensa muscular.

deferent *adj.* deferente.

defibrillation *n.* desfibración, desfibrilación.

defibrillator *n.* desfibrilador.

deficiency *n.* carencia, deficiencia.

immune deficiency deficiencia de inmunidad, deficiencia inmune, deficiencia inmunitaria, deficiencia inmunológica.

deficit *n.* déficit.

sensory deficit déficit sensitivo.

vitamin deficit déficit vitamínico.

definition *n.* definición.

definitive *adj.* definitivo, -va.

deflection *n.* deflexión, desflexión.

deformation *n.* deformación.

deforming *adj.* deformante.

deformity *n.* deformidad.

rotational deformity decalaje.

degeneratio *n.* degeneración, degeneratio.

degeneration *n.* degeneración.

macular degeneration degeneración macular.

deglutition *n.* deglución.

degradation *n.* degradación.

degree *n.* grado.

degree of freedom grado de libertad.

degrowth *n.* decrecimiento.

degustation *n.* degustación.

dehiscence *n.* dehiscencia.

wound dehiscence dehiscencia de una herida.

dehydrate *v.* deshidratar.

dehydration *n.* dehidración, deshidratación.

delacrimation *n.* deslagrimación, lagrimeo.

delactation *n.* delactación, deslactación.

deletion *n.* deleción, pérdida.

chromosomal deletion deleción cromosómica.

delimitation *n.* delimitación.

deliriant *adj.* delirante.

delivery *n.* extracción, parto.

abdominal delivery extracción abdominal, parto abdominal.

premature delivery parto prematuro.

spontaneous delivery extracción expontánea, parto espontáneo, parto eutícico, parto eutócico.

vaginal delivery parto vaginal.

deltoide *adj.* deltoide, deltoideo, -a.

delusion *n.* delirio.

traumatic delusion delirio traumático.

demented *adj.* demente.

dementia *n.* demencia.

Alzheimer's dementia demencia de Alzheimer.

senile dementia demencia senil.

vascular dementia demencia vascular.

demineralization *n.* desmineralización.

demography *n.* demografía.

demyelination *n.* desmielinación.

segmentary demyelination desmielinación segmentaria.

demyelinization *n.* desmielinización.

denaturation *n.* desnaturalización.

protein denaturation desnaturalización de proteínas.

denatured *adj.* desnaturalizado, -da.

dendrite *n.* dendrita.

denial *n.* denegación, negación.

dens *n.* dens, diente.

dens lacteus diente de leche.

densitometer *n.* densitómetro.

densitometry *n.* densitometría.

bone densitometry densitometría ósea.

density *n.* densidad.

dentatum *adj.* dentado, -da.

dentin *n.* dentina.

dentist *n.* dentista.

dentistry *n.* odontología.
dentition *n.* dentición.
  first dentition dentición primaria, primera dentición.
  primary dentition dentición primaria, primera dentición.
  secondary dentition dentición secundaria, segunda dentición.
denture *n.* dentadura.
denturism *n.* ortodoncia.
denturist *adj.* ortodoncista.
denutrition *n.* desnutrición.
deodorant *n.* desodorante.
deodorize *v.* desodorizar.
deodorizer *n.* desodorizante.
department *n.* servicio.
  emergency department servicio de urgencias.
dependence *n.* dependencia.
depersonalization *n.* despersonalización.
depigmentation *n.* depigmentación, despigmentación.
depilation *n.* depilación.
deplete *v.* agotar.
depletion *n.* deplección.
depolarization *n.* despolarización.
  slow diastolic depolarization despolarización diastólica lenta.
depolarize *v.* despolarizar.
depolarizer *n.* despolarizador.
depopulation *n.* despoblación.
deposit *n.* depósito.
depressant *n.* depresor, -ra.
depressed *adj.* deprimido, -da.
depression *n.* abatimiento, depresión.
  mental depression depresión mental.

  postnatal depression depresión posparto.
deprivation *n.* deshabituación, privación.
depth *n.* profundidad.
derangement *n.* desarreglo.
dereistic *adj.* dereístico, -ca, irreal.
derivation *n.* derivación.
dermabrasion *n.* dermabrasión, dermoabrasión.
dermatitis *n.* dermatitis.
  allergic dermatitis dermatitis alérgica.
  atopic dermatitis dermatitis atópica.
  napkin dermatitis dermatitis del área del pañal.
dermatologic *adj.* dermatológico, -ca.
dermatologist *n.* dermatólogo, -ga.
dermatology *n.* dermatología.
dermatosis *n.* dermatosis.
  acarine dermatosis dermatosis acarina.
  seborrheic dermatosis dermatosis seborreica.
  ulcerative dermatosis dermatosis ulcerosa.
dermic *adj.* dérmico, -ca.
dermis *n.* dermis.
dermographism *n.* dermografismo.
dermoid *n.* dermoide.
desaturation *n.* desaturación.
descending *adj.* descendente.
descensus *n.* descenso, descensus.
descent *n.* descenso.
desensitization *n.* desensibilización.
desensitize *v.* desensibilizar.
desiccation *n.* desecación.
desquamation *n.* descamación.
desquamative *adj.* descamativo, -va.

destructive *adj.* destructivo, -va.

detachment *n.* desprendimiento.

choroidal detachment desprendimiento de coroides.

detachment of members desprendimiento de los miembros.

detachment of the placenta desprendimiento de la placenta, desprendimiento placentario.

detachment of the retina desprendimiento de la retina, desprendimiento de retina, desprendimiento retiniano.

epiphytical detachment desprendimiento epifisario.

exudative retinal detachment desprendimiento de retina exudativo, desprendimiento exudativo de la retina.

placental detachment desprendimiento de la placenta, desprendimiento placentario.

posterior vitreous detachment desprendimiento posterior del vítreo.

retinal detachment desprendimiento de la retina, desprendimiento de retina, desprendimiento retiniano.

rhegmatogenous retinal detachment desprendimiento regmatógeno de la retina.

vitreous detachment desprendimiento vítreo.

detect *v.* detectar.

detection *n.* detección.

detector *n.* detector.

detergent *adj., n.* detergente.

deterioration *n.* deterioro.

alcoholic deterioration deterioro alcohólico.

senile deterioration deterioro senil.

determinant *n.* determinante.

antigenic determinant determinante antigénico.

determinant of occlusion determinante de oclusión.

disease determinant determinante de enfermedad.

gait determinant determinante de la marcha.

genetic determinant determinante genético.

hidden determinant determinante oculto.

immunogenic determinant determinante inmunogénico.

isoallotypic determinant determinante isoalotípico.

psychic determinant determinante psíquico.

sequential determinant determinante secuencial.

determination *n.* determinación.

blood gas determination determinación de gases en sangre.

sex determination determinación del sexo, determinación sexual.

determinism *n.* determinismo.

psychic determinism determinismo psíquico.

detoxicate *v.* desintoxicar, destoxicar.

detoxication *n.* desintoxicación, destoxicación.

detoxification *n.* desintoxicación, destoxificación.

detoxify *v.* desintoxicar, destoxificar, detoxificar.

detrition *n.* desgaste, detrición.

detritus *n.* desecho, detrito, detritus.

detrusor *adj.* detrusor.

detubation *n.* destubación.

development *n.* desarrollo.

child development desarrollo infantil.

embryologic development desarrollo embrionario.

prenatal development desarrollo prenatal.

psychomotor and physical development of infants desarrollo físico y psicomotor de los lactantes.

psychosocial development desarrollo psicosocial.

deviance *n.* desviación.

deviant *adj.* desviado, -da.

sexual deviant desviado sexual.

deviation *n.* desviación.

complement deviation desviación del complemento.

deviation from normal desviación de la norma.

deviation of the teeth desviación de los dientes.

deviation of the tongue desviación de la lengua.

deviation to the left desviación a la izquierda, desviación hacia la izquierda.

deviation to the right desviación a la derecha, desviación hacia la derecha.

dissociated vertical deviation desviación vertical disociada.

eye deviation desviación del ojo.

immune deviation desviación inmunitaria, desviación inmunológica.

latent deviation desviación latente.

left axis deviation (LAD) desviación izquierda del eje.

manifest deviation desviación manifiesta.

minimal deviation desviación mínima.

minimum deviation desviación mínima.

organic deviation desviación orgánica.

primary deviation desviación primaria.

right axis deviation (RAD) desviación derecha del eje.

sample standard deviation desviación estándar de una muestra.

secondary deviation desviación secundaria.

sexual deviation desviación sexual.

skew deviation desviación oblicua, desviación sesgada.

social deviation desviación social.

spinal column deviation desviación de la columna vertebral.

squint deviation desviación estrábica.

standard deviation (SD) desviación estándar (DE).

strabismal deviation desviación estrábica.

strabismic deviation desviación estrábica.

uterine deviation desviación uterina.

device *n.* dispositivo.

contraceptive device dispositivo anticonceptivo, dispositivo contraceptivo.

devisceration *n.* desvisceración.

devitalization *n.* desvitalización.

pulp devitalization desvitalización pulpar.

devitalize *v.* desvitalizar.

devitalized *adj.* desvitalizado, -da.

dextrocardia *n.* dextrocardia.

corrected dextrocardia dextrocardia corregida.

dextrocardia with situs inversus dextrocardia con situs inversus.

false dextrocardia dextrocardia falsa.

isolated dextrocardia dextrocardia aislada.

mirror-image dextrocardia dextrocardia en imagen en espejo.

secondary dextrocardia dextrocardia secundaria.

type 1 dextrocardia dextrocardia tipo 1.

type 2 dextrocardia dextrocardia tipo 2.

type 3 dextrocardia dextrocardia tipo 3.

type 4 dextrocardia dextrocardia tipo 4.

dextrocardiogram *n.* dextrocardiograma.

dextrocerebral *adj.* dextrocerebral.

dextromanual *adj.* dextromano, -na, dextromanual, diestro, -tra.

dextroversion *n.* dextroversión.

dextroversion of the heart dextroversión del corazón.

diabetes *n.* diabetes.

adult-onset diabetes diabetes de comienzo en la edad adulta.

alimentary diabetes diabetes alimentaria.

artificial diabetes diabetes artificial.

bronze diabetes diabetes bronceada.

calcinuric diabetes diabetes calcinúrica.

cerebrospinal diabetes diabetes cerebroespinal.

clinical diabetes diabetes clínica.

diabetes albuminurinicus diabetes albuminúrica.

diabetes insipidus diabetes insípida.

diabetes mellitus (DM) diabetes azucarada, diabetes glucémica, diabetes mellitus (DM), diabetes sacarina.

endocrine diabetes mellitus diabetes mellitus endocrina.

gestational diabetes mellitus (GDM) diabetes mellitus gestacional (DMG).

growth-onset diabetes diabetes de comienzo en el crecimiento.

insulin-deficient diabetes diabetes con deficiencia de insulina.

insulin-dependent diabetes diabetes insulinodependiente.

insulin-dependent diabetes mellitus (IDDM) diabetes mellitus insulinodependiente (DMID).

juvenile diabetes diabetes juvenil.

juvenile onset diabetes diabetes de comienzo en la juventud.

masked diabetes diabetes disimulada.

maturity-onset diabetes diabetes de comienzo en la madurez.

maturity-onset diabetes of youth (MODY) diabetes de comienzo en la madurez de la juventud.

nephrogenic diabetes insipidus diabetes insípida nefrogénica.

non-insulin dependent diabetes diabetes no insulinodependiente.

non-insulin dependent diabetes (NIDD) diabetes no insulinodependiente (DNID).

non-insulin-dependent diabetes mellitus (NIDDM) diabetes mellitus no insulinodependiente (DMNID).

overflow diabetes diabetes por derramamiento.

pregnancy diabetes diabetes del embarazo.

skin diabetes diabetes cutánea.

type I diabetes diabetes tipo I.

type II diabetes diabetes del adulto, diabetes tipo II.

diabetic *adj.* diabético, -ca.

diabetology *n.* diabetología.

diagnose *v.* diagnosticar.

diagnosis *n.* diagnóstico.

antenatal diagnosis diagnóstico antenatal.

clinical diagnosis diagnóstico clínico.

cytohistologic diagnosis diagnóstico citohistológico, diagnóstico citológico.

diagnosis by exclusion diagnóstico por exclusión.

differential diagnosis diagnóstico diferencial.

direct diagnosis diagnóstico directo.

laboratory diagnosis diagnóstico de laboratorio.

neonatal diagnosis diagnóstico neonatal.

pathologic diagnosis diagnóstico patológico.

physical diagnosis diagnóstico físico.

prenatal diagnosis diagnóstico prenatal.

serum diagnosis diagnóstico serológico.

topographic diagnosis diagnóstico topográfico.

diagram *n.* diagrama.

dialysate *n.* dializador, -ra.

dialysis *n.* diálisis.

continuous ambulatory peritoneal dialysis (CAPD) diálisis peritoneal ambulatoria continua (DPAC).

renal dialysis diálisis renal.

dialyze *v.* dializar.

dialyzer *n.* dializadorr.

diameter *n.* diámetro.

diapason *n.* diapasón.

diaphragm *n.* diafragma.

arcing spring contraceptive diaphragm diafragma anticonceptivo de espiral.

coil-spring contraceptive diaphragm diafragma anticonceptivo de muelle espiral.

contraceptive diaphragm diafragma anticonceptivo.

flat spring contraceptive diaphragm diafragma anticonceptivo de resorte plano.

vaginal diaphragm diafragma vaginal.

diaphragmatic *adj.* diafragmático, -ca.

diarrhea *n.* diarrea.

acute diarrhea diarrea aguda.

diarrhea ablactatorum diarrea del destete.

diarrhea chylosa diarrea quilosa.

dysentric diarrhea diarrea disentérica.

enteral diarrhea diarrea entérica, diarrea intestinal.

epidemic diarrhea of the newborn diarrea epidémica del recién nacido.

fatty diarrhea diarrea grasa.

gastrogenous diarrhea diarrea gastrógena.

infantile diarrhea diarrea infantil.

irritative diarrhea diarrea irritativa.

lienteric diarrhea diarrea lientérica.

mecanical diarrhea diarrea mecánica.

membranous diarrhea diarrea membranosa.

morning diarrhea diarrea matinal.

mucous diarrhea diarrea mucosa.

neonatal diarrhea diarrea neonatal.

nocturnal diarrhea diarrea nocturna.

osmotic diarrhea diarrea osmótica.

pancreatogenous diarrhea diarrea pancreatógena.

paradoxical diarrhea diarrea paradójica.

parenteral diarrhea diarrea parenteral.

purulent diarrhea diarrea purulenta.

putrefactive diarrhea diarrea putrefactiva.

simple diarrhea diarrea simple.

summer diarrhea diarrea estival.

traveler's diarrhea diarrea del viajero.

tropical diarrhea diarrea tropical.

watery diarrhea diarrea acuosa.

diarrheal *adj.* diarreico, -ca.

diarrheic *adj.* diarreico, -ca.

diarthrosis *n.* diartrosis.

diastema *n.* diastema.

diastole *n.* diástole.

cardiac diastole diástole cardíaca.

diastolic *adj.* diastólico, -ca.

diathermal *adj.* diatérmico, -ca.

diathermocoagualtion *n.* diatermocoagulación.

diathermy *n.* diatermia.

surgical diathermy diatermia quirúrgica.

diathesis *n.* diátesis.

die *v.* morir.

diet *n.* dieta, régimen.

absolute diet dieta absoluta.

adequate diet dieta adecuada.

alkali-ash diet dieta alcalina, dieta de cenizas alcalinas.

balanced diet dieta equilibrada.

basal diet dieta basal.

basic diet dieta básica.

challenge diet dieta de provocación.

clear liquid diet dieta hídrica, dieta líquida clara.

diabetic diet dieta diabética, dieta para diabéticos, régimen diabético.

elimination diet dieta de eliminación, régimen de eliminación.

full diet dieta completa.

full liquid diet dieta líquida completa.

gluten-free diet dieta libre de gluten, dieta sin gluten.

gouty diet dieta para gotosos.

high calorie diet dieta rica en calorías.

high fat diet dieta rica en grasas.

high fiber diet dieta rica en fibra.

high protein diet dieta rica en proteínas.

high-potassium diet dieta rica en potasio.

high-vitamin diet dieta rica en vitaminas.

ketogenic diet dieta cetógenica.

light diet dieta libre de purinas ligera, dieta ligera.

liquid diet dieta líquida.

low calorie diet dieta baja en calorías, dieta pobre en calorías.

low fat diet dieta pobre en grasas.

low oxalate diet dieta pobre en oxalato.

low purine diet dieta pobre en purina.

low residue diet dieta pobre en residuos.

low-calcium diet dieta pobre en calcio.

low-caloric diet dieta hipocalórica.

low-cholesterol diet dieta pobre en colesterol.

low-saturated-fat diet dieta pobre en grasas saturadas.

milk diet dieta láctea.

mixed diet dieta mixta.

optimal diet dieta óptima.

protein sparing diet dieta de conservación de proteínas.

purine restricted diet dieta con restricción de purina.

rachitic diet dieta raquítica.

reducing diet dieta reductora.

reduction diet dieta de adelgazamiento.

regular diet dieta regular.

rice diet dieta de arroz.

salt-free diet dieta sin sal.

soft diet dieta blanda.

dietetic *adj.* dietético, -ca.

dietetics *n.* dietética.

dietitian *n.* dietetista, dietista.

difference *n.* diferencia.

individual difference diferencia individual.

light difference diferencia luminosa.

differentiated *adj.* diferenciado, -da.

differentiation *n.* diferenciación.

diffusion *n.* difusión.

digestant *adj.* digestivo, -va.

digestion *n.* digestión.

digital *adj.* digital.

dilatation *n.* dilatación.

dilation *n.* dilatación.

diopter *n.* dioptría.

diphtheria *n.* difteria.

cutaneous diphtheria difteria cutánea, difteria dérmica.

diphtheria gravis difteria grave.

gangrenous diphtheria difteria gangrenosa.

laryngeal diphtheria difteria laríngea, garrotillo.

malignant diphtheria difteria maligna.

nasal diphtheria difteria nasal.

nasopharyngeal diphtheria difteria nasofaríngea.

pharyngeal diphtheria difteria faríngea.

septic diphtheria difteria séptica.

surgical diphtheria difteria quirúrgica.

umbilical diphtheria difteria umbilical.

diplopia *n.* diplopía, diploscopía.

directive *n.* instrucción.

disability *n.* discapacidad, incapacidad.

mental disability incapacidad mental.

disarticulation *n.* desarticulación.

disc *n.* disco.

protruded disc disco protruido.

discharge *n.* alta, descarga.

absolute discharge alta definitiva.

epileptic discharge descarga epiléptica.

involuntary discharge alta involuntaria.

discordance *n.* discordancia.

discus *n.* disco, discus.

disease *n.* enfermedad.

Addison's disease enfermedad de Addison.

Alzheimer's disease enfermedad de Alzheimer.

autoimmune disease enfermedad autoinmune.

aviator's disease enfermedad de los aviadores.

celiac disease celiaquía, enfermedad celíaca.

Chagas' disease enfermedad de Chagas, enfermedad de Chagas-Cruz.

Chagas-Cruz disease enfermedad de Chagas, enfermedad de Chagas-Cruz.

chronic hypertensive disease enfermedad hipertensiva crónica.

contagious disease enfermedad contagiosa.

Crohn's disease enfermedad de Crohn.

Cushing's disease enfermedad de Cushing.

deficiency disease enfermedad por deficiencia.

exanthematous disease enfermedad exantemática.

graft versus host disease enfermedad de injerto versus huésped.

infectious disease enfermedad infecciosa.

infective disease enfermedad infecciosa.

mental disease enfermedad mental.

molecular disease enfermedad molecular.

notifiable disease enfermedad notificable.

occupational disease enfermedad ocupacional.

organic disease enfermedad orgánica.

parasitic disease enfermedad parasitaria.

pelvic inflammatory disease enfermedad inflamatoria de la pelvis.

periodic disease enfermedad periódica.

Pott's disease enfermedad de Pott.

primary disease enfermedad primaria.

radiation disease enfermedad por radiaciones.

sexually transmitted disease (STD) enfermedad de transmisión sexual (ETS).

sickle cell disease enfermedad drepanocítica.

specific disease enfermedad específica.

storage disease enfermedad por almacenamiento.

valvular heart disease valvulopatía cardíaca.

venereal disease enfermedad venérea.

von Willebrand's disease enfermedad de von Willebrand.

disequilibrium *n.* desequilibrio.

disinfect *v.* desinfectar.

disinfectant *n.* desinfectante.

disinfection *n.* desinfección.

disinfestation *n.* desinfestación.

disinhibition *n.* desinhibición.

disk *n.* disco.

dislocation *n.* descoyuntamiento, dislocación, lluxatio, luxación.

complete dislocation luxación completa.

congenital dislocation luxación congénita.

dislocation of the clavicle luxación de la clavícula.

dislocation of the hip luxación de cadera.

dislocation of the knee luxación de la rodilla.

dislocation of the lens luxación del cristalino.

dislocation of the shoulder luxación del hombro.

fractura dislocation luxación y fractura.

habitual dislocation luxación habitual, luxación iterativa.

incomplete dislocation luxación incompleta.

simple dislocation luxación simple.

disorder *n.* desorden, trastorno.

acute stress disorder trastorno por estrés agudo.

adjustment disorder trastorno adaptativo.

affective disorder trastorno afectivo.

antisocial personality disorder trastorno antisocial de la personalidad.

anxiety disorder trastorno de ansiedad.

attention-deficit hyperactive disorder trastorno por déficit de atención con hiperactividad.

autistic disorder trastorno autista, trastorno autístico.

behavior disorder trastorno del comportamiento.

bipolar disorder trastorno bipolar.

cyclotimic disorder trastorno ciclotímico.

developmental disorder trastorno del desarrollo.

eating disorder trastorno de la conducta alimentaria.

functional disorder trastorno funcional.

gait disorder trastorno de la marcha.

hypochondriac disorder trastorno hipocondríaco.

immunodeficiency disorder trastorno por inmunodeficiencia.

inherited disorder trastorno hereditario.

learning disorder trastorno del aprendizaje.

major depressive disorder trastorno depresivo mayor.

maniac-depressive disorder trastorno maniacodepresivo.

mental disorder trastorno mental.

metabolic disorder trastorno metabólico.

mood disorder trastorno del estado del ánimo.

multifactorial disorder trastorno multifactorial.

neurotic disorder trastorno neurótico.

pain disorder trastorno por dolor.

panic disorder trastorno de pánico.

post-traumatic stress disorder trastorno por estrés postraumático.

schizoaffective disorder trastorno esquizoafectivo.

schizoid personality disorder trastorno esquizoide de la personalidad.

sexual disorder trastorno sexual.

sexual identity disorder trastorno de la identidad sexual.

sleep disorder trastorno del sueño.

disorganization *n.* desorganización.

disorientation *n.* desorientación.

dispareunia *n.* dispareunia.

disparity *n.* disparidad.

displacement *n.* decalaje, desplazamiento.

condylar displacement desplazamiento condíleo.

fetal displacement desplazamiento fetal.

lateral pelvic displacement desplazamiento pélvico lateral.

tissue displacement desplazamiento hístico, desplazamiento tisular.

disproportion *n.* desproporción.

cephalopelvic disproportion (CPD) desproporción cefalopélvica (DCP).

disruption *n.* disrupción.

dissection *n.* disección.

aortic dissection disección aórtica.

dissociation *n.* disociación.

dissolvent *n.* disolvente.

distal *adj.* distal, distalis.

distalis *adj.* distal, distalis.

distance *n.* distancia.

distensibility *n.* distensibilidad.

distension *n.* distensión.

distention *n.* distensión.

distillation *n.* destilación.

distortion *n.* distorsión.

distress *n.* distrés, sufrimiento.

adult respiratory distress distrés respiratorio del adulto.

fetal distress sufrimiento fetal.

distribution *n.* distribución.

drug distribution distribución del fármaco.

normal distribution distribución normal.

diuresis *n.* diuresis.

diverticulitis *n.* diverticulitis.

diverticulum *n.* divertículo, diverticulum.

divisio *n.* división.

division *n.* división.

cell division división celular.

dizziness *n.* aturdimiento, desvanecimiento, mareo.

doctor *n.* doctor, -ra.

dolor *n.* dolor.

dolor capitis dolor capitis, dolor de cabeza.

dolorific *adj.* dolorífico, doloroso.

dominance *n.* dominancia.
 genetic dominance dominancia genética.
dominant *adj.* dominante.
donor *n.* dador, donador, -ra, donante.
 blood donor donante de sangre.
 cadaveric donor donante de cadáver.
 living donor donante vivo.
 xenogenic donor donante xenogénico.
Doppler *n.* Doppler.
dorsalgia *n.* dorsalgia.
dorsum *n.* dorso, dorsum.
dosage *n.* dosificación.
dose *n.* dosis.
 equivalent dose dosis equivalente.
 initial dose dosis inicial.
 loading dose dosis de ataque.
 maximal dose dosis máxima.
 minimal dose dosis mínima.
 minimum dose dosis mínima.
dosis *n.* dosis.
dot *n.* mancha.
double *adj.* doble.
drainage *n.* drenaje.
dream *n.* ensueño, sueño.
drepanocyte *n.* drepanocito.
drepanocytemia *n.* drepanocitemia.
drepanocytic *adj.* drepanocítico, -ca.
dressing *n.* apósito, vendaje.
drift *n.* deriva, desplazamiento, desviación.
 antigenic drift deriva antigénica, desplazamiento antigénico, desviación antigénica.

genetic drift deriva genética, desplazamiento genético, desviación genética.
 ulnar drift desviación cubital.
drifting *n.* desplazamiento.
drip *n.* goteo.
 intravenous drip goteo intravenoso.
 postnasal drip goteo posnasal.
drive *n.* impulso, pulsión.
 aggressive drive impulso agresivo, pulsión agresiva, pulsión destructiva.
 sexual drive impulso sexual, pulsión sexual.
drop *n.* gota.
 ear drop gota para el oído.
 eye drop gota ocular, gota para los ojos.
dropper *n.* cuentagotas, gotero.
dropsy *n.* hidropepsia, hidropesia.
drowning *n.* ahogamiento.
 near drowning ahogamiento incompleto.
 secondary drowning ahogamiento secundario.
drowsiness *n.* modorra, sopor.
drug *n.* droga, drogar, fármaco, medicamento.
 drug dependence drogodependencia.
 sulfa drug sulfamida.
drunkenness *n.* embriaguez.
dry *adj.* seco, -ca.
dualism *n.* dualismo.
duct *n.* conducto.
 aberrant duct conducto aberrante.
 hypophyseal duct conducto hipofisario.

thyroglossal duct conducto tirogloso.

thyrolingual duct conducto tirolingual.

ductus *n.* conducto, ductus.

dumb *adj.* mudo, -da.

duodenum *n.* duodeno.

duplication *n.* duplicación.

duplication of chromosomes duplicación cromosómica.

dwarf *n.* enano, -na.

achondroplasic dwarf enano acondroplásico.

dwarfism *n.* enanismo.

achondroplastic dwarfism enanismo acondroplásico.

hypophyseal dwarfism enanismo hipofisario.

dyad *n.* díada.

dyeing *adj.* colorante.

dying *adj.* moribundo, -da.

dysarthria *n.* disartria.

dyscontrol *n.* descontrol.

dysentery *n.* disentería.

dysfunction *n.* disfunción.

erectile dysfunction disfunción eréctil.

sexual dysfunction disfunción sexual.

dyslexia *n.* dislexia.

dyslexic *adj.* disléxico, -ca.

dyslipidemia *n.* dislipidemia.

dysmenorrhea *n.* dismenorrea.

dyspepsia *n.* dispepsia.

dysphagia *n.* disfagia.

dysphagy *n.* disfagia.

dysphonia *n.* disfonía.

dysplasia *n.* displasia.

dyspnea *n.* disnea.

dysthymia *n.* distimia.

dystocia *n.* distocia.

dystonia *n.* distonía.

dystonia deformans progressiva distonía deformante muscular, distonía deformante progresiva.

dystonia musculorum deformans distonía deformante muscular, distonía deformante progresiva, distonía muscular deformante.

dystrophia *n.* distrofia.

dystrophia endothelialis corneae distrofia endotelial de la córnea.

dystrophy *n.* distrofia.

Duchenne's muscular dystrophy distrofia muscular de Duchenne.

endothelial dystrophy of the cornea distrofia endotelial de la córnea.

muscular dystrophy distrofia muscular.

dysuria *n.* alginuresis, disuria.

dysury *n.* disuria.

E

ear *n.* oído, oreja.

external ear auris externa, oído externo.

inner ear auris interna, oído interno.

internal ear auris interna, oído interno.

lop ear oreja caída.

middle ear auris media, oído medio.

outer ear auris externa, oído externo.

swimmer's ear oído de nadador.

eardrum *n.* tambor, tímpano.

ebrious *adj.* ebrio, -a.

ecchymosis *n.* equimosis.

echographer *n.* ecógrafo.

echographist *n.* ecografista.

echography *n.* ecografía.

echolalia *n.* ecolalia.

eclampsia *n.* eclampsia.

ecstasy *n.* éxtasis.

ectasia *n.* ectasia,, ectasis.

ectasis *n.* ectasia,, ectasis.

ectopia *n.* ectopia.

ectopic *adj.* ectópico, -ca.

ectopy *n.* ectopia.

ectropion *n.* ectropía, ectropión.

eczema *n.* eccema, eczema.

atopic eczema eccema atópico, eccema constitucional.

contact eczema eccema de contacto.

seborrheic eczema eccema seborreico.

edema *n.* edema.

edge *n.* borde.

cutting edge borde cortante.

effect *n.* efecto.

secundary effect efecto secundario.

side effect efecto colateral.

effectiveness *n.* efectividad, eficacia.

contraceptive effectiveness eficacia anticonceptiva.

efferent *adj.* eferente.

effusion *n.* derrame, efusión.

articular effusion derrame articular.

cerebral effusion derrame cerebral.

joint effusion derrame articular, derrame sinovial.

ego *n.* ego, yo.

ejaculatio *n.* eyaculación.

ejaculation *n.* eyaculación.

ejection *n.* eyección.

elasticity *n.* elasticidad.

elbow *n.* codo.

baseball pitcher's elbow codo de lanzador.

dropped elbow codo péndulo.

golfer's elbow codo de golfista.

miner's elbow codo de los mineros.

nursemaid's elbow codo de las niñeras.

pulled elbow codo dislocado.

student elbow codo del estudiante.

tennis elbow codo de tenista.

electrocardiogram (ECG) *n.* electrocardiograma (ECG).

electrocardiography *n.* electrocardiografía.

elephantiasis *n.* elefantiasis.

elevator *n.* elevador.

embole *n.* embolia.

embolectomy *n.* emboliectomía.

embolic *adj.* embólico, -ca.

embolism *n.* embolia.

cerebral embolism embolia cerebral.

pulmonary embolism embolia pulmonar.

venous embolism embolia venosa.

embolization *n.* embolización.

embolus *n.* émbolo.

emboly *n.* embolia.

embriopathy *n.* embriopatía.

embryo *n.* embrión.

embryology *n.* embriología.

embryopathia *n.* embriopatía.

emergence *n.* despertar.

emergency *n.* emergencia, urgencia.

emesia *n.* emesia, emesis.

emesis *n.* emesia, emesis.

emetic *adj.* emético, -ca, emetizante.

emollient *adj.* emoliente.

emotional *adj.* emocional.

emotivity *n.* emotividad.

emphysema *n.* enfisema.

 pulmonary emphysema enfisema pulmonar.

emphysematous *adj.* enfisematoso, -sa.

empiric *adj.* empírico, -ca.

empirical *adj.* empírico, -ca.

empyema *n.* empiema.

enamel *n.* esmalte.

encapsulated *adj.* encapsulado, -da.

encapsuled *adj.* encapsulado, -da.

encephalic *adj.* encefálico, -ca.

encephalitis *n.* encefalitis.

encephalomyelitis *n.* encefalomielitis.

encephalon *n.* encéfalo.

encephalopathia *n.* encefalopatía.

encephalopathy *n.* encefalopatía.

encysted *adj.* enquistado, -da.

end *n.* extremo.

endemic *adj.* endémico, -ca.

ending *n.* terminación.

 nerve ending terminación nerviosa.

endocarditis *n.* endocarditis.

endocrinologist *n.* endocrinólogo, -a.

endocrinology *n.* endocrinología.

endodontia *n.* endodoncia.

endodontics *n.* endodoncia.

endodontist *n.* endodoncista, endodontista.

endoenteritis *n.* endoenteritis.

endometriosis *n.* endometriosis.

endometritis *n.* endometritis.

endometrium *n.* endometrio.

endoscope *n.* endoscopio.

endoscopist *n.* endoscopista.

endoscopy *n.* endoscopia.

endothelial *adj.* endotelial.

endothelium *n.* endotelio.

enema *n.* enema, lavativa.

 barium enema enema baritado, enema de bario.

energy *n.* energía.

engagement *n.* encajamiento.

engine *n.* machina, máquina.

 surgical engine máquina quirúrgica.

engorged *adj.* ingurgitado, -da.

engorgement *n.* ingurgitación, ingurgitación.

enkephalin *n.* encefalina.

enophthalmos *n.* enoftalmos.

enrichment *n.* enriquecimiento.

enteral *adj.* enteral.

enteric *adj.* entérico, -ca.

enteritis *n.* enteritis.

enterocolitis *n.* enterocolitis.

enterocyte *n.* enterocito.

enterotoxin *n.* enterotoxina.

enterovirus *n.* enterovirus.

entity *n.* entidad.

enuresis *n.* enuresis.

 diurnal enuresis enuresis diurna.

 nocturnal enuresis enuresis nocturna.

envelope *n.* cubierta, envoltura.

environment *n.* ambiente.

enzyme *n.* enzima.

eosinophil *n.* eosinófilo.

eosinophile *n.* eosinófilo.

eosinophilia *n.* eosinofilia.

ependyma *n.* epéndimo.

ependymitis *n.* ependimitis.

epicardia *n.* epicardias.

epicarditis *n.* epicarditis.

epicardium *n.* epicardio.

epicondylian *adj.* epicondilar, epicondíleo, -a.

epicondylic *adj.* epicondilar, epicondíleo, -a.

epicondylitis *n.* epicondilitis.

epidemic *n.* epidemia, epidémico, -ca.

epidemiology *n.* epidemiología.

epiderm *n.* epidermis, epidermo.

epidermic *adj.* epidérmico, -ca.

epidermis *n.* epidermis, epidermo.

epidermolysis *n.* epidermólisis.

epididymis *n.* epidídimo.

epididymitis *n.* epididimitis.

epidural *adj.* epidural.

epigaster *n.* epigáster.

epigastric *adj.* epigástrico, -ca.

epiglottis *n.* epiglotis.

epilepsia *n.* epilepsia.

epilepsy *n.* epilepsia.

   focal epilepsy epilepsia focal.

   generalized epilepsy epilepsia generalizada.

   grand mal epilepsy epilepsia de gran mal, epilepsia de grand mal.

   hysterical epilepsy epilepsia histérica.

   partial epilepsy epilepsia parcial.

   petit mal epilepsy epilepsia de pequeño mal, epilepsia de petit mal.

epileptic *adj.* epiléptico, -ca.

epiphysis *n.* epífisis.

episiotomy *n.* episiotomía.

episode *n.* episodio.

epistaxis *n.* epistaxis.

epithelium *n.* epitelio, epithelium.

equilibrium *n.* equilibrio.

   acid-base equilibrium equilibrio ácido-base, equilibrio acidobásico.

erection *n.* erección.

erosion *n.* erosión.

error *n.* error.

   medical error error médico.

erubescence *n.* erubescencia, rubefacción.

eruption *n.* erupción.

erysipelas *n.* erisipela.

erythema *n.* eritema.

erythroblast *n.* eritroblasto, hemonormoblasto.

erythrocyte *n.* eritrocito.

erythrocytopoiesis *n.* eritrocitopoyesis.

erythrocytosis *n.* eritrocitosis.

erythroderma *n.* eritrodermia.

erythropoiesis *n.* eritropoyesis.

erythropoietic *adj.* eritropoyético, -ca.

esophagitis *n.* esofagitis.

esophagus *n.* esófago.

essential *adj.* esencial.

estimate *n.* estimación.

estriol *n.* estriol.

estrogen *n.* estrógeno.

estrogenic *adj.* estrogénico, -ca.

ethics *n.* ética.

ethmoid *adj.* etmoide, etmoideo, -a.

   ethmoid bone etmoides.

ethmoidal *adj.* etmoidal.

ethmoidale *adj.* etmoidal.

ethological *adj.* etológico, -ca.

ethology *n.* etología.

ethylism n. etilismo.

etiologic adj. etiológico, -ca.

etiological adj. etiológico, -ca.

etiology n. etiología.

  etiology and pathogenesis etiopatogenia.

etiopathic adj. etiopático, -ca.

etiopathogenesis n. etiopatogenia.

eucaryote n. eucariota.

eukaryote n. eucariota.

eunuch n. eunuco.

euphoria n. euforia.

euthanasia n. eutanasia.

eutonic adj. eutónico, -ca.

evacuation n. evacuación.

evaluation n. evaluación.

evaporation n. evaporación.

eventration n. eventración.

eversion n. eversión.

evisceration n. evisceración.

evolution n. evolución.

evolutive adj. evolutivo, -va.

exacerbation n. exacerbación.

examination n. examen.

  cytologic examination examen citológico.

  mini mental state examination mini examen del estado mental.

  Papanicolaou examination examen de Papanicolaou.

  postmortem examination examen post mortem.

exanthema n. exantema.

excess n. exceso.

exchange n. intercambio.

excision n. escisión, excisión, rescisión.

  wound excision desbridamiento.

excrescence n. excrecencia.

excretion n. excreción.

exenteration n. evisceración, exenteración.

exfoliation n. exfoliación.

exhaustion n. agotamiento, extenuación.

  heat exhaustion agotamiento por calor.

  nervous exhaustion agotamiento nervioso.

exocervix n. exocérvix.

exodontics n. exodoncia.

exophthalmus n. exoftalmos.

exophthalmia n. exoftalmía.

exophthalmos n. exoftalmos.

exostosis n. exostosis.

expander n. expansor.

  plasma expander expansor del plasma.

expectorant n. expectorante.

expectoration n. expectoración.

experience n. experiencia.

  internal experience vivencia.

expiration n. espiración, expiración.

exploration n. exploración.

  gynecological exploration exploración ginecológica.

  physical exploration exploración física.

exposure n. exposición.

expulsion n. expulsión.

expulsive adj. expulsivo, -va.

exsanguination n. exanguinación.

exsiccation n. desecación.

extension n. extensión.

exterior n. exterior.

externalization n. externalización.

extracorporeal adj. extracorporal, extracorpóreo, -a.

extracorpored *adj.* extracorporal, extracorpóreo, -a.

extraction *n.* extracción.

⋯raneous *adj.* extraño, ña.

⋯systole *n.* extrasístole, extra-sístolia.

extravasation *n.* extravasación.

extreme *n.* extremo.

extrusion *n.* extrusión.

extubate *v.* extubar.

exudate *n.* exudado.

exudation *n.* exudación.

eye *n.* ojo.

  aphakic eye ojo afáquico.

  artificial eye ojo artificial.

  bank eye banco de ojo.

  bleary eye ojo blefarítico, ojo lega-ñoso.

  cyclopean eye ojo de cíclope.

  cyclopian eye ojo de cíclope.

  deviating eye ojo desviado.

  dominant eye ojo dominante.

  following eye ojo errante.

  schematic eye ojo esquemático.

  scotopic eye ojo escotópico.

  squinting eye ojo bizco, ojo estrá-bico.

eyebrow *n.* ceja.

eyelash *n.* pestaña.

eyelid *n.* párpado.

eyepiece *n.* ocular.

F

fabulation *n.* fabulación.

face *n.* cara, facies, faz.

  bird face braquignatia, cara de pájaro.

  cow face cara de vaca, facies bovina, facies de vaca.

  dish face cara de plato.

  frog face cara de sapo.

  hippocratic face cara hipocrática, facies agónica, facies descompósita, facies hipocrática.

  masklike face facies de máscara, cara de máscara.

  moon face cara de luna llena, facies de luna, facies lunar.

facies *n.* facies.

facing *n.* carilla.

factitial *adj.* facticio, -cia.

factitious *adj.* facticio, -cia.

factor *n.* factor.

faculty *n.* facultad.

  rational faculty razón.

failure *n.* fallo, insuficiencia.

  circulatory failure insuficiencia circulatoria.

  congestive heart failure (CHF) insuficiencia cardíaca congestiva (ICC).

  heart failure insuficiencia cardíaca.

  mitral failure insuficiencia mitral.

  renal failure insuficiencia renal.

  respiratory failure insuficiencia respiratoria.

faint *n.* desfallecimiento, desmayo.

false *adj.* falso, -sa.

family *n.* familia.

farcy *n.* farcinosis, muermo.

fascia *n.* fascia.

fasciitis *n.* fascitis.

fat *n.* grasa.

  polyunsaturated fat grasa poliinsaturada.

  unsaturated fat grasa insaturada.

fate *n.* destino.

fatherhood *n.* paternidad.

fatigue *n.* fatiga.

fatty *adj.* graso, -sa.

fear *n.* miedo, temor.

fecal *adj.* fecal.

fecaloma *n.* fecaloma.

feces *n.* heces.

feculent *adj.* feculento, -ta.

fecundate *v.* fecundar.

fecundatio *n.* fecundación.

fecundation *n.* fecundación.

fecundity *n.* fecundidad.

feedback *n.* feedback, retroacción, retroalimentación.

feeding *n.* alimentación.

   artificial feeding alimentación artificial.

   bottle feeding alimentación con biberón.

   breast feeding alimentación al pecho.

   forced feeding alimentación forzada.

   forcible feeding alimentación forzada.

   gastric feeding alimentación gástrica.

   gastrostomy feeding alimentación mediante gastrostomía.

   nasogastric feeding alimentación nasogástrica.

feeling *n.* sentimiento.

   feeling of guilt sentimiento de culpabilidad.

   feeling of inferiority sentimiento de inferioridad.

female *n.* hembra.

femenine *adj.* femenino, -na.

feminization *n.* feminización.

femoral *adj.* femoral.

femur *n.* fémur.

fenestra *n.* fenestra, ventana.

fenestration *n.* fenestración.

fermentation *n.* fermentación.

ferritin *n.* ferritina.

ferrule *n.* casquillo, gatillo.

ferrum *n.* ferrum, hierro.

fertile *adj.* fértil.

fertility *n.* fertilidad.

fetal *adj.* fetal.

fetid *adj.* fétido, -da.

fetishism *n.* fetichismo.

fetopathy *n.* fetopatía.

fetoprotein *n.* fetoproteína.

fetoscope *n.* fetoscopio.

fetoscopy *n.* fetoscopia.

fetus *n.* feto.

fever *n.* fiebre.

   Argentine hemorrhagic fever fiebre argentina hemorrágica.

   periodic fever fiebre periódica.

   recurrent fever fiebre recurrente.

   relapsing fever fiebre recidivante.

fibrillation *n.* fibrilación.

fibrin *n.* fibrina.

fibrinogen *n.* fibrinógeno.

fibrinogenesis *n.* fibrinogénesis.

fibrinolysis *n.* fibrinólisis.

fibroblast *n.* fibroblasto.

fibrogenesis *n.* fibrogénesis.

fibroma *n.* fibroma.

   fibroma myxomatodes fibroma mixomatodes, fibroma mixomatoide, fibroma mixomatoso.

fibromatosis *n.* fibromatosis.

fibromatous *adj.* fibromatoso, -sa.

fibromyoma *n.* fibromioma.

fibrosis *n.* fibrosis.

fibula *n.* fíbula, peroné.

field *n.* campo.
  auditory field campo auditivo.
  visual field campo de visión, campo visual.

figure *n.* figura.

filariasis *n.* filariasis, filariosis.

file *n.* lima.
  endodontic file lima endodóntica.

filiation *n.* filiación.

filling *n.* obturación.

film *n.* película.
  dental film película dental.

finger *n.* dedo.
  hammer finger dedo en llave, dedo en martillo, dedo trabado.
  ring finger anular.
  spring finger dedo en resorte.

fingernail *n.* uña.

fingerprint *n.* huella digital.

first-aid kit *n.* botiquín.

fissura *n.* fisura, hendidura.

fissure *n.* cisura, fisura, hendidura.

fistula *n.* fístula.
  blind fistula fístula ciega.
  complete fistula fístula completa.
  external fistula fístula externa.
  internal fistula fístula interna.
  intestinal fistula fístula intestinal.

fistulization *n.* fistulización.

fixation *n.* contención, fijación.

flaccid *adj.* fláccido, -da, flácido, -da.

flange *n.* aleta.
  buccal flange aleta bucal.
  labial flange aleta labial.
  lingual flange aleta lingual.

flap *n.* colgajo.

flare *n.* enrojecimiento.

flatulence *n.* flatulencia.

flatulent *adj.* flatulento, -ta.

flatus *n.* flato.

flavor *n.* sabor.

flex *v.* flexionar.

flexibility *n.* flexibilidad.

flexible *adj.* flexible.

flexion *n.* flexión.

flexura *n.* flexión, flexura.

flexure *n.* flexión.

flicker *n.* destello.

floor *n.* suelo.

flora *n.* flora.
  intestinal flora flora intestinal.

flow *n.* flujo.

flu *n.* gripe.
  avian flu gripe aviar.
  bird flu gripe aviar.
  swine flu gripe A, gripe porcina.

fluctuant *adj.* fluctuante.

fluctuation *n.* fluctuación.

fluid *n.* fluido, líquido.
  amniotic fluid líquido amniótico.
  ascitic fluid líquido ascítico.
  cerebrospinal fluid líquido cefalorraquídeo.
  extravascular fluid líquido extravascular.
  interstitial fluid líquido intersticial.
  intracellular fluid líquido intracelular.
  intraocular fluid líquido intraocular.
  pericardial fluid líquido pericárdico.
  peritoneal fluid líquido peritoneal.
  pleural fluid líquido pleural.
  prostatic fluid líquido prostático.

seminal fluid líquido seminal.
synovial fluid líquido sinovial.
tissue fluid líquido hístico, líquido tisular.
flush *n.* rubor, sofoco.
flutter *n.* aleteo, flúter.
auricular flutter aleteo auricular.
ocular flutter aleteo ocular.
flux *n.* flujo.
menstrual flux flujo menstrual.
focus *n.* foco.
fold *n.* pliegue.
follicle *n.* folículo.
follicular *adj.* folicular.
folliculitis *n.* foliculitis.
fomite *n.* fomite.
fontanel *n.* fontanela.
food *n.* alimento, comida.
dietetic food alimento dietético.
foot *n.* pie.
athlete's foot pie de atleta.
club foot pie zambo.
drop foot pie caído.
flat foot pes planus, pie plano.
foramen *n.* agujero, foramen.
force *n.* fuerza.
vital force fuerza vital.
forceps *n.* fórceps, pinzas.
cup biopsy forceps pinzas para biopsias.
cutting forceps pinzas para cortar.
obstetrical forceps fórceps obstétrico.
forearm *n.* antebrachium, antebrazo.
forehead *n.* frente.
foreign *adj.* extraño, -ña.
forensic *adj.* forense.
forensic scientist forense.
forgetting *n.* olvido.

form *n.* forma.
formation *n.* formación.
fosso *n.* fosa.
fovea *n.* fóvea.
fraction *n.* fracción.
ejection fraction (EF) fracción de eyección (FE), fracción de eyección sistólica.
filtration fraction (FF) fracción de filtración (FF).
systolic ejection fraction fracción de eyección (FE), fracción de eyección sistólica.
fracture *n.* fractura.
fragilitas *n.* fragilidad, fragilitas.
fragility *n.* fragilidad.
fragility of bone fragilidad de los huesos, fragilitas ossium.
fragment *n.* fragmento.
fragmentation *n.* fragmentación.
framework *n.* esqueleto.
frank *adj.* franco, -ca.
freckle *n.* peca.
freeze-drying *n.* congelación-desecación, criodesecación.
freezing *n.* congelación.
fremitus *n.* frémito.
frequency *n.* frecuencia.
fretting *n.* desgaste.
friction *n.* fricción, friega.
fright *n.* susto.
frigid *adj.* frígido, -da.
frigidity *n.* frigidez.
frostbite *n.* congelación.
deep frostbite congelación profunda.
superficial frostbite congelación superficial.
fulminant *adj.* fulminante.

funcigide *n.* fungicida.
function *n.* función.
functional *adj.* funcional.
fundamental *adj.* fundamental.
fundus *n.* fondo, fundus.
 fundus oculi fondo de ojo.
 fundus of the uterus fondo del útero, fondo uterino.
 fundus of the vagina fondo de la vagina.
 fundus uteri fondo del útero, fondo uterino.
 fundus vaginae fondo de la vagina.
fungus *n.* fungus, hongo.
furrow *n.* surco.
furuncle *n.* furúnculo.
furunculosis *n.* furunculosis.
fusiform *adj.* fusiforme.
fusion *n.* fusión.

G

GABAergic *adj.* gabaminérgico, -ca.
gadfly *n.* tábano.
gain *n.* beneficio, ganancia.
 primary gain beneficio primario de la enfermedad, ganancia primaria.
 secondary gain beneficio secundario de la enfermedad, ganancia secundaria.
gait *n.* marcha.
 antalgic gait marcha antálgica.
 ataxic gait marcha atáxica.
 cerebellar gait marcha cerebelosa, marcha oscilante.
 spastic gait marcha espasmódica, marcha espástica.

 Trendelenburg gait marcha de Trendelenburg.
galactorrhea *n.* galactia, galactorrea.
gall *n.* rozadura.
gallop *n.* galope.
 atrial gallop galope auricular.
gallstone *n.* cálculo.
gambling *n.* ludopatía.
gamete *n.* gameto.
gametogenesis *n.* gametogénesis, gametogenia.
gammagraphy *n.* gammagrafía.
gammopathy *n.* gammapatía.
gangliectomy *n.* gangliectomía.
gangliitis *n.* gangliítis, ganglitis.
ganglion *n.* ganglio, ganglión.
ganglionic *adj.* ganglionar.
gangosa *n.* gangosa.
gangrene *n.* gangrena.
 gas gangrene gangrena gaseosa.
 gaseous gangrene gangrena gaseosa.
 progressive gangrene gangrena progresiva.
gap *n.* brecha, intervalo.
 DNA gap brecha de ADN, brecha de DNA.
gargarism *n.* gargarismo.
gargoylysm *n.* gargoilismo, gargolismo.
gas *n.* gas.
 intestinal gas gas intestinal.
gasometry *n.* gasometría.
gastric *adj.* gástrico, -ca.
gastritis *n.* gastritis.
gastroduodenal *adj.* gastroduodenal.
gastroenteritis *n.* gastroenteritis.

gastroplasty *n.* gastroplastia.
gastroxynsis *n.* gastroxinsis.
gauge *n.* calibrador.
gauze *n.* gasa.
gel *n.* gel.
gelatin *n.* gelatina.
gemellary *adj.* gemelar.
geminus *n.* gemelo, -la, gémino, -na.
gender *n.* género.
gene *n.* gen.
  autosomal gene gen autosómico.
  dominant gene gen dominante.
  X-linked gene gen ligado a X.
  Y-linked gene gen ligado a Y.
general *adj.* general.
  general practitioner generalista.
generation *n.* generación.
genesis *n.* génesis.
genetic *adj.* genético, -ca.
geneticist *n.* genetista.
genetics *n.* genética.
  molecular genetics genética molecular.
genital *adj.* genital.
genitalia *n.* genitales, genitalia.
  external genitalia genitales externos.
  internal genitalia genitales internos.
genitals *n.* genitales, genitalia.
genome *n.* genoma.
genomic *adj.* genómico, -ca.
genotype *n.* genotipo.
genu *n.* genu, rodilla.
genus *n.* género, genus.
geode *n.* geoda.
geriatric *adj.* geriátrico, -ca.
geriatrician *n.* geriatra.
geriatrics *n.* geriatría.
germ *n.* germen.
germicidal *adj.* germicida.

germicide *n.* germicida.
gerontal *adj.* geriátrico, -ca, geróntico, -ca.
gerontologist *n.* gerontólogo, -ga.
gerontology *n.* gerontología.
gestagen *n.* gestágeno.
gestagenic *adj.* gestágeno, -na.
gestation *n.* gestación.
gestational *adj.* gestacional.
giant *n.* gigante.
giddiness *n.* mareo, vahído.
gigantism *n.* gigantismo.
ginger *adj.* pelirrojo, -ja, taheño, -ña, tajeño, -ña.
gingiva *n.* encía, gingiva.
gingival *adj.* gingival.
gingivitis *n.* gingivitis.
girdle *n.* cintura.
  shoulder girdle cintura escapular.
  thoracic girdle cintura torácica.
glabella *n.* glabela.
glabellum *n.* glabela.
gland *n.* glándula.
  apocrine gland glándula apocrina.
  eccrine gland glándula ecrina.
  exocrine gland glándula abierta, glándula anacrina, glándula de secreción externa, glándula exocrina.
  heterocrine gland glándula heterocrina.
  holocrine gland glándula holocrina.
  lacrimal gland glándula lagrimal.
  lactiferous gland glándula mamaria.
  mammary gland glándula mamaria.
  milk gland glándula mamaria.
  parotid gland glándula parótida.
  pituitary gland glándula pituitaria.

prostate gland glándula prostática.

salivary gland glándula salival.

sexual gland glándula sexual.

sudoriferous gland glándula sudorípara.

sudoriparous gland glándula sudorípara.

sweat gland glándula sudorípara.

glanders *n.* muermo.

glandula *n.* glándula.

glandula lacrimalis glándula lagrimal.

glandula mammaria glándula mamaria.

glandula parotidea glándula parótida.

glandula parotis glándula parótida.

glandula prostatica glándula prostática.

glandular *adj.* glandular.

glans *n.* glande, glans.

glass *n.* cristal, vidrio.

glasses *n.* gafas.

bifocal glasses gafas bifocales.

Franklin glasses gafas bifocales.

glaucoma *n.* glaucoma.

angle-closure glaucoma glaucoma de ángulo cerrado.

chronic glaucoma glaucoma crónico.

congenital glaucoma glaucoma congénito.

malignant glaucoma glaucoma maligno.

open-angle glaucoma glaucoma de ángulo abierto.

glia *n.* glía.

glioma *n.* glioma.

gliosis *n.* gliosis.

globule *n.* glóbulo.

globulin *n.* globulina.

serum globulin globulina séricas.

varicella-zoster immune globulin (VZIG) globulina inmune contra la varicela zóster, globulina inmunitaria contra la varicela zóster.

globulinemia *n.* globulinemia.

globus *n.* globo, globus.

globus of the eye globo del ojo, globo ocular.

glomerular *adj.* glomerular.

glomerule *n.* glomérulo.

glomerulitis *n.* glomerulitis.

glomerulonephritis *n.* glomerulonefritis.

glomerulonephropathy *n.* glomerulonefropatía.

glomerulopathy *n.* glomerulopatía.

glomerulus *n.* glomérulo.

glomus *n.* glomo, glomus.

glossitis *n.* glosistis.

glottic *adj.* glótico, -ca.

glottis *n.* glotis.

glucagon *n.* glucagón.

glucagonoma *n.* glucagonoma.

glucide *n.* glúcido.

glucogen *n.* glucógeno.

glucolysis *n.* glucólisis.

glucose *n.* glucosa.

glucosuria *n.* glucosuria.

gluteal *adj.* glúteo, -a.

gluten *n.* gluten.

glycemia *n.* glicemia, glucemia.

glycerin *n.* glicerina.

glycerinum *n.* glicerina, glicerinum.

glycerol *n.* glicerol.

glycogenosis *n.* glucogenosis.

glycoprotein *n.* glicoproteína, glucoproteína.

glycosuria *n.* glucosuria.

glykemia *n.* glicemia, glucemia.

gnosia *n.* gnosia.

goal *n.* meta.

goiter *n.* bocio.
  acute goiter bocio agudo.
  Basedow's goiter bocio de Basedow.
  colloid goiter bocio coloidal, bocio coloide.
  congenital goiter bocio congénito.
  diffuse goiter bocio difuso.
  ectopic goiter bocio ectópico.
  endemic goiter bocio endémico.
  exophthalmic goiter bocio exoftálmico.
  familial goiter bocio familiar.
  follicular goiter bocio folicular.
  intrathoracic goiter bocio intratorácico.
  iodide goiter bocio por yoduro.
  lingual goiter bocio lingual.
  multinodular goiter bocio multinodular.
  nodular goiter bocio nodular.
  non-toxic goiter bocio no tóxico.
  simple goiter bocio simple.
  thoracic goiter bocio torácico.
  toxic goiter bocio tóxico.
  toxic multinodular goiter bocio multinodular tóxico.
  toxic nodular goiter bocio nodular tóxico.
  vascular goiter bocio vascular.

gold *n.* oro.

gonad *n.* gónada.

gonadectomy *n.* gonadectomía.

gonarthritis *n.* gonartritis.

gonarthrosis *n.* gonartrosis.

gonorrhea *n.* gonorrea.

gout *n.* gota.
  articular gout gota articular.
  tophaceous gout gota tofácea.

grade *n.* grado.
  Gleason's tumor grade grado tumoral de Gleason.

gradient *n.* gradiente.

graduated *adj.* graduado, -da.

graft *n.* injertar, injerto.
  autogenous graft injerto autógeno.
  autologous graft injerto autólogo.
  cadaver graft injerto de cadáver.
  corneal graft injerto corneal.
  heterologous graft injerto heterólogo.
  homologous graft injerto homólogo.
  skin graft injerto cutáneo, injerto de piel.

grain *n.* grano.

granular *adj.* granular.

granulatio *n.* granulación.

granulation *n.* granulación.

granule *n.* gránulo.

granulocyte *n.* granulocito.
  band form granulocyte granulocito en banda.
  immature granulocyte granulocito inmaduro.
  segmented granulocyte granulocito segmentado.

granulocytic *adj.* granulocitario, -ria, granulocítico, -ca.

granulocytosis *n.* granulocitosis.

granuloma *n.* granuloma.

granulomatous *adj.* granulomatoso.

granum *n.* grano, granum.

graph *n.* gráfica, gráfico.

grave *adj.* grave.

gravid *n.* grávida.

gravida *n.* grávida.

graviditas *n.* gravidez, graviditas.

gravidity *n.* gravidez.

gravis *adj.* grave.

gravity *n.* gravedad.

green *adj.* verde.

grief *n.* aflicción, duelo, pena.

grinding *n.* abrasio, abrasión, desgaste, lijado, trituración.

gripe *n.* retortijón.

grippal *adj.* gripal.

grippe *n.* gripe.

groin *n.* ingle.

groove *n.* corredera, surco.

group *n.* grupo.
  control group grupo de control.
  therapeutic group grupo terapéutico.

grouping *n.* agrupamiento.
  blood grouping agrupamiento sanguíneo.

growth *n.* crecimiento.
  absolute growth crecimiento absoluto.
  catch-up growth crecimiento compensador.
  condylar growth crecimiento condíleo.
  differential growth crecimiento diferencial.
  intrauterine retarded growth crecimiento intrauterino retardado.
  new growth crecimiento nuevo.
  relative growth crecimiento relativo.

grunting *n.* quejido.

guanidine *n.* guanidina.

guidance *n.* guía.

guide *n.* guía.

guideline *n.* guía.

gum *n.* encía, goma.

gustatory *adj.* gustativo, -va.

gut *n.* intestino, intestinum.
  blind gut intestino ciego.

gutta *n.* gota, gutta.

gymnastics *n.* gimnasia.

gynecologic *adj.* ginecológico, -ca.

gynecological *adj.* ginecológico, -ca.

gynecologist *n.* ginecólogo, -ga.

gynecology *n.* ginecología.

gynecomania *n.* ginecomanía.

gypsum *n.* yeso.

H

habit *n.* hábito, rutina.

haemorrhagia *n.* hemorragia.

hair *n.* cabello, capillus, pelo, vello.
  ingrown hair pelo encarnado, pelo invaginado.
  pubic hair vello pubiano, vello púbico.

hairy *adj.* peludo, -da.

half-caste *adj.* mestizo, -za.

half-life *n.* semidesintegración, semivida.

halitosis *n.* halitosis.

hallucination *n.* alucinación.
  alcoholic hallucination alucinación alcohólica.
  auditory hallucination alucinación auditiva.

olfactory hallucination alucinación olfatoria.

somatic hallucination alucinación somática.

tactile hallucination alucinación táctil.

visual hallucination alucinación visual.

hallucinogen *n.* alucinógeno.

hallucinosis *n.* alucinosis.

halo *n.* halo.

hand *n.* mano.

accoucheur's hand mano de comadrón, mano de partero.

claw hand mano en garra.

club hand mano zamba.

crab hand mano de cangrejo.

dead hand mano muerta.

drop hand mano caída, mano péndula.

frozen hand mano congelada.

obstetrical hand mano obstétrica.

skeleton hand mano de esqueleto, mano esquelética.

writing hand mano de escritor.

handicap *n.* impedimento.

mental handicap minusvalía mental.

handicapped *adj.* inválido, -da, minusválido, -da.

handle *n.* mango.

hangnail *n.* padrastro.

hapten *n.* hapteno.

haptene *n.* hapteno.

hardening *n.* endurecimiento.

hardness *n.* dureza.

head *n.* cabeza.

medusa head cabeza de medusa.

headache *n.* cefalea.

cluster headache cefalea acuminada, cefalea en grupo.

Horton's headache cefalea de Horton.

migraine headache cefalea migrañosa.

tension headache cefalea tensional.

tension-type headache cefalea tensional.

healing *n.* curación.

healing by first intention curación por primera intención.

healing by second intention curación por segunda intención.

healing by third intention curación por tercera intención.

health *n.* salud, sanitas.

community mental health salud mental comunitaria.

environmental health salud medioambiental.

family health salud familiar.

industrial health salud laboral.

mental health salud mental.

occupational health salud profesional.

sexual health salud sexual.

healthy *adj.* sano, -na.

hear *v.* oír.

hearing aid *n.* audífono.

heart *n.* cor, corazón.

artificial heart corazón artificial.

athlete's heart corazón atlético, corazón de atleta.

athletic heart corazón atlético, corazón de atleta.

fat heart corazón adiposo, corazón graso.

fatty heart corazón adiposo, corazón graso.

frosted heart corazón congelado, corazón recubierto.

hanging heart corazón colgante.

horizontal heart corazón horizontal.

hypoplastic heart corazón hipoplásico.

left heart corazón izquierdo.

movable heart corazón móvil.

pulmonary heart corazón pulmonar.

right heart corazón derecho.

sabot heart corazón en zueco.

suspended heart corazón suspendido.

systemic heart corazón sistémico.

three-chambered heart cor triloculare, corazón de tres cavidades.

venous heart corazón venoso.

vertical heart corazón vertical.

wandering heart corazón errante.

heat *n.* calor.

heel *n.* talón, tacón.

anterior heel talón anterior.

painful heel talón doloroso.

height *n.* altura, estatura, talla.

helminth *n.* helminto.

hemachromatosis *n.* hemacromatosis, hemocromatosis.

hemagglutination *n.* hemaglutinación.

hemangioma *n.* hemangioma.

hemapoiesis *n.* hemapoyesis.

hemapoietic *adj.* hemapoyético, -ca.

hematemesis *n.* hematemesis.

hematic *adj.* hemático, -ca.

hematin *n.* hematina, hemocroína.

hematocrit *n.* hematocrito.

hematocyte *n.* hematocito.

hematokrit *n.* hematocrito.

hematoma *n.* hematoma.

intracranial hematoma hematoma intracraneal.

hematopoiesis *n.* hematopoyesis.

hematopoietic *adj.* hematopoyético.

hematuria *n.* hematuria.

macroscopic hematuria hematuria macroscópica.

microscopic hematuria hematuria microscópica.

renal hematuria hematuria renal.

hemianopia *n.* hemianopía, hemianopsia.

hemianopsia *n.* hemianopía, hemianopsia, hemianopsis.

hemiartrhosis *n.* hemiartrosis.

hemicranial *adj.* hemicraneal.

hemiglobin *n.* hemiglobina, hemoglobina.

hemiplegia *n.* hemiplejía.

hemiplegic *adj.* hemipléjico, -ca.

hemispherium *n.* hemisferio.

hemochromatosis *n.* hemocromatosis.

hemodialysis *n.* hemodiálisis.

home hemodialysis hemodiálisis domiciliaria.

hospital hemodialysis hemodiálisis hospitalaria.

hemodialyzer *n.* hemodializador.

hemodynamics *n.* hemodinámica.

hemoglobin *n.* hemoglobina.

hemoglobinemia *n.* hemoglobinemia.

hemoglobinuria *n.* hemoglobinuria.

hemogram *n.* hemograma.

hemolysis *n.* hemólisis.
hemolytic *adj.* hemolítico, -ca.
hemophilia *n.* hemofilia.
hemophiliac *n.* hemofílico.
hemophilic *adj.* hemofílico, -ca.
hemoptysis *n.* hemoptisis.
hemorrhage *n.* hemorragia.
  cerebral hemorrhage hemorragia cerebral.
  dysfunctional uterine hemorrhage (DUB) hemorragia uterina disfuncional (HUD).
  internal hemorrhage hemorragia interna.
  intestinal hemorrhage hemorragia intestinal.
  intracerebral hemorrhage hemorragia intracerebral.
  intracranial hemorrhage hemorragia intracraneal.
  massive hemorrhage hemorragia masiva.
  nasal hemorrhage hemorragia nasal.
  postpartum hemorrhage hemorragia posparto.
  recurring hemorrhage hemorragia recidivante, hemorragia recurrente.
  uterine hemorrhage hemorragia uterina.
  vaginal hemorrhage hemorragia vaginal.
hemorrhagic *adj.* hemorrágico, -ca.
hemorrhoids *n.* hemorroides.
hemosiderosis *n.* hemosiderosis.
hemostasia *n.* hemostasia, hemostasis.
hemostasis *n.* hemostasis.
hemostatic *adj.* hematostático, -ca, hemostático, -ca.

hepar *n.* hígado.
heparin *n.* heparina.
  heparin calcium heparina cálcica.
  heparin sodium heparina sódica.
heparinization *n.* heparinización.
heparinize *v.* heparinizar.
hepatic *adj.* hepático, -ca.
hepatitic *adj.* hepatítico, -ca.
hepatitis *n.* hepatitis.
hepatobiliary *adj.* hepatobiliar.
hepatocyte *n.* hepatocito.
hepatoma *n.* hepatoma, hepatonco.
hepatomegalia *n.* hepatomegalia.
hepatomegaly *n.* hepatomegalia.
hepatopathy *n.* hepatopatía.
hepatosplenomegaly *n.* hepatoesplenomegalia, hepatosplenomegalia.
hepatotoxicity *n.* hepatotoxicidad.
hereditary *adj.* hereditario, -ria.
heredity *n.* herencia.
  autosomal heredity herencia autosómica.
  recessive heredity herencia recesiva.
  sex-linked heredity herencia ligada al sexo.
  X-linked heredity herencia ligada al cromosoma X.
  Y-linked heredity herencia ligada al cromosoma Y.
heritability *n.* heredabilidad, herencia.
hermaphrodite *n.* hermafrodita.
hermaphroditism *n.* hermafroditismo.
hernia *n.* hernia.
  abdominal hernia hernia abdominal.
  diaphragmatic hernia hernia diafragmática.

incomplete hernia hernia incompleta.

inguinal hernia hernia inguinal.

strangulated hernia hernia estrangulada.

herniated *adj.* herniado, -da.

herniation *n.* herniación.

cerebral herniation herniación cerebral.

herniation of the intervetebral disk herniación de disco intervetebral.

herpes *n.* herpes.

genital herpes herpes genital.

herpes genitalis herpes genital.

herpes gestationis herpes gestacional, herpes gravídico.

herpes recurrens herpes recurrente.

herpes simplex herpes simple.

herpes zoster herpes zoster.

recurrent herpes herpes recurrente.

relapsing herpes herpes recidivante.

herpetic *adj.* herpético, -ca.

herpetiform *adj.* herpetiforme.

heterogeneity *n.* heterogeneidad, heterogenicidad.

genetic heterogeneity heterogeneidad genética.

heterogeneous *adj.* heterogéneo, -a.

heterogenous *adj.* heterogéneo, -a, heterogénico, -ca, heterógeno, -na.

heterosexual *adj.* heterosexual.

heterosexuality *n.* heterosexualidad.

heterozygote *n.* heterocigoto, heterozigoto.

hiatus *n.* hiato.

hiccough *n.* hipo.

hiccup *n.* hipo.

hidradenitis *n.* hidradenitis.

hip *n.* cadera.

hippocampus *n.* hipocampo, hippocampus.

hirsutism *n.* hirsutismo.

histamine *n.* histamina.

histic *adj.* hístico, -ca.

histiocytosis *n.* histiocitosis.

histochemistry *n.* histoquímica.

histocompatibility *n.* histocompatibilidad.

histocompatible *adj.* histocompatible.

histocytosis *n.* histiocitosis, histocitosis.

histology *n.* histología.

normal histology histología normal.

pathologic histology histología patológica.

histoplasmosis *n.* histoplasmosis.

history *n.* antecedentes, historia.

case history historia personal y familiar.

clinical history historia clínica.

family history historia familiar.

health history historia clínica.

personal and social history antecedentes personales y sociales.

hive *n.* habón.

hoarse *adj.* ronco, -ca.

hoarseness *n.* ronquera.

holder *n.* soporte.

homeopath *n.* homeópata.

homeopathic *adj.* homeopático, -ca.

homeopathist *n.* homeópata.

homeopathy *n.* homeopatía.

homeostasis *n.* homeostasia, homeostasis.
homicide *n.* homicidio.
homocystinemia *n.* homocistinemia.
homocystinuria *n.* homocistinuria.
homogenicity *n.* homogenicidad.
homonymous *adj.* homónimo, -ma.
homosexual *adj.* homosexual.
homosexuality *n.* homosexualidad.
homozygosis *n.* homocigosis.
homozygosity *n.* homocigosidad.
homozygote *adj.* homocigoto, -ta, homozigoto.
honey *n.* miel.
hordeolum *n.* orzuelo.
  hordeolum externum orzuelo externo.
  hordeolum internum orzuelo interno.
hormonal *adj.* hormonal.
hormone *n.* hormona.
horn *n.* cuerno.
horsefly *n.* tábano.
hospital *n.* hospital.
  general hospital hospital general.
  geriatric day care hospital hospital geriátrico de día.
  maternity hospital hospital de maternidad, hospital materno.
  mental hospital manicomio.
  psychiatric hospital hospital psiquiátrico.
hospitalization *n.* hospitalización.
host *n.* hospedador, huésped.
hum *n.* zumbido.
  venous hum zumbido venoso.
humectant *adj.* humectante.
humerus *n.* húmero.

humidifier *n.* humidificador.
humidity *n.* humedad.
humor *n.* humor.
  humor vitreus humor vítreo.
  vitreous humor humor vítreo.
humoral *adj.* humoral.
hump *n.* giba, joroba.
humpback *n.* corcova, gibosidad, joroba.
hunger *n.* hambre.
hyaline *adj.* hialino, -na.
hybrid *n.* híbrido, -da.
hybridization *n.* hibridación.
hydrated *adj.* hidratado, -da.
hydration *n.* hidratación.
hydrocele *n.* hidrocele.
hydrocephalia *n.* hidrocefalia.
  congenital hydrocephalia hidrocefalia congénita.
  external hydrocephalia hidrocefalia externa.
  internal hydrocephalia hidrocefalia interna.
  normal-pressure hydrocephalia hidrocefalia normotensa.
  obstructive hydrocephalia hidrocefalia obstructiva.
hydroma *n.* hidroma, higroma.
hydronephrosis *n.* hidronefrosis.
hydrophobia *n.* fobodipsia, hidrofobia.
hydrops *n.* hidropepsía, hidropesia.
hydrosoluble *adj.* hidrosoluble.
hydrotherapeutics *n.* hidroterapia.
hydrotherapy *n.* hidroterapia.
hydrous *adj.* hidratado, -da, hidroso, -sa.
hygiene *n.* higiene.
  dental hygiene higiene dental.

hygienic *adj.* higiénico, -ca.

hygroma *n.* higroma.

hymen *n.* himen.

  hymen septate himen tabicado.

  imperforated hymen himen imperforado.

hymenal *adj.* himenal.

hyoid *adj.* hioide, hioideo, -a, hioides.

hypacusia *n.* hipacusia, hipoacusia, hipoacusis.

hypacusis *n.* hipacusis, hipoacusia, hipoacusis.

hypalbuminemia *n.* hipalbuminemia, hipoalbuminemia.

hyperactive *adj.* hiperactivo, -va.

hyperactivity *n.* hiperactividad.

hyperalgesia *n.* hiperalgesia.

hyperazotemia *n.* hiperazoemia.

hyperbaric *adj.* hiperbárico, -ca.

hyperbetalipoproteinemia *n.* hiperbetalipoproteinemia.

hyperbilirubinemia *n.* hiperbilirrubinemia.

  neonatal hyperbilirubinemia hiperbilirrubinemia neonatal.

hypercalcemia *n.* hipercalcemia.

hypercalciuria *n.* hipercalciuria.

hypercellularity *n.* hipercelularidad.

hyperchloremia *n.* hipercloremia.

hyperchlorhydria *n.* hiperclorhidria.

hypercholesterolemia *n.* hipercolesterolemia.

  familial hypercholesterolemia hipercolesterolemia familiar.

hypercholesterolemic *adj.* hipercolesterolémico, -ca.

hyperchylomicronemia *n.* hiperquilomicronemia.

hypercoagulability *n.* hipercoagulabilidad.

hypercorticism *n.* hipercorticismo.

hyperechogenicity *n.* hiperecogenicidad.

hyperemesis *n.* hiperemesis.

  hyperemesis gravidarum hiperemesis del embarazo, hiperemesis gravídica.

hyperemia *n.* hiperemia.

hyperesthesia *n.* hiperestesia.

hyperextension *n.* hiperextensión.

hyperflexion *n.* hiperflexión.

hyperfunction *n.* hiperfunción.

hypergammaglobulinemia *n.* hipergammaglobulinemia.

  monoclonal hypergammaglobulinemia hipergammaglobulinemia monoclonal.

hyperglycemia *n.* hiperglicemia, hiperglucemia.

hypergonadism *n.* hipergonadismo.

hyperhidrosis *n.* hiperhidrosis, hiperidrosis.

hyperinsulinism *n.* hiperinsulinismo.

hyperkalemia *n.* hipercaliemia.

hyperkaliemia *n.* hipercaliemia.

hyperkeratinization *n.* hiperqueratinización.

hyperkeratosis *n.* hiperqueratosis.

hyperkinesia *n.* hipercinesia, hiperquinesia.

hyperkinesis *n.* hipercinesia, hipercinesis.

hyperlaxicity *n.* hiperlaxitud.

hyperlipemia *n.* hiperlipemia.

hyperlipidemia *n.* hiperlipidemia.

hyperlipoidemia *n.* hiperlipidemia, hiperlipoidemia.

hyperlipoproteinemia *n.* hiperlipoproteinemia.

hypermenorrhea *n.* hipermenorrea.

hypermetrope *n.* hipermétrope.

hypermetropia *n.* hipermetropía.

hypermetropy *n.* hipermetropía.

hypermotility *n.* hipermotilidad.

hypernatremia *n.* hipernatremia.

hyperostosis *n.* hiperostosis.

hyperparathyroidism *n.* hiperparatiroidismo.

hyperphosphatemia *n.* hiperfosfatemia.

hyperphosphaturia *n.* hiperfosfaturia.

hyperpigmentation *n.* hiperpigmentación.

hyperplasia *n.* hiperplasia.

  benign prostatic hyperplasia hiperplasia prostática benigna (HBP).

  cystic hyperplasia of the breast hiperplasia quística de la mama.

hyperptyalism *n.* hiperptialismo.

hyperreactive *adj.* hiperreactivo, -va.

hyperreactivity *n.* hiperreactividad.

  bronchial hyperreactivity hiperreactividad bronquial.

hyperreflexia *n.* hiperreflexia.

hypersalivation *n.* hipersalivación.

hypersecretion *n.* hipersecreción.

hypersensitivity *n.* hipersensibilidad.

  contact hypersensitivity hipersensibilidad por contacto.

  delayed hypersensitivity (DH) de tipo retardado (HTR), hipersensibilidad retardada (HR).

  delayed-type hypersensitivity (DTH) de tipo retardado (HTR), hipersensibilidad retardada (HR).

  immediate hypersensitivity hipersensibilidad inmediata.

  immune complex hypersensitivity hipersensibilidad por inmunocomplejos.

  tuberculin-type hypersensitivity hipersensibilidad tipo tuberculina.

hypersensitization *n.* hipersensibilización.

hypersomnolence *n.* hipersomnolencia.

hypersystole *n.* hipersístole, hipersistolia.

hypertelorism *n.* hipertelorismo.

hypertension *n.* hipertensión.

  adrenal hypertension hipertensión suprarrenal.

  arterial hypertension hipertensión arterial.

  essential hypertension hipertensión esencial.

  essential arterial hypertension hipertensión arterial esencial.

  idiopathic hypertension hipertensión idiopática.

  intracranial hypertension hipertensión intracraneal.

  malignant hypertension hipertensión maligna.

  ocular hypertension hipertensión ocular.

  pulmonary hypertension hipertensión pulmonar.

pulmonary arterial hypertension hipertensión arterial pulmonar.

renal hypertension hipertensión renal.

secondary hypertension hipertensión secundaria.

secondary arterial hypertension hipertensión arterial secundaria.

symptomatic hypertension hipertensión sintomática.

systemic arterial hypertension hipertensión arterial sistémica.

vascular hypertension hipertensión vascular.

white coat arterial hypertension hipertensión arterial de bata blanca.

hypertensive *adj.* hipertensivo, -va, hipertenso, -sa.

hypertensor *adj.* hipertensor, -ra.

hyperthermia *n.* hipertermia.

hyperthyroid *adj.* hipertiroide, hipertiroideo, -a.

hyperthyroidism *n.* hipertiroidismo.

ophthalmic hyperthyroidism hipertiroidismo oftálmico.

primary hyperthyroidism hipertiroidismo primario.

secondary hyperthyroidism hipertiroidismo secundario.

hypertonia *n.* hipertonía.

hypertonic *adj.* hipertónico, -ca.

hypertonicity *n.* hipertonicidad.

hypertrichosis *n.* hipertricosis.

hypertrophic *adj.* hipertrófico, -ca.

hypertrophy *n.* hipertrofia.

prostatic hypertrophy hipertrofia prostática.

ventricular hypertrophy hipertrofia ventricular.

hypertryglyceridemia *n.* hipertrigliceridemia.

hyperuricemia *n.* hiperuricemia.

hyperventilation *n.* hiperventilación.

hypervitaminosis *n.* hipervitaminosis.

hypervolemia *n.* hipervolemia.

hypervolemic *adj.* hipervolémico, -ca.

hypnosis *n.* hipnosis.

hypnotic *adj.* hipnótico, -ca.

hypoactivity *n.* hipoactividad.

hypoacusia *n.* hipoacusia, hipoacusis.

hypoacusis *n.* hipoacusia, hipoacusis.

hypoalbuminemia *n.* hipoalbuminemia.

hypoaldosteronemia *n.* hipoaldosteronemia.

hypoaldosteronism *n.* hipoaldosteronismo.

hypoallergenic *adj.* hipoalérgenico, -ca.

hypocalciuria *n.* hipocalciuria.

hypocellular *adj.* hipocelular.

hypochondria *n.* hipocondría.

hypochondriac *n.* hipocondríaco, -ca.

hypochondriacal *adj.* hipocondríaco, -ca.

hypocorticoidism *n.* hipocorticoismo.

hypodinamia *n.* hipodinamia.

hypoechogenic *adj.* hipoecogénico, -ca.

hypoechogenicity *n.* hipoecogenicidad.

hypoestrogenism *n.* hipoestrogenismo.

hypofunction *n.* hipofunción, hipofuncionamiento.

hypogammaglobulinemia *n.* hipogammaglobulinemia.

  physiologic hypogammaglobulinemia hipogammaglobulinemia fisiológica.

  X-linked infantile hypogammaglobulinemia hipogammaglobulinemia infantil ligada a X, hipogammaglobulinemia ligada a X.

hypogastric *adj.* hipogástrico, -ca.

hypogastrium *n.* hipogastrio.

hypoglycemia *n.* hipoglucemia.

  fasting hypoglycemia hipoglucemia en ayunas.

  ketotic hypoglycemia hipoglucemia cetósica.

hypoglycemic *adj.* hipoglucémico, -ca.

hypogonadism *n.* hipogonadismo.

hypokalemia *n.* hipocalemia, hipocaliemia.

hypokaliemia *n.* hipocaliemia.

hypomania *n.* hipomanía.

hypomaniac *n.* hipomaníaco, -ca.

hyponatremia *n.* hiponatremia.

hypoparathyroidism *n.* hipoparatiroidia, hipoparatiroidismo.

  familial hypoparathyroidism hipoparatiroidismo familiar.

hypoperfusion *n.* hipoperfusión.

hypopharyngeal *adj.* hipofaríngeo, -a.

hypopharynx *n.* hipofaringe.

hypophosphatemia *n.* hipofosfatemia.

hypophosphaturia *n.* hipofosfaturia.

hypopituitarism *n.* hipopituitarismo.

hypoplasia *n.* hipoplasia.

hypoplasty *n.* hipoplasia.

hypoprolactinemia *n.* hipoprolactinemia.

hypoproteinemia *n.* hipoproteinemia.

hyposecretion *n.* hiposecreción.

hyposensitivity *n.* hiposensibilidad.

hyposensitization *n.* hiposensibilización.

hypospadias *n.* hipospadia, hipospadias.

hypotension *n.* hipotensión.

  arterial hypotension hipotensión arterial.

  chronic idiopathic orthostatic hypotension hipotensión ortostática crónica, hipotensión ortostática idiopática crónica.

  chronic orthostatic hypotension hipotensión ortostática crónica, hipotensión ortostática idiopática crónica.

  postural hypotension hipotensión postural.

hypotensive *adj.* hipotensivo, -va, hipotenso, -sa.

hypotensor *adj.* hipotensor, -ra.

hypothalamus *n.* hipotálamo.

hypothenar *n.* hipotenar.

hypothesis *n.* hipótesis.

hypothyroid *adj.* hipotiroideo, -a.

hypothyroidism *n.* hipotiroidía, hipotiroidismo.

hypotonic *adj.* hipotónico, -ca.

hypotony *n.* hipotonía.

hypovolemia *n.* hipovolemia.
hypovolemic *adj.* hipovolémico, -ca.
hypoxemia *n.* hipoxemia.
hypoxia *n.* hipoxia.
hypoxic *adj.* hipóxico, -ca.
hysterectomy *n.* histerectomía, metrostéresis.
hysteria *n.* histeria.
hysteric *adj.* histérico, -ca.
hysterical *adj.* histérico, -ca.
hysterosalpingography *n.* histerosalpingografía.
hysteroscope *n.* histeroscopio.
hysteroscopy *n.* histeroscopia.

I

iatrogenesis *n.* yatrogénesis.
iatrogenia *n.* iatrogenia.
iatrogenic *adj.* iatrogénico, -ca, iatrógeno, -na, yatrogénico, -ca, yatrógeno, -na.
iatrogeny *n.* yatrogenia.
ichthyosis *n.* ictiosis.
icteric *adj.* ictérico, -ca.
icterus *n.* ictericia, icterus.
 congenital hemolytic icterus ictericia hemolítica congénita, icterus hemolítico congénito.
 icterus neonatorum ictericia del neonato, ictericia neonatal, icterus neonatal.
ictus *n.* ictus.
idiocy *n.* idiocia, idiotez.
idiopathic *adj.* idiopático, -ca.
idiot *n.* idiota.
ileal *adj.* ileal.

ileectomy *n.* ileectomía.
ileitis *n.* ileítis.
ileostomate *adj.* ileostomizado, -da.
ileostomy *n.* ileostomía.
 urinary ileostomy ileostomía urinaria.
ileum *n.* íleon.
ileus *n.* íleo, íleus.
iliac *adj.* ilíaco, -ca.
ill *adj.* enfermo, -ma.
illness *n.* enfermedad.
 mental illness enfermedad mental.
image *n.* imagen.
 body image imagen corporal.
 visual image imagen visual.
imagination *n.* imaginación.
imbalance *n.* desequilibrio, imbalance.
imbalanced *adj.* desequilibrado, -da.
immature *adj.* inmaduro, -ra.
immaturity *n.* inmadurez.
immediate *adj.* inmediato, -ta.
immobility *n.* inmovilidad.
immobilization *n.* inmovilización.
immobilize *v.* inmovilizar.
immune *adj.* inmune.
immunity *n.* inmunidad.
 acquired immunity inmunidad adquirida.
 active immunity inmunidad activa.
 adoptive immunity inmunidad adoptiva.
 cell-mediated immunity (CMI) inmunidad de mediación celular, inmunidad mediada por células (IMC), inmunidad mediada por células T (IMCT).
 cellular immunity inmunidad celular.

cross immunity inmunidad cruzada.

familial immunity inmunidad familiar.

humoral immunity inmunidad humoral.

inherited immunity inmunidad hereditaria.

maternal immunity inmunidad materna.

non-specific immunity inmunidad inespecífica.

T cell-mediated immunity (TCMI) inmunidad de mediación celular, inmunidad mediada por células (IMC), inmunidad mediada por células T (IMCT).

immunization *n.* inmunización.

active immunization inmunización activa.

passive immunization inmunización pasiva.

immunize *v.* inmunizar.

immunoassay *n.* inmunoanálisis, inmunoensayo, inmunovaloración.

immunocompetence *n.* inmunocompetencia, inmunosuficiencia.

immunocompetent *adj.* inmunocompetente, inmunosuficiente.

immunocomplex *n.* inmunocomplejo.

immunocompromised *adj.* inmunocomprometido, -da.

immunodeficiency *n.* inmunodeficiencia.

immunodeficient *adj.* inmunodeficiente.

immunodepression *n.* inmunodepresión.

immunofluorescence *n.* inmunofluorescencia.

immunoglobulin *n.* inmunoglobulina.

immunohistochemistry *n.* inmunohistoquímica.

immunologic *adj.* inmunológico, -ca.

immunological *adj.* inmunológico, -ca.

immunologist *n.* inmunólogo, -ga.

immunology *n.* inmunología.

immunoperoxidase *n.* inmunoperoxidasa.

immunoproliferative *adj.* inmunoproliferativo, -va.

immunostimulant *adj.* inmunoestimulante.

immunosuppresant *n.* inmunosupresor.

immunosuppression *n.* inmunosupresión.

immunotherapy *n.* inmunoterapia.

impact *n.* impacto.

impaction *n.* impacción.

impairment *n.* deterioro.

mental impairment deterioro mental.

impermeability *n.* impermeabilidad.

impetigo *n.* impétigo.

implant *n.* implante.

dental implant implante dental.

impotence *n.* impotencia, impotentia.

impotency *n.* impotencia, impotentia.

impotentia *n.* impotencia, impotentia.

impulsiveness *n.* impulsividad.

impulsivity *n.* impulsividad.
inactivation *n.* inactivación.
inanition *n.* inanición.
inappetence *n.* inapetencia.
incision *n.* incisión.
incisive *adj.* incisivo, -va.
inclinatio *n.* inclinación.
inclination *n.* inclinación.
incline *n.* inclinación.
inclusion *n.* inclusión.
incompatibility *n.* incompatibilidad.
  Rh incompatibility incompatibilidad Rh.
incompatible *adj.* incompatible.
incompetence *n.* incompetencia.
incompetency *n.* incompetencia.
incompetent *adj.* incompetente.
incontinence *n.* incontinencia.
  anal incontinence incontinencia anal.
  fecal incontinence incontinencia fecal.
  incontinence of urine incontinencia urinaria.
  urinary incontinence incontinencia urinaria.
incontinentia *n.* incontinencia, incontinentia.
  incontinentia urinae incontinencia urinaria.
increment *n.* incremento.
incus *n.* incus, yunque.
index *n.* índice.
  saturation index índice de saturación.
indicatio *n.* indicación.
indication *n.* indicación.
indicator *n.* indicador, -ra.

indifference *n.* indiferencia.
indigestion *n.* indigestión.
indirect *adj.* indirecto, -ta.
indolent *adj.* indolente, indoloro, -ra.
induced *adj.* inducido, -da.
induction *n.* inducción.
induration *n.* induración.
inebriation *n.* embriaguez, inebriación.
inertia *n.* inercia.
infancy *n.* infancia, lactancia.
infant *n.* lactante.
infanticide *n.* infanticida, infanticidio.
infantile *adj.* infantil.
infantilism *n.* infantilismo.
infarct *n.* infarto.
infarction *n.* infarto.
  cardiac infarction infarto cardíaco.
  cerebral infarction infarto cerebral.
  intestinal infarction infarto intestinal.
  mesenteric infarction infarto mesentérico.
  myocardial infarction (MI) infarto del miocardio (IM).
infect *v.* infectar.
infection *n.* infección.
  airborne infection infección aérea, infección transmitida por el aire.
  cross infection infección cruzada.
  droplet infection infección por gotillas, infección transmitida por gotitas.
  hospital-acquired infection infección adquirida en el hospital.
  iatrogenic infection infección iatrogénica, infección yatrogénica.

nosocomial infection infección nosocomial.

opportunistic infection infección oportunista.

systemic infection infección sistémica.

urinary infection infección urinaria.

vector-borne infection infección transmitida por un vector.

viral infection infección vírica, viriasis.

water-borne infection infección transmitida por agua.

infectious *adj.* infeccioso, -sa.

inferior *adj.* inferior.

infertility *n.* infertilidad.

infiltration *n.* infiltración.

infirm *adj.* enfermizo, -za, infirme.

infirmity *n.* achaque, dolencia.

inflammation *n.* inflamación.

inflammatory *adj.* inflamatorio, -ria.

influenza *n.* influenza.

infraction *n.* infracción.

infradiaphragmatic *adj.* infradiafragmático, -ca.

infrared *adj.* infrarrojo, -ja.

infusion *n.* infusión.

ingesta *n.* ingesta.

ingrowing toenail *n.* uñero.

ingrowth *n.* increscencia.

inguen *n.* ingle.

inguinal *adj.* inguinal.

inhalation *n.* inhalación.

inhale *v.* inhalar.

inheritance *n.* herencia.

autosomal dominant inheritance herencia autosómica dominante.

autosomal inheritance herencia autosómica.

autosomal recessive inheritance herencia autosómica recesiva.

crisscross inheritance herencia cruzada.

polygenic inheritance herencia poligénica.

X-linked dominant inheritance herencia dominante ligada al cromosoma X.

X-linked inheritance herencia ligada al cromosoma X.

X-linked recessive inheritance herencia recesiva ligada al cromosoma X.

inhibition *n.* inhibición.

inhibitive *adj.* inhibidor, -ra.

inhibitor *n.* inhibidor.

angiotensin converting enzyme inhibitor (ACE) inhibidor de la enzima convertidora de angiotensina, inhibidor de la enzima de conversión, inhibidor de la enzima de conversión de la angiotensina (ECA).

appetite inhibitor inhibidor del apetito.

inhibitory *adj.* inhibidor, -ra, inhibitorio, -ria.

initial *adj.* inicial.

initiation *n.* iniciación.

inject *v.* inyectar.

injection *n.* inyección.

booster injection inyección de recuerdo.

insulin injection inyección de insulina.

intraarticular injection inyección intraarticular.

intramuscular injection inyección intramuscular.

intravascular injection inyección intravascular.

intravenous injection inyección intravenosa.

injury *n.* injuria, lesión.

blast injury lesión por explosión.

deceleration injury lesión por desaceleración.

injury of the intervertebral disk lesión del disco intervertebral.

vital injury lesión vital.

inlet *n.* entrada.

innervation *n.* inervación.

innidation *n.* anidación, innidación.

innocuous *adj.* innocuo, -cua, inocuo, -cua.

innoxious *adj.* innocuo, -cua.

inoculation *n.* inoculación.

inorganic *adj.* inorgánico, -ca.

inotropic *adj.* inotrópico, -ca, inótropo, -pa.

negatively inotropic inotrópico negativo.

positively inotropic inotrópico positivo.

inpatient *adj.* hospitalizado, -da.

insalubrious *adj.* insalubre.

insane *adj.* insano, -na, loco, -ca.

insanitary *adj.* antihigiénico, -ca, insanitario, -ria.

inscriptio *n.* inscripción.

inscription *n.* inscripción.

insemination *n.* inseminación.

artificial insemination inseminación artificial.

insensibility *n.* insensibilidad.

insert *n.* inserción, insertar.

insertio *n.* inserción.

insertion *n.* inserción.

insolation *n.* insolación.

insoluble *adj.* insoluble.

insomnia *n.* insomnio.

insomniac *adj.* insomne.

insomnic *adj.* insomne.

inspection *n.* inspección.

inspirate *v.* inspirar.

inspiration *n.* inspiración.

instability *n.* inestabilidad.

instillation *n.* instilación.

eardrop instillation instilación de gotas óticas.

nasal instillation of medication instilación nasal de medicamentos.

instinct *n.* instinto, pulsión.

aggressive instinct instinto agresivo, pulsión agresiva, pulsión destructiva.

institutionalize *v.* hospitalizar.

instrument *n.* instrumento.

instrumental *adj.* instrumental.

instrumentation *n.* instrumentación.

insufficiency *n.* insuficiencia.

cardiac insufficiency insuficiencia cardíaca.

circulatory insufficiency insuficiencia circulatoria.

coronary insufficiency insuficiencia coronaria.

mitral insufficiency insuficiencia mitral.

renal insufficiency insuficiencia renal.

respiratory insufficiency insuficiencia respiratoria.

insufflation *n.* insuflación.

insulation *n.* aislamiento.

insulator *n.* aislante.

insulin *n.* insulina.

  globin zinc insulin insulina cíncica globina, insulina con cinc y globina.

  intermediate-acting insulin insulina de acción intermedia.

  long-acting insulin insulina de acción prolongada.

  rapid-acting insulin insulina de acción rápida.

  short-acting insulin insulina de acción corta.

  slow-acting insulin insulina de acción lenta.

intake *n.* ingesta, ingreso.

  caloric intake ingesta calórica.

integration *n.* integración.

intelligence *n.* inteligencia.

intensity *n.* intensidad.

interaction *n.* interacción.

  drug-drug interaction interacción medicamentosa.

  food and drug interaction interacción entre alimentos y fármacos.

interchange *n.* intercambio.

intercourse *n.* intercambio.

intercross *n.* entrecruzamiento.

intern *n.* interno, -na.

internal *adj.* interno, -na.

interne *n.* interno, -na.

interval *n.* intervalo.

intervention *n.* intervención.

interview *n.* entrevista.

intestinal *adj.* intestinal.

intestine *n.* intestino, intestinum.

  blind intestine intestino ciego.

  ileum intestine intestino íleon.

  jejunum intestine intestino yeyuno.

  large intestine intestino grueso.

  small intestine intestino delgado.

intestinum *n.* intestino, intestinum.

  intestinum caecum intestino ciego.

  intestinum cecum intestino ciego.

  intestinum crassum intestino grueso.

  intestinum ileum intestino íleon.

  intestinum jejunum intestino yeyuno.

  intestinum tenue intestino delgado.

intima *adj.* íntima.

intolerance *n.* intolerancia.

  drug intolerance intolerancia a fármacos.

  gluten intolerance intolerancia al gluten.

  lactose intolerance intolerancia a la lactosa.

intoxation *n.* intoxación.

intoxication *n.* intoxicación.

intra-abdominal *adj.* intraabdominal.

intracellular *adj.* intracelular.

intrascrotal *adj.* intraescrotal, intrascrotal.

introitus *n.* introito.

introversion *n.* introversión.

intrusion *n.* intrusión.

intubate *v.* intubar.

intubation *n.* intubación.

  gastric intubation sondaje gástrico.

  intratracheal intubation intubación intratraqueal.

  nasal intubation intubación nasal.

  nasogastric intubation intubación nasogástrica.

nasotracheal intubation intubación nasotraqueal.

oral intubation intubación bucal, intubación oral.

orotracheal intubation intubación bucotraqueal, intubación orotraqueal.

invagination *n.* invaginación.

invalid *n.* inválido, -da.

invalidism *n.* invalidez.

invertebrate *n.* invertebrado, -da.

investigation *n.* investigación.

clinical investigation investigación clínica.

involuntary *adj.* involuntario, -ria.

involution *n.* involución.

involution of the uterus involución del útero, involución uterina.

uterine involution involución del útero, involución uterina.

iodic *adj.* yódico, -ca.

iodide *n.* yoduro.

iodinate *v.* yodar.

iodinated *adj.* yodado, -da.

iodine *n.* iodo, yodo.

iodize *v.* yodar, yodizar.

iodized *adj.* yodado, -da.

iodopsin *n.* yodopsina.

iodotherapy *n.* yodoterapia.

ion *n.* ión.

ionization *n.* dialectolisis, ionización.

ionophoresis *n.* ionoforesis.

ipsilateral *adj.* ipsilateral, ipsolateral.

iridectomize *v.* iridectomizar.

iridectomy *n.* iridectomía.

iridoplegia *n.* iridoplejía.

iris *n.* iris.

iritic *adj.* irítico, -ca.

iritis *n.* iritis.

iron *n.* hierro.

irradiate *adj.* irradiado, -da, irradiar.

irradiation *n.* irradiación.

irreducible *adj.* irreducible.

irregular *adj.* irregular.

irreversible *adj.* irreversible.

irrigation *n.* irrigación.

bladder irrigation irrigación vesical.

irritability *n.* irritabilidad.

irritable *adj.* irritable.

irritant *n.* irritante.

irritation *n.* irritación.

ischemia *n.* isquemia.

cerebral ischemia isquemia cerebral.

chronic intestinal ischemia isquemia intestinal crónica.

ischemia retinae isquemia retinae.

myocardial ischemia isquemia del miocardio, isquemia miocárdica.

renal ischemia isquemia renal.

silent ischemia isquemia silenciosa, isquemia SUBclínica.

ischemic *adj.* isquémico, -ca.

ischiatic *adj.* isquiádico, -ca, isquiático, -ca.

ischiotibial *adj.* isquiotibial.

ischium ischium, isquion.

islet *n.* islote.

islet of Langerhans islote de Langerhans.

pancreatic islet islote pancreático.

isoallele *n.* isoalelo.

isoallelism *n.* isoalelismo.

isoantibody *n.* isoanticuerpo.

isoantigen n. isoantígeno.
isoenzyme n. isoenzima.
isoimmunization n. isoinmunización.
isolated adj. aislado, -da.
isolation n. aislamiento.
  infectious isolation aislamiento infeccioso.
  social isolation aislamiento social.
isolator n. aislante.
  surgical isolator aislante quirúrgico.
isoleucine n. isoleucina.
isosensitization n. isosensibilización.
isthmus n. istmo.
itch n. comezón, prurito.
itching n. picazón.
Ixodes Ixodes.
  Ixodes bicornis Ixodes bicornis.

non-hemolytic jaundice ictericia no hemolítica.
jaw n. maxilar, quijada.
jejunal adj. yeyunal.
jejunectomy n. yeyunectomía.
jejunitis n. yeyunitis.
jejunum n. yeyuno.
jelly n. gelatina, jalea.
jerk n. sacudida.
jugular adj. yugular.
juice n. jugo.
  gastric juice jugo gástrico.
  intestinal juice jugo intestinal.
  pancreatic juice jugo pancreático.
  prostatic juice jugo prostático.
junction n. unión.
juxta-articular adj. yuxtaarticular.

J

jacket n. chaleco, corsé, funda.
jaundice n. ictericia.
  acholuric jaundice ictericia acolúrica.
  choleric jaundice ictericia colérica.
  cholestatic jaundice ictericia colestática.
  congenital hemolytic jaundice ictericia hemolítica congénita, icterus hemolítico congénito.
  congenital jaundice ictericia congénita.
  jaundice of the newborn ictericia del recién nacido.
  neonatal jaundice ictericia neonatal, icterus neonatal.

K

kaliemia n. caliemia.
karyotype n. cariotipo.
keloid n. queloide, queloides.
keratan sulfate n. queratán-sulfato.
keratectomy n. keratectomía, queratectomía.
keratin n. queratina.
keratinization n. queratinización.
keratinize v. queratinizar.
keratinized adj. queratinizado, -da.
keratinocyte n. queratinocito.
keratitis n. queratitis.
keratoacanthoma n. queratoacantoma.
keratoconjunctivitis n. queratoconjuntivitis.
keratoconus n. queratocono.

keratocyte *n.* queratocito.

keratoderma *n.* queratodermia.

keratoiditis *n.* queratoiditis.

keratopathy *n.* queratopatía.

keratoplasia *n.* queratoplasia.

keratosis *n.* queratosis.

  actinic keratosis queratosis actínica.

  keratosis palmaris et plantaris queratosis palmar y plantar.

  keratosis seborrheica queratosis seborreica.

  keratosis senilis queratosis senil.

  seborrheic keratosis queratosis seborreica.

  senile keratosis queratosis senil.

  solar keratosis queratosis solar.

kernicterus *n.* kerníctero, kernicterus, querníctero.

ketoacidosis *n.* acidocetosis, cetoacidosis.

ketoaciduria *n.* cetoaciduria.

ketone *n.* cetona.

ketonemia *n.* cetonemia.

ketonic *adj.* cetónico, -ca.

ketonuria *n.* cetonuria.

ketosis *n.* cetosis.

kidney *n.* riñón.

  floating kidney riñón ectópico, riñón flotante.

  horseshoe kidney riñón en herradura.

  polycystic kidney riñón poliquístico.

  pyelonephritic kidney riñón pielonefrítico.

kinesia *n.* cinesia, cinesis.

kinesiology *n.* cinesiología, kinesiología.

kinesis *n.* cinesia, cinesis, kinesis.

kinesthesia *n.* cinestesia, kinestesia.

kinesthetic *adj.* cinestésico, -ca, kinestésico, -ca.

kinetics *n.* cinética.

kleptomaniac *n.* cleptomaníaco, cleptómano.

knee *n.* rodilla.

  locked knee rodilla bloqueada.

kneeguard *n.* rodillera.

knife *n.* bisturí, cuchilla, cuchillo.

knock-kneed *n.* patizambo, -ba, zambo, -ba.

knot *n.* nudo.

  surgeon's knot nudo de cirujano.

  surgical knot nudo quirúrgico.

kolytic *adj.* colítico, -ca.

kraurosis *n.* craurosis.

kyllosis *n.* quilosis.

kyphoscoliosis *n.* cifoescoliosis, cifoscoliosis.

kyphosis *n.* cifosis.

L

label *n.* marcaje.

  radioactive label marcaje radiactivo.

labial *adj.* labial.

labile *adj.* lábil.

  heat labile termolábil.

lability *n.* labilidad.

labium *n.* labio.

labor *n.* parto.

  artificial labor parto artificial.

  complicated labor parto complicado.

induced labor parto inducido, parto provocado.

instrumental labor parto instrumental.

multiple labor parto múltiple.

prolonged labor parto prolongado.

laboratory *n.* laboratorio.

clinical laboratory laboratorio clínico.

labyrinth *n.* laberinto.

labyrinthectomy *n.* laberintectomía.

labyrinthitis *n.* laberintitis.

labyrinthotomy *n.* laberintotomía.

labyrinthus *n.* laberinto.

lacerated *adj.* lacerado, -da, rasgado, -da.

laceration *n.* laceración.

brain laceration laceración cerebral.

scalp laceration laceración del cuero cabelludo.

vaginal laceration laceración vaginal.

lachrymal *adj.* lacrimal, lagrimal.

lacrimal *n.* lacrimal, lagrimal.

lacrimation *n.* lacrimación, lagrimación, lagrimeo.

lacrimonasal *adj.* lacrimonasal.

lactate *v.* lactar.

lactation *n.* lactación, lactancia.

lacteal *adj.* lácteo, -a.

lactic *adj.* láctico, -ca.

lactose *n.* lactosa.

lactosidosis *n.* lactosidosis.

laeve *adj.* leve.

lame *adj.* cojo -ja.

lameness *n.* cojera.

lamina *n.* lámina.

laminectomy *n.* laminectomía.

lancet *n.* lanceta, sangradera.

language *n.* lenguaje.

body language lenguaje corporal.

sensory-based language lenguaje sensitivo.

sign language lenguaje de signos.

verbal language lenguaje verbal.

lanugo *n.* lanugo.

laparotomy *n.* laparotomía.

exploration laparotomy laparotomía exploradora.

staging laparotomy laparotomía de estadiaje.

lapsus *n.* lapsus.

laryngeal *adj.* laríngeo, -a.

laryngectomee *n.* laringuectomizado, -da.

laryngectomized *adj.* laringuectomizado, -da.

laryngectomy *n.* laringuectomía.

laryngitis *n.* laringitis.

acute catarrhal laryngitis laringitis aguda, laringitis catarral aguda.

chronic catarrhal laryngitis laringitis catarral crónica.

croupous laryngitis laringitis crupal, laringitis cruposa.

diphtheritic laryngitis laringitis diftérica.

laryngitis stridulosa laringitis estridulosa.

spasmodic laryngitis laringitis espasmódica.

laryngopharyngitis *n.* laringofaringitis.

laryngoscope *n.* laringoscopio.

laryngoscopy *n.* laringoscopia.

direct laryngoscopy laringoscopia directa.

indirect laryngoscopy laringoscopia de espejo, laringoscopia indirecta.

laryngospasm *n.* laringoespasmo, laringospasmo.

laryngotomy *n.* laringotomía.

larynx *n.* laringe.

artificial larynx laringe artificial.

laser *n.* láser.

late *adj.* tardío, -a.

latenciation *n.* latenciación.

latency *n.* latencia.

lateral *adj.* lateral.

laterality *n.* lateralidad.

latitude *n.* latitud.

laugh *n.* risa.

lavage *n.* lavado.

blood lavage lavado de la sangre, lavado general, lavado sanguíneo.

bronchial lavage lavado bronquial.

bronchopulmonary lavage lavado broncopulmonar, lavado gástrico.

gastric lavage lavado del estómago.

peritoneal lavage lavado peritoneal.

pleural lavage lavado pleural.

vesical lavage lavado vesical.

law *n.* ley.

Mendel's law ley de Mendel.

lax *adj.* laxo, -xa.

laxative *n.* laxante.

laxity *n.* laxitud.

layer *n.* capa.

lead *n.* derivación.

aVf lead derivación aVF.

leanness *n.* delgadez.

learning *n.* aprendizaje.

psychomotor learning aprendizaje psicomotor.

left-handed *n.* zurdo, -da.

leg *n.* pierna.

legionellosis *n.* legionelosis.

leiomyoma *n.* leiomioma, liomioma.

leishmaniasis *n.* leishmaniasis, leishmaniosis.

leishmaniosis *n.* leishmaniosis.

length *n.* longitud.

lens *n.* cristalino, lente.

bifocal lens lente bifocal.

contact lens lente de contacto, lentilla.

leper *adj.* leproso, -sa.

lepra *n.* lepra.

lepromatous *adj.* lepromatoso, -sa.

leprosary *n.* leprosería.

leprose *adj.* leproso, -sa.

leprosy *n.* lepra.

cutaneous leprosy lepra cutánea.

lepromatous leprosy lepra lepromatosa.

leprous *adj.* leproso, -sa.

leptomeninges *n.* leptomeninges.

leptomeningitis *n.* leptomeningitis.

leptospirosis *n.* leptospirosis.

lesbian *adj.* lesbiana.

lesbianism *n.* lesbianismo.

lesion *n.* lesión.

degenerative lesion lesión degenerativa.

discharging lesion lesión de descarga.

gross lesion lesión macroscópica, lesión manifiesta.

histologic lesion lesión histológica.

medullar lesion lesión medular.

organic lesion lesión orgánica.

lethal *adj.* letal.

lethargy *n.* letargia, letargo.

leucine *n.* leucina, leukina.

leukemia *n.* leucemia.

acute leukemia leucemia aguda.

acute lymphoblastic leukemia leucemia linfoblástica aguda.

acute lymphocytic leukemia leucemia linfocítica aguda.

acute myeloid leukemia leucemia mieloide aguda.

acute non-lymphocytic leukemia leucemia aguda no linfocítica.

chronic lymphocytic leukemia (LLC) leucemia linfocítica crónica (LLC).

chronic myelocytic leukemia leucemia mielocítica crónica, leucemia mieloide crónica (LMC).

granulocytic leukemia leucemia granulocítica.

lymphatic leukemia leucemia linfática.

lymphoblastic leukemia leucemia linfoblástica.

lymphocytic leukemia leucemia linfocítica.

lymphoid leukemia leucemia linfoide.

megakarycytic leukemia leucemia megacariocítica.

mixed leukemia leucemia mixta.

monocytic leukemia leucemia monocítica.

myeloblastic acute leukemia leucemia aguda mieloblástica.

myeloblastic leukemia leucemia mieloblástica.

myelocytic leukemia leucemia mielocítica.

plasmacytic leukemia leucemia plasmática.

leukemic *adj.* leucémico, -ca.

leukencephalitis *n.* leucencefalitis, leucoencefalitis.

leukina *n.* leucina, leukina.

leukoblast *n.* leucoblasto.

leukocytal *adj.* leucocitario, -a, leucocítico, -ca.

leukocyte *n.* leucocito.

basophilic leukocyte leucocito basófilo.

eosinophilic leukocyte leucocito eosinófilo.

lymphoid leukocyte leucocito linfoide.

mast leukocyte leucocito cebado.

multinuclear leukocyte leucocito multinuclear.

neutrophilic leukocyte leucocito neutrófilo.

non-motile leukocyte leucocito inmóvil, leucocito no mótil.

polymorphonuclear leukocyte leucocito polimorfonuclear.

polynuclear leukocyte leucocito polinuclear.

segmented leukocyte leucocito segmentado.

leukocytic *adj.* leucocitario, -a, leucocítico, -ca.

leukocytolysis *n.* leucocitólisis.

leukocytosis *n.* leucocitosis.

absolute leukocytosis leucocitosis absoluta.

leukocytosis of the newborn leucocitosis del neonato.

lymphocytic leukocytosis leucocitosis linfocítica.

monocytic leukocytosis leucocitosis monocítica.

mononuclear leukocytosis leucocitosis mononuclear.

neutrophilic leukocytosis leucocitosis neutrófila.

pathologic leukocytosis leucocitosis patológica.

leukocyturia *n.* leucocituria.

leukoderma *n.* leucodermia.

leukodermia *n.* leucodermia.

leukodystrophy *n.* leucodistrofia.

leukoencephalopathy *n.* leucoencefalopatía.

leukogram *n.* leucograma.

leukopenia *n.* leucopenia.

leukoplasia *n.* leucoplasia.

leukorrhea fluor albus, leucorrea, uterorrea.

leukosis *n.* leucosis.

levator *n.* elevador, levator.

level *n.* nivel.

blood level nivel sanguíneo.

blood level of glucose nivel sanguíneo de glucosa.

hearing level nivel auditivo.

level of consciousness nivel de consciencia.

operant level nivel operativo.

serum creatinine level nivel de creatinina en suero.

lever *n.* palanca.

levocardia *n.* levocardia.

libido *n.* líbido.

lichen *n.* liquen.

lichen planus liquen plano.

lien *n.* bazo, lien.

lien mobilis bazo movible, bazo móvil.

life *n.* vida.

artificial life vida artificial.

average life vida media.

plasma half life vida media plasmática.

postnatal life vida posnatal.

prenatal life vida antenatal, vida intrauterina, vida prenatal, vida uterina.

sexual life vida sexual.

vegetative life vida vegetativa.

lifting *n.* lifting.

facial lifting lifting facial.

ligament *n.* ligamento.

ligamentum *n.* ligamento, ligamentum.

ligation *n.* ligación, ligadura.

ligature *n.* ligadura.

surgical ligature ligadura quirúrgica.

light *n.* lux, luz.

infrared light luz infrarroja.

ultraviolet light luz ultravioleta.

limb *n.* extremidad, miembro.

inferior limb miembro inferior.

lower limb miembro inferior.

superior limb miembro superior.

thoracic limb miembro torácico.

upper limb miembro superior.

limbic *adj.* límbico, -ca.

limp *n.* cojera.

line *n.* línea.

cell line línea celular.

epiphysial line línea epifisaria.

linea *n.* línea.

lineage *n.* descendencia, linaje.

cell lineage linaje celular.

linear *adj.* lineal.

lingua *n.* lengua, lingua.

  lingua fissurata lengua fisurada, lingua fissurata.

lingual *adj.* lingual.

lingualis *adj.* lingual.

lining *n.* revestimiento.

linked *adj.* ligado, -da.

lip *n.* labio.

  cleft lip labio fisurado, labio hendido.

lipase *n.* lipasa.

lipemia *n.* lipemia.

lipid *n.* lípido.

lipidic *adj.* lipídico, -ca.

lipidosis *n.* lipidosis.

lipoatrophia *n.* lipoatrofia.

lipodystrophia *n.* lipodistrofia.

lipodystrophy *n.* lipodistrofia.

lipoid *adj.* lipoidal, lipoide.

lipoidosis *n.* lipoidosis.

lipoma *n.* lipoma.

lipomatosis *n.* lipomatosis.

lipoprotein *n.* lipoproteína.

liposoluble *adj.* liposoluble.

liposome *n.* liposoma.

liposuction *n.* lipoaspiración.

lipothymia *n.* lipotimia.

liquid *adj.* líquido, -da.

liquor *n.* licor, líquido, liquor.

  liquor cerebrospinalis líquido cefalorraquídeo, líquido cerebrospinal, liquor cerebrospinalis.

lissive *adj.* miorrelajante.

lithiasis *n.* litiasis.

  pancreatic lithiasis litiasis pancreática.

  urinary lithiasis litiasis urinaria.

lithotomy *n.* litotomía.

lithotrity *n.* litotricia.

liveborn *adj.* nacido, -da vivo, -va.

liver *n.* hígado.

  biliary cirrhotic liver hígado cirrótico biliar.

  cirrhotic liver hígado cirrótico.

  fatty liver hígado adiposo, hígado graso.

livid *adj.* lívido, -da, plomizo, -za.

lividity *n.* lividez.

  postmortem lividity lividez postmortem.

livor *n.* livor.

  livor mortis livor mortis.

lobation *n.* lobulación.

lobe *n.* lóbulo, lobus.

lobotomy *n.* lobotomía.

lobulation *n.* lobulación.

lobus *n.* lóbulo, lobus.

local *adj.* local.

localization *n.* localización.

lochia *n.* lochia, loquios.

locus *n.* locus, lugar.

logopedia *n.* logopedia.

logopedics *n.* logopedia.

longevity *n.* longevidad.

longitudinal *adj.* longitudinal.

longitudinalis *adj.* longitudinal.

loop *n.* asa, bucle.

lordoscoliosis *n.* lordoescoliosis.

lordosis *n.* lordosis.

loss *n.* deterioro.

  hearing loss deterioro auditivo.

lotio *n.* loción.

lotion *n.* loción.

louse *n.* piojo.

lucid *adj.* lúcido, -da.

lucidity *n.* lucidez.

lues *n.* lúe, lúes.

lumbago n. lumbago.

lumbar adj. lumbar.

lumbricus n. lombriz.

lung n. pulmón.

  coalminer's lung pulmón de los mineros del carbón.

  farmer's lung pulmón de granjero.

  honeycomb lung pulmón en panal, pulmón en panal de abeja.

lupus n. lupus.

  systemic lupus erythematosus (SLE) lupus eritematoso sistémico (LES).

luteal adj. lúteo, -a.

lutein n. luteína.

luteinization n. luteinización.

lux n. lux, luz.

luxatio n. luxatio, luxación.

luxation n. lluxatio, luxación.

  complicated luxation luxación complicada.

  dental luxation luxación dentaria.

luxus n. lujo, luxus.

lymph n. linfa.

lymphadenitis n. linfadenitis.

lymphadenopathy n. linfadenopatía.

lymphangioma n. linfangioma.

lymphangitis n. linfangitis.

lymphatic adj. linfático, -ca.

lymphocitosis n. linfocitosis.

lymphocyte n. linfocito.

  amplifier T lymphocyte linfocito T amplificador.

  B lymphocyte linfocito B.

  cytotoxic T lymphocyte linfocito T citotóxicos.

  helper T lymphocyte linfocito T ayudador.

  killer lymphocyte linfocito asesino.

  T lymphocyte linfocito T.

  transformed lymphocyte linfocito transformado.

lymphocytic adj. linfocítico, -ca.

lymphoid adj. linfoide, linfoideo, -a.

lymphoma n. linfoma.

  Hodgkin's lymphoma linfoma de Hodgkin.

lymphopathia n. linfopatía.

lymphopathy n. linfopatía.

lysate n. lisado, lisado, -da.

lysosome n. lisosoma.

lyssa n. lisa.

M

machine n. machina, máquina.

  heart-lung machine máquina cardiopulmonar, máquina corazón-púlmon.

  kidney machine máquina renal.

macroangiopathy n. macroangiopatía.

macrobiotic adj. macrobiótico, -ca.

macrobiotics n. macrobiótica.

macrocyte n. macrocito.

macrocytosis n. macrocitosis.

macroglobulin n. macroglobulina.

macroglobulinemia n. macroglobulinemia.

macroglossia n. macroglosia.

macrognathia n. macrognatia, macrognatismo.

macrolide n. macrólido.

macrophage n. macrófago.

macroscopic adj. macroscópico, -ca.

macroscopical *adj.* macroscópico, -ca.

macroscopy *n.* macroscopia.

macrosigmoid *n.* macrosigmoide.

macrosis *n.* macrosis.

macula *n.* macula, mácula.

macula corneae mácula corneal.

macula retinae mácula blanca de la retina, mácula de la retina, mácula lútea de la retina.

mongolian macula mácula mongólica.

maculopapule *n.* maculopápula.

mad *adj.* loco, -ca.

magma *n.* magma.

magnesium *n.* magnesio, magnesium.

magnification *n.* magnificación.

maim *v.* mutilar.

main *n.* mano.

main d'accoucheur mano de comadrón, mano de partero.

main en squelette mano de esqueleto, mano esquelética.

mal *n.* mal.

petit mal mal pequeño, pequeño mal.

malabsorption *n.* malabsorción.

congenital lactose malabsorption malabsorción congénita de lactosa.

maladjusted *adj.* maladaptado, -da.

maladjustment *n.* inadaptación, maladaptación.

malaise *n.* malestar.

malar *adj.* malar.

malaria *n.* helópira, malaria, paludismo.

malarious *adj.* malárico, -ca.

maldevelopment *n.* maldesarrollo.

maldigestion *n.* maladigestión, maldigestión.

male *n.* macho, varón.

maleruption *n.* malaerupción, malerupción.

malformation *n.* malformación.

malignancy *n.* malignidad.

malignant *adj.* maligno, -na.

mallear *adj.* malear.

malleolar *adj.* maleolar.

malleolus *n.* maléolo.

malnutrition *n.* desnutrición, malnutrición.

energy-protein malnutrition malnutrición proteicocalórica.

malocclusion *n.* maloclusión.

close-bite malocclusion maloclusión de mordida cerrada.

open-bite malocclusion maloclusión de mordida abierta.

malpractice *n.* mala práctica.

malpraxis *n.* malpraxis.

malpresentation *n.* malapresentación.

maltreatment *n.* maltrato.

mamalgia *n.* mamalgia.

mamillitis *n.* mamilitis.

mammaplasty *n.* mamaplastia.

mammillitis *n.* mamilitis.

mammitis *n.* mamitis.

mammogram *n.* mamograma.

mammograph *n.* mamógrafo.

mammographic *adj.* mamográfico, -ca.

mammography *n.* mamografía.

film screen mammography mamografía de barrido.

mammoplasty *n.* mamoplasia, mamoplastia.

augmentation mammoplasty mamoplastia de aumento, mamoplastia de incremento.

reconstructive mammoplasty mamoplastia reconstructiva.

reduction mammoplasty mamoplastia de reducción.

mandible *n.* mandíbula.

lower mandible mandíbula inferior.

upper mandible mandíbula superior.

mandibular *adj.* mandibular.

maneuver *n.* maniobra.

aspirant maneuver maniobra de aspiración.

Valsalva's maneuver maniobra de Valsalva.

mania *n.* manía.

maniac *adj.* maníaco, -ca.

maniac-depressive *adj.* maniaco-depresivo, -va.

manifestation *n.* manifestación.

manipulation *n.* manipulación.

genetic manipulation manipulación genética.

spinal manipulation manipulación vertebral.

manometer *n.* manómetro.

aneroid manometer manómetro aneroide.

dial manometer manómetro de dial.

differential manometer manómetro diferencial.

mercurial manometer manómetro de mercurio, manómetro mercurial.

manometry *n.* manometría.

manual *adj.* manual.

manus mano, manus.

manus extensa mano extendida.

manus flexa mano en flexión.

manus vara mano vara.

map *n.* mapa.

bone map mapa óseo.

brain electric activity map (BEAM) mapa de actividad eléctrica cerebral (MAEC).

chromosomal map mapa cromosómico.

cognitive map mapa cognitivo.

cytologic map mapa citológico.

linkage map mapa de ligadura, mapa de ligamiento.

physical map mapa físico.

marasmus *n.* marasmo.

marble *adj.* marmóreo, -a.

margin *n.* borde, margen.

anterior margin margen anterior.

inferior margin margen inferior.

margin of safety margen de seguridad.

superior margin margen superior.

marginal *adj.* marginal, marginalis.

margination *n.* marginación.

margo *n.* borde, margen, margo.

mark *n.* marca.

birth mark marca de nacimiento.

strawberry mark marca de fresa, marca en frambuesa.

marker *n.* marcador.

biochemical marker marcador bioquímico.

cell-surface marker marcador celular de superficie.

genetic marker marcador genético.

tumor marker marcador tumoral.

marmoreal *adj.* marmóreo, -a.

marrow n. médula.
masculinity n. masculinidad.
masculinization n. masculinización.
masculinize v. masculinizar.
masked adj. enmascarado, -da.
massage n. masaje.
  cardiac massage masaje cardíaco.
  electrovibratory massage masaje electrovibratorio.
  external cardiac massage masaje cardíaco externo.
  gingival massage masaje gingival.
  heart massage masaje cardíaco.
  prostatic massage masaje prostático.
  vibratory massage masaje vibratorio, vibroterapéutica.
masseur n. masajista.
massotherapy n. masoterapia.
mastadenitis n. mastadenitis.
mastalgia n. mastalgia.
mast-cell n. mastocito.
mastectomy n. mastectomía.
  extended radical mastectomy mastectomía radical ampliada.
  mastectomy lumpectomy mastectomía lumpectomía.
  modified radical mastectomy mastectomía radical modificada.
  radical mastectomy mastectomía radical.
  simple mastectomy mastectomía simple.
  total mastectomy mastectomía total.
mastication n. masticación.
masticatory adj. masticatorio, -ria.
mastitis n. mastitis.
  acute mastitis mastitis aguda.

  cystic mastitis mastitis quística.
  mastitis neonatorum mastitis del recién nacido, mastitis neonatal.
  retromammary mastitis mastitis retromamaria.
mastocyte n. mastocito.
mastocytoma n. mastocitoma.
mastocytosis n. mastocitosis.
mastodynia n. mastodinia.
mastogram n. mastograma.
mastography n. mastografía.
mastoid adj. mastoideo, -a.
mastoidectomy n. mastoidectomía.
mastoiditis n. mastoiditis.
mastopathy n. mastopatía.
masturbation n. masturbación.
materia n. materia.
material n. material.
  dental material material dental.
  genetic material material genético.
  suture material material de sutura.
maternal adj. maternal, materno, -na.
maternity n. maternidad.
mating n. apareamiento.
  assortative mating apareamiento concordante, apareamiento selectivo.
  assorted mating apareamiento concordante, apareamiento selectivo.
  assortive mating apareamiento concordante, apareamiento selectivo.
matrix n. matriz.
  matrix unguis matriz de la uña, matriz ungueal, matriz ungular.
  nail matrix matriz de la uña, matriz ungueal, matriz ungular.
matter n. materia.
maturation n. maduración.

bone maturation maduración ósea.

cervical maturation maduración cervical.

mature *adj.* madurar, maduro, -ra.

maxilla *n.* maxilar.

maxillary *adj.* maxilar.

maxillodental *adj.* maxilodental, maxilodentario, -ria.

maximum *n.* máximo.

meal *n.* comida.

mean *n.* media.

arithmetic mean media aritmética.

population mean media de la población.

sample mean media muestral.

standard error of the mean error estándar de la media.

measles *n.* sarampión.

measure *n.* medida.

measurement *n.* determinación, medición, valoración.

direct measurement of blood pressure determinación directa de la tensión arterial.

meatus *n.* meato, meatus.

mechanics *n.* mecánica.

mechanism *n.* mecanismo.

defense mechanism mecanismo de defensa.

immunological mechanism mecanismo inmunológico.

mechanism of labor mecanismo del parto.

mental mechanism mecanismo mental.

pain mechanism mecanismo del dolor.

proprioceptive mechanism mecanismo propioceptivo.

mechanoreceptor *n.* mecanorreceptor.

meconium *n.* meconio.

medial *adj.* medial.

medialis *adj.* medial.

median *adj.* mediana, mediano, -na.

mediastinal *adj.* mediastínico, -ca.

mediastinitis *n.* mediastinitis.

mediastinum *n.* mediastino.

mediator *n.* mediador.

medicable *adj.* medicable.

medical *adj.* médico, -ca.

medicamentous *adj.* medicamentoso, -sa.

medicated *adj.* medicado, -da.

medication *n.* medicación.

conservative medication medicación conservadora.

hypodermic medication medicación hipodérmica.

intravenous medication medicación intravenosa.

ionic medication medicación iónica.

preanesthetic medication medicación preanestésica.

transduodenal medication medicación transduodenal.

medicine *n.* medicamento, medicina.

alternative medicine medicina alternativa.

clinical medicine medicina clínica.

comparative medicine medicina comparada.

compound medicine medicamento compuesto.

emergency medicine medicina de urgencia.

evidence based medicine medicina basada en la evidencia.

experimental medicine medicina experimental.

family medicine medicina de familia, medicina familiar.

fetal medicine medicina fetal.

forensic medicine medicina forense.

geriatric medicine medicina geriátrica.

internal medicine medicina interna.

legal medicine medicina legal.

medicine community medicina comunitaria.

neonatal medicine medicina neonatal.

occupational medicine medicina del trabajo.

osteopathic medicine medicina osteopática.

patent medicine medicamento sin receta.

pediatric medicine medicina pediátrica.

perinatal medicine medicina perinatal.

preventive medicine medicina preventiva.

proprietary medicine medicamento patentado.

psychosomatic medicine medicina psicosomática.

scientific medicine medicina cléntífica.

sports medicine medicina del deporte, medicina deportiva.

tropical medicine medicina tropical.

medium *n.* medio, medium.

contrast medium medio de contraste.

culture medium medio de cultivo.

external medium medio externo.

radioactive contrast medium medio de contraste radiactivo.

medulla *n.* médula.

megacolon *n.* megacolon, megalocolia.

megakaryocite *n.* megacariocito.

megalomania *n.* megalomanía.

melanin *n.* melanina.

melanocyte *n.* melanocito.

melanocytoma *n.* melanocitoma.

melanoma *n.* melanoma.

benign juvenile melanoma melanoma juvenil, melanoma juvenil benigno.

choroidal melanoma melanoma de úvea.

in situ malignant melanoma melanoma maligno in situ.

juvenile melanoma melanoma juvenil, melanoma juvenil benigno.

malignant melanoma melanoma maligno, melanoscirro.

nodular melanoma melanoma nodular.

primary cutaneous melanoma melanoma cutáneo primario.

melanosis *n.* melanosis.

melasma *n.* melasma.

melasma gravidarum melasma gravídico, melasma uterino.

melasma suprarenale melasma suprarenal.

melatonin *n.* melatonina.

melena *n.* melena.

melena neonatorum melena del recién nacido, melena neonatal.

melena vera melena verdadera.

member *n.* miembro.

phantom member miembro fantasma.

virile member miembro viril.

membrana *n.* membrana.

membranae deciduae decidua.

membrane *n.* membrana.

arachnoid membrane membrana aracnoidea.

cell membrane membrana celular.

diphtheritic membrane membrana diftérica.

egg membrane membrana del huevo.

embryonic membrane membrana embrionaria.

hyaline membrane membrana hialina.

nuclear membrane membrana nuclear.

placental membrane membrana placentaria.

plasma membrane membrana plasmática.

viteline membrane membrana vitelina.

membranous *adj.* membranoso, -sa.

membrum *n.* miembro.

membrum inferius miembro inferior.

membrum muliebre miembro de la mujer.

membrum superius miembro superior.

membrum virile miembro viril.

memory *n.* memoria.

anterograde memory memoria anterógrada.

inmunologic memory memoria inmunológica.

long term memory (LTM) memoria a largo plazo (MLP).

retrograde memory memoria retrógrada.

selective memory memoria selectiva.

senile memory memoria senil.

short-term memory (STM) memoria a corto plazo (MCP).

visual memory memoria visual.

menarche *n.* menarca, menarquia, menarquía.

Mendelian *adj.* mendeliano, -na.

meningeal *adj.* meníngeo, -a.

meningeoma *n.* meningeoma, meningioma.

meningitis *n.* meningitis.

meningioma *n.* meningioma.

meningism *n.* meningismo.

meningitic *adj.* meningítico, -ca.

meningitis *n.* meningitis.

acute aseptic meningitis meningitis aséptica, meningitis aséptica aguda.

aseptic meningitis meningitis aséptica, meningitis aséptica aguda.

bacterial meningitis meningitis bacteriana.

cerebral meningitis meningitis cerebral.

cerebrospinal meningitis meningitis cefalorraquídea, meningitis cerebroespinal.

meningitis serosa circumscripta meningitis serosa circunscrita, meningitis serosa circunscrita quística.

meningococcal meningitis meningitis meningocócica.

neoplastic meningitis meningitis neoplásica.

pneumococcal meningitis meningitis neumocócica.

traumatic meningitis meningitis traumática.

viral meningitis meningitis viral, meningitis virásica.

meningocele *n.* meningocele.

meningococcemia *n.* meningococemia, meningococia.

acute fulminating meningococcemia meningococemia fulminante aguda.

meningococci *n.* meningococo.

meningoencephalitis *n.* meningoencefalitis.

meningoma *n.* meningioma, meningoma.

meninx *n.* meninge.

meniscal *adj.* meniscal.

meniscectomy *n.* meniscectomía.

meniscitis *n.* meniscitis.

meniscus *n.* menisco.

menopausal *adj.* menopáusico, -ca.

menopause *n.* menopausia, menopausis.

artificial menopause menopausia artificial.

male menopause menopausia masculina.

menopause praecox menopausia precoz, menopausia prematura.

surgical menopause menopausia quirúrgica.

menorrhea *n.* menorrea.

menorrheal *adj.* menorreico, -ca.

menstrual *adj.* menstrual, menstrualis.

menstruate *v.* menstruar.

menstruation *n.* menstruación.

anovular menstruation menstruación anovular, menstruación anovulatoria.

anovulatory menstruation menstruación anovular, menstruación anovulatoria.

delayed menstruation menstruación retrasada.

non-ovulational menstruation menstruación no ovulatoria, menstruación sin ovulación.

regurgitant menstruation menstruación regurgitante, menstruación retrógrada.

retrograde menstruation menstruación regurgitante, menstruación retrógrada.

suppressed menstruation menstruación suprimida.

vicarious menstruation menstruación sustitutiva, menstruación vicariante.

menstruum *n.* menstruo.

mental *adj.* mental, mentoniano, -na.

mentality *n.* mentalidad.

menton *n.* mentón.

mentoplasty *n.* mentoplastia.

mentum *n.* mentón.

mephitis *n.* fetidez.

meralgia *n.* meralgia.

mercury *n.* mercurio.

mesangial *adj.* mesangial.

mesangium *n.* mesangio.

mesencephalitis *n.* mesencefalitis.

mesencephalon *n.* mesencéfalo, mesoencéfalo.

mesenchyma *n.* mesénquima.

mesenchymal *adj.* mesenquimático, -ca, mesenquimatoso, -sa.

mesenchymoma *n.* mesenquimoma.

mesenteric *adj.* mesentérico, -ca.

mesenterium mesenterio, mesenterium.

mesentery *n.* mesenterio.

mesh *n.* malla.

mesial *adj.* mesial.

mesially *adj.* mesial.

mesocardium *n.* mesocardio.

mesoderm *n.* mesodermo.

intraembryonic mesoderm mesodermo intraembrionario.

mesothelial *adj.* mesotelial.

mesothelioma *n.* mesotelioma.

mesothelium *n.* mesotelio.

messenger *n.* mensajero.

second messenger segundo mensajero.

metabolic *adj.* metabólico, -ca.

metabolism *n.* metabolismo.

acid-base metabolism metabolismo acidobásico.

anaerobic metabolism metabolismo anaeróbico.

basal metabolism metabolismo basal.

carbohydrate metabolism metabolismo de carbohidratos, metabolismo de los hidratos de carbono.

cholesterol metabolism metabolismo del colesterol.

drug metabolism metabolismo farmacológico.

electrolyte metabolism metabolismo de los electrólitos.

endogenous metabolism metabolismo endógeno.

energy metabolism metabolismo energético.

exogenous metabolism metabolismo exógeno.

fat metabolism metabolismo de las grasas, metabolismo graso.

intermediary metabolism metabolismo intermediario.

iron metabolism metabolismo del hierro.

protein metabolism metabolismo de las proteínas, metabolismo proteico.

renal metabolism metabolismo renal.

respiratory metabolism metabolismo respiratorio.

metabolite *n.* metabolito.

metabolizable *adj.* metabolizable.

metabolize *v.* metabolizar.

metacarpal *adj.* metacarpiano, -na.

metacarpophalangeal *adj.* metacarpofalángico, -ca.

metacarpus *n.* metacarpo.

metal *n.* metal.

metalbumin *n.* metaalbúmina.

metallic *adj.* metálico, -ca.

metamorphosis *n.* metamorfosis.

metaphase *n.* metafase.

metaphyseal *adj.* metafisario, -ria.

metaphysial *adj.* metafisario, -ria.

metaphysis *n.* metáfisis.

metaphysitis *n.* metafisitis.

metaplasia *n.* metaplasia.

metaplastic *adj.* metaplásico, -ca.

metastasis *n.* metaptosis, metástasis.

  biochemical metastasis metástasis bioquímica.

  calcareous metastasis metástasis calcárea.

  contact metastasis metástasis de contacto.

  crossed metastasis metástasis cruzada.

  direct metastasis metástasis directa.

  paradoxical metastasis metástasis paradójica.

  pulsating metastasis metástasis pulsátil.

  retrograde metastasis metástasis retrógrada.

  satellite metastasis metástasis satélite.

metastatic *adj.* metastásico, -ca, metastático, -ca.

metatarsal *adj.* metatarsiano, -na.

metatarsalgia *n.* metatarsalgia.

metatarsectomy *n.* metatarsectomía.

metatarsus *n.* metatarso, metatarsus.

meter *n.* metro.

methadone *n.* metadona.

methemoglobin *n.* metahemoglobina.

methemoglobinemia *n.* metahemoglobinemia.

method *n.* método.

  basal body temperature method of family planning método de planificación familiar mediante la temperatura basal.

  basal temperature method método de temperatura basal.

  calendar method of family planning método del calendario de planificación familiar.

  cervical mucus method of family planning método de planificación familiar del moco cervical.

  contraceptive method método contraceptivo.

  correlational method método correlativo.

  cross-sectional method método de cortes transversales.

  diffusion method método de difusión.

  direct method método directo.

  experimental method método experimental.

  natural family planning method método de planificación familiar natural.

  natural method método natural.

  ovulation method of family planning método de la ovulación para planificación familiar.

  rhythm method método del ritmo.

  trial and error method método empírico.

  withdrawal method método de la retirada.

methodology *n.* metodología.

methylated *adj.* metilado, -da.

methylation *n.* metilación.

methylcellulose *n.* metilcelulosa.

metritis *n.* metritis.

metrorrhea *n.* metrorrea.

micella *n.* micela.

micelle *n.* micela.

micranatomy *n.* microanatomía.
microabscess *n.* microabsceso.
microadenoma *n.* microadenoma.
microadenopathy *n.* microadenopatía.
microalbuminuria *n.* microalbuminuria.
microanatomist *n.* microanatomista.
microbe *n.* microbio.
microbicidal *adj.* microbicida.
microbicide *n.* microbicida.
microbiological *adj.* microbiológico, -ca.
microbiologist *n.* microbiólogo, -ga.
microbiology *n.* microbiología.
microcephalia *n.* microcefalia.
microcephalic *adj.* microcefálico, -ca.
microcephalous *adj.* microcefálico.
microcephalus *n.* microcéfalo.
microcephaly *n.* microcefalia.
microcirculation *n.* microcirculación.
microcyst *n.* microquiste.
microcytic *adj.* microcítico, -ca.
micrognathia *n.* micrognacia, micrognatia.
micrograft *n.* microinjerto.
microinfarct *n.* microinfarto.
micromanipulation *n.* micromanipulación.
microphone *n.* micrófono.
microphthalmos *n.* microftalmía,
microftalmos.
microphthalmus *n.* microftalmía,
microftalmos.
microscope *n.* microscopio.
  compound microscope microscopio compuesto.

  dark-field microscope microscopio de campo oscuro.
  electron microscope microscopio
electrónico.
  laser microscope microscopio láser.
  light microscope microscopio de
luz.
  operating microscope microscopio de operaciones, microscopio
operatorio, microscopio quirúrgico.
  polarizing microscope microscopio de luz polarizada.
  *scanning electron microscope
(SEM)* microscopio electrónico de
barrido (MEG).
  scanning microscope microscopio
de barrido.
  slit lamp microscope microscopio
de lámpara de hendidura.
  *transmission scanning electron
microscope* microscopio electrónico de barrido de transmisión.
microscopic *adj.* microscópico, -ca.
microscopical *adj.* microscópico,
-ca.
microscopist *n.* microscopista.
microscopy *n.* microscopía.
  clinical microscopy microscopía
clínica.
  electron microscopy microscopía
electrónica.
  fluorescence microscopy microscopía de fluorescencia, microscopía
fluorescente.
  fundus microscopy microscopía de
fondo, microscopía fúndica.
  immersion microscopy microscopía de inmersión.

immune electron microscopy microscopía inmunoelectrónica.

immunofluorescence microscopy microscopía de inmunofluorescencia, microscopía inmunofluorescente.

scanning electron microscopy microscopía electrónica de barrido.

transmission scanning electron microscopy (TSEM) microscopía electrónica de barrido de transmisión (MEBT).

ultraviolet microscopy microscopía ultravioleta.

microsection *n.* microsección.

microsurgery *n.* microcirugía.

microsuture *n.* microsutura.

microtome *n.* microtomo.

miction *n.* micción.

midget *n.* enano, -na.

midwife *n.* comadrona, matrona.

migraine *n.* jaqueca, migraña.

accompanied migraine migraña acompañada.

classic migraine migraña clásica.

common migraine migraña común.

fulgurating migraine jaqueca fulgurante, migraña fulgurante.

hemiplegic migraine jaqueca hemipléjica, migraña hemipléjica.

migraine with aura migraña con aura.

migraine without aura migraña sin aura.

ophthalmic migraine jaqueca oftálmica, migraña oftálmica.

ophthalmoplegic migraine jaqueca oftalmopléjica, migraña oftalmopléjica.

migrainous *adj.* migrañoso, -sa.

migranoid *adj.* jaquecoso, -sa.

migranous *adj.* jaquecoso, -sa.

migration *n.* migración.

mild *adj.* leve.

miliary *adj.* miliar.

milk *n.* leche.

mimic *adj.* mímica, mímico, -ca.

mimicry *n.* mimetismo.

mind *n.* mente.

mineral *n.* mineral.

mineralcorticoid *n.* mineralcorticoide, mineralocorticoide.

mineralization *n.* mineralización.

mineralized *adj.* mineralizado, -da.

minilaparatomy *n.* minilaparatomía.

minim *n.* mínima.

minimization *n.* minimización.

minimum *n.* mínimo.

light minimum mínimo de luz.

minimum audibile mínimo audible.

minimum cognoscibile mínimo cognoscible.

minimum legibile mínimo legible.

minimum separabile mínimo separable.

visibile minimum mínimo visible.

miosis *n.* miosis.

mirror *n.* espejo.

misogyny *n.* misoginia.

mite *n.* ácaro.

mitigate *v.* mitigar.

mitochondria *n.* mitocondria.

mitochondrial *adj.* mitocondrial.

mitosis *n.* mitosis.

pathologic mitosis mitosis patológica.

mitral *adj.* mitral.

mixed *adj.* mixto, -ta.

mixture *n.* mezcla, mixtura.

mnemotechnics *n.* mnemotecnia.

mobility *n.* movilidad.

mobilization *n.* movilización.

mobilize *v.* movilizar.

modality *n.* modalidad.

model *n.* modelar.
  medical model modelo médico.

modification *n.* modificación.
  behavior modification modificación de conducta.

molar *adj.* molar, muela.
  first molar primer molar.
  second molar segundo molar.
  sixth-year molar molar de los seis años, molar del sexto años.
  third molar tercer molar.
  twelfth-year molar molar de los doce años.

molarity *n.* molaridad.

mole *n.* mola.
  hydatid mole mola hidatídica, mole hidatiforme.
  hydatidiform mole mola hidatídica, mole hidatiforme.
  malignant mole mola maligna, mola metastatizante.
  vesicular mole mola vesicular.

molecular *adj.* molecular.

molecule *n.* molécula.
  adhesion molecule molécula de adhesión.

molluscum *n.* molusco.
  molluscum contagiosum molusco contagioso.

mongolism *n.* mongolismo.
  translocation mongolism mongolismo por traslocación.

monitor *n.* monitor, monitorizar.
  blood pressure monitor monitor de presión arterial.
  cardiac monitor monitor cardíaco.
  central venous pressure monitor monitor de presión venosa central.
  CVP monitor monitor de PVC.
  electronic fetal monitor monitor fetal electrónico.
  Holter monitor monitor Holter.

monoarticular *adj.* monoarticular.

monochromatic *adj.* monocromático, -ca.

monoclonal *adj.* monoclonal, monoclónico, -ca.

monocyte *n.* monocito.

monocytopenia *n.* monocitopenia.

monolayer *n.* monocapa.

mononuclear *adj.* mononuclear.

mononucleosis *n.* mononucleosis.
  cytomegalovirus mononucleosis mononucleosis por citomegalovirus.
  infectious mononucleosis mononucleosis infecciosa.

mononucleotide *n.* mononucleótido.

monoxide *n.* monóxido.

monoxygenase *n.* monoxigenasa.

monozygotic *adj.* monocigótico, -ca.

monozygous *adj.* monocigoto, -ta.

mons mons, monte.
  mons veneris monte de venus.

monster *n.* monstruo.

monstrosity *n.* monstruosidad.

monstrum monstrum, monstruo.

morbid *adj.* mórbido, -da, morboso, -sa.

morbidity *n.* morbididad, morbosidad.

morbility *n.* morbilidad.

morgue *n.* morgue.

moribund *adj.* moribundo, -da.

morphea *n.* morfea.

morphine *n.* morfina.

morphological *adj.* morfológico, -ca.

morphology *n.* morfología.

mortality *n.* mortalidad.

  fetal mortality mortalidad fetal.

  infant mortality mortalidad infantil.

  maternal mortality mortalidad maternal.

  neonatal mortality mortalidad neonatal.

  perinatal mortality mortalidad perinatal.

  prenatal mortality mortalidad prenatal.

mort-aux-rats *n.* raticida.

morula *n.* mórula.

morulation *n.* morulación.

mosaic *n.* mosaico.

  colposcopic mosaic mosaico cervical.

  sex chromosomic mosaic mosaico de cromosomas sexuales.

  sex mosaic mosaico sexual.

mosaicism *n.* mosaicismo, mosaiquismo.

  cellular mosaicism mosaicismo celular.

  chromosome mosaicism mosaicismo cromosómico.

  gene mosaicism mosaicismo de genes.

mother *n.* madre.

  surrogate mother madre de alquiler, madre sustituta.

motherhood *n.* maternidad.

  genetic motherhood maternidad genética.

  gestational motherhood maternidad gestacional.

  legal motherhood maternidad legal.

  surrogate motherhood maternidad de alquiler, maternidad SUBrogada.

motile *adj.* mótil, movible, móvil.

motility *n.* motilidad.

motivation *n.* motivación.

motive *adj.* motivo.

motoneuron *n.* motoneurona.

motoricity *n.* motricidad.

moulting *n.* muda.

mount *n.* monte.

  mount of venus monte de venus.

mourning *n.* duelo.

mouse *n.* ratón.

  nu/nu mouse ratón nu/nu.

mouth *n.* boca.

  denture sore mouth boca lastimada por prótesis, boca ulcerada por dentadura.

  dry mouth boca seca.

  saburral mouth boca saburral.

  sore mouth boca ulcerada.

mouthwash *n.* colutorio, gargarismo.

movement *n.* movimiento.

  active movement movimiento activo.

  associated movement movimiento asociado.

automatic movement movimiento automático.

body movement movimiento corporal.

choreic movement movimiento coreico, movimiento coreiforme.

ciliary movement movimiento ciliar.

circus movement movimiento circular, movimiento de circo.

conjugate movement of the eyes movimiento conjugado de los ojos.

contralateral associated movement movimiento contralateral asociado.

decorticated movement movimiento de decorticación.

decorticated posturing movement movimiento de decorticación.

disconjugate movement of the eyes movimiento no conjugado de los ojos.

dystonic movement movimiento distónico.

fetal movement movimiento fetal.

fixational ocular movement movimiento ocular de fijación.

forced movement movimiento forzado.

hinge movement movimiento en bisagra.

jaw movement movimiento del maxilar inferior, movimiento mandibular.

lateral movement movimiento lateral.

mandibular movement movimiento del maxilar inferior, movimiento mandibular.

masticatory movement movimiento masticatorio.

muscular movement movimiento muscular.

non-rapid eye movement movimiento ocular no rápido.

paradoxical movement of the eyelids movimiento paradójico de los párpados.

passive movement movimiento pasivo.

pendular movement movimiento pendular.

precordial movement movimiento precordial.

rapid eye movement (REM) movimiento ocular rápido.

reflex movement movimiento reflejo.

resistive movement movimiento de resistencia, movimiento resistido.

spontaneous movement movimiento espontáneo.

streaming movement movimiento de corriente, movimiento de flujo.

translatory movement movimiento de traslación, movimiento traslatorio.

mucin *n.* mucina.

mucinosis *n.* mucinosis.

mucionoid *adj.* mucinoide.

mucocele *n.* mucocele.

mucoid *adj.* mucoide.

mucolytic *adj.* mucolítico, -ca.

mucopurulent *adj.* mucopurulento, -ta.

mucosa *n.* mucosa.

mucositis *n.* mucositis.

mucous *adj.* mucoso, -sa.

mucus *n.* moco, mucosidad, mucus.

mulatto *adj., n.* mulato, -ta.

multiarticular *adj.* multiarticular.

multicellular *adj.* multicelular.

multifactorial *adj.* multifactorial.

multifocal *adj.* multifocal.

multigravida *adj.* multigrávida.

multilobar *adj.* multilobular.

multilobular *adj.* multilobulillar.

multipara *adj.* multípara.

multiparity *n.* multiparidad.

multiparous *adj.* multíparo, -ra.

multiple *adj.* múltiple.

multiplication *n.* multiplicación.

multisensitivity *n.* multisensibilidad.

mumps *n.* paperas.

murmur *n.* murmullo, soplo.
  heart murmur soplo cardíaco.

muscarinic *adj.* muscarínico, -ca.

muscarinique *n.* muscarina.

muscle *n.* músculo.
  agonistic muscle músculo agonista.
  antigravity muscle músculo antigravitatorio.
  antagonistic muscle músculo antagonista.
  articular muscle músculo articular.
  extrinsic muscle músculo extrínseco.
  intrafusal muscle músculo intrafusal.
  intrinsic muscle músculo intrínseco.
  involuntary muscle músculo involuntario.
  isometric muscle músculo isométrico.

  myotomic muscle músculo miotómico.
  nonstriated muscle músculo liso.
  prime muscle músculo principal.
  smooth muscle músculo de fibra lisa, músculo liso.
  striated muscle músculo de fibra estriada, músculo estriado.
  synergitic muscle músculo sinérgico.
  voluntary muscle músculo voluntario.

muscular *adj.* muscular.

musculature *n.* musculatura.

musculoaponeurotic *adj.* musculoaponeurótico, -ca.

musculocutaneous *adj.* musculocutáneo, -a.

musculoskeletal *adj.* musculoesquelético, -ca.

musculotendinous *adj.* musculotendinoso, -sa.

musculus *n.* músculo.

musicotherapy *n.* musicoterapia.

mutagen *n.* mutágeno.

mutagenesis *n.* mutagénesis.

mutagenic *adj.* mutagénico, -ca.

mutant *n.* mutante.

mutation *n.* mutación.
  addition-deletion mutation mutación por inserción-deleción.
  allelic mutation mutación alélica.
  back mutation mutación retrógrada.
  chromosomal mutation mutación cromosómica.
  constitutive mutation mutación constitutiva.
  induced mutation mutación inducida.

lethal mutation mutación letal, mutación mortal.

natural mutation mutación natural.

neutral mutation mutación neutra.

reverse mutation mutación corregida, mutación inversa.

silent mutation mutación silente.

somatic mutation mutación somática.

spontaneous mutation mutación espontánea.

supressor mutation mutación supresora.

visible mutation mutación visible.

mute *adj.* mudo, -da.

mutilation *n.* mutilación.

mutism *n.* mutismo.

mutualist *adj.* mutualista.

myalgia *n.* mialgia.

epidemic myalgia mialgia epidémica.

lumbar myalgia mialgia lumbar.

myalgia abdominis mialgia abdominal.

myalgia capitis mialgia cefálica, mialgia craneal.

myalgia cervicalis mialgia cervical.

myalgia thermica mialgia térmica.

myasthenia *n.* miastenia.

myasthenia gravis miastenia grave, miastenia grave seudoparalítica.

myasthenia gravis pseudoparalytica miastenia grave, miastenia grave seudoparalítica.

neonatal myasthenia miastenia neonatal.

myasthenic *adj.* miasténico, -ca.

mycelium *n.* micelio.

aerial mycelium micelio aéreo.

mycobacteria *n.* micobacteria.

mycologist *n.* micólogo, -ga.

mycology *n.* micetología, micología.

mycosis *n.* micetosis, micosis.

mycosis chronica micosis crónica.

mycosis fungoides micosis fungoides.

mycosis intestinalis micosis intestinal, micosis intestinalis.

mycotic *adj.* micótico, -ca.

mydriasis *n.* midriasis, platicoria.

alternating mydriasis midriasis alternante.

amaurotic mydriasis midriasis amaurótica.

paralytic mydriasis midriasis paralítica.

pharmacologic mydriasis midriasis artificial, midriasis farmacológica.

spasmodic mydriasis midriasis espasmódica.

spastic mydriasis midriasis espástica.

spinal mydriasis midriasis espinal.

mydriatic *adj.* midriático, -ca.

myelin *n.* mielina.

myelinated *adj.* mielinado, -da, mielinizado, -da.

myelinic *adj.* mielínico, -ca.

myelinization *n.* mielinización.

myelitis *n.* mielitis.

acute ascending myelitis mielitis ascendente, mielitis ascendente aguda.

acute myelitis mielitis aguda.

acute transverse myelitis mielitis transversa aguda, mielitis transversal aguda.

ascending myelitis mielitis ascendente, mielitis ascendente aguda.

bulbar myelitis mielitis bulbar.

central myelitis mielitis central.

chronic myelitis mielitis crónica.

compression myelitis mielitis por compresión.

concussion myelitis mielitis por concusión, mielitis por conmoción.

descending myelitis mielitis descendente.

diffuse myelitis mielitis difusa.

disseminated myelitis mielitis diseminada.

hemorrhagic myelitis mielitis hemorrágica.

myelitis vaccinia mielitis por vacuna.

neuro-optic myelitis mielitis neuroóptica.

postvaccinal myelitis mielitis por vacuna.

transverse myelitis mielitis transversa, mielitis transversal.

traumatic myelitis mielitis traumática.

myeloblast *n.* mieloblasto.

myelocyte *n.* mielocito.

myeloid *adj.* mieloide, mieloideo, -a.

myeloma *n.* mieloma.

multiple myeloma mieloma múltiple.

plasma cell myeloma mieloma de células plasmáticas.

myelopathy *n.* mielopatía.

myelopoietic *adj.* mielopoyético, -ca.

myeloproliferative *adj.* mieloproliferativo, -va.

myelosis *n.* mielosis.

myelosuppression *n.* mielosupresión.

myelosuppressive *adj.* mielosupresor, -ra.

myoblast *n.* mioblasto.

myocardiac *adj.* miocárdico, -ca.

myocardial *adj.* miocárdico, -ca.

myocardiopathy *n.* miocardiopatía.

alcoholic myocardiopathy miocardiopatía alcohólica.

congestive myocardiopathy miocardiopatía congestiva.

constrictive myocardiopathy miocardiopatía constrictiva.

diabetic myocardiopathy miocardiopatía diabética.

dilated myocardiopathy miocardiopatía dilatada.

hypertrophic myocardiopathy miocardiopatía hipertrófica.

hypertrophic obstructive myocardiopathy miocardiopatía hipertrófica obstructiva.

idiopathic myocardiopathy miocardiopatía idiopática.

infiltrative myocardiopathy miocardiopatía infiltrante.

peripartum myocardiopathy miocardiopatía periparto.

post partum myocardiopathy miocardiopatía posparto.

primary myocardiopathy miocardiopatía primaria.

restrictive myocardiopathy miocardiopatía restrictiva.

secondary myocardiopathy miocardiopatía secundaria.

myocarditis *n.* miocarditis.

acute septic myocarditis miocarditis séptica aguda.

chronic myocarditis miocarditis crónica.

fibrous myocarditis miocarditis fibrosa.

idiopathic myocarditis miocarditis idiopática.

interstitial myocarditis miocarditis intersticial.

rheumatic myocarditis miocarditis reumática.

toxic myocarditis miocarditis tóxica.

tuberculous myocarditis miocarditis tuberculosa.

myocardium *n.* miocardio.

myoclonia *n.* mioclonía.

cortical myoclonia mioclonía cortical.

disseminated myoclonia mioclonía generalizada.

fibrillary myoclonia mioclonía fibrilar.

focal myoclonia mioclonía focal.

multiplex myoclonia mioclonía múltiple.

myoclonia epileptica mioclonía epiléptica.

spinal myoclonia mioclonía espinal.

stimulus sensitive myoclonia mioclonía sensible a los estímulos.

myoclonic *adj.* mioclónico, -ca.

myoclonus *n.* mioclono.

nocturnal myoclonus mioclono nocturno.

myocyte *n.* miocito.

myodystrophia *n.* miodistrofia.

myodystrophy *n.* miodistrofia.

myoglobin *n.* mioglobina.

myoglobinuria *n.* mioglobinuria.

myoglobulin *n.* mioglobulina.

myoglobulinuria *n.* mioglobulinuria.

myogram *n.* miograma.

myoma *n.* mioma.

myopathy *n.* miopatía.

alcoholic myopathy miopatía alcohólica.

mitochondrial myopathy miopatía mitocondrial.

myopathy cordis miopatía cardíaca.

ocular myopathy miopatía ocular.

thyrotoxic myopathy miopatía tirotóxica.

myope *adj.* miope.

myopericarditis *n.* miopericarditis.

myopia *n.* miopía.

chromatic myopia miopía cromática.

curvature myopia miopía de curvatura.

degenerative myopia miopía degenerativa.

malignant myopia miopía maligna, miopía perniciosa.

night myopia miopía nocturna.

pathologic myopia miopía patológica.

premature myopia miopía prematura.

primary myopia miopía primaria.

progressive myopia miopía progresiva.

simple myopia miopía simple.

space myopia miopía espacial.

transient myopia miopía transitoria.

myosis *n.* miosis.
myositis *n.* miositis.
myringitis *n.* miringitis.
myringoplasty *n.* miringoplastia.
myringotomy *n.* miringotomía.
mythomania *n.* mitomanía.
myxedema *n.* mixedema.
pretibial myxedema mixedema pretibial.
myxoma *n.* mixoma.
atrial myxoma mixoma auricular.

N

nacreous *adj.* nacarado, -da.
naevus *n.* naevus, nevo.
naevus cavernosus nevo cavernoso.
naevus pigmentosus nevo pigmentado, nevo pigmentario, nevo pigmentoso.
naevus spilus nevo plano.
nail *n.* clavo, uña.
pitted nail uña con hoyuelos.
spoon nail uña en cuchara.
nailing *n.* enclavamiento.
name *n.* nombre.
generic name nombre genérico.
non-proprietary name nombre no patentado, nombre no registrado.
proprietary name nombre patentado, nombre registrado.
systematic name nombre sistemático.
trivial name nombre trivial, nombre vulgar.

nanism *n.* nanismo.
nape *n.* nuca.
narcissism *n.* narcisismo.
narcissistic *adj.* narcisista.
narcolepsia *n.* narcolepsia.
narcolepsy *n.* narcolepsia.
narcoleptic *adj.* narcoléptico, -ca.
narcosis *n.* narcosis.
narcotic *adj.* narcótico, -ca.
narcotic hypnoytic narcótico hipnótico.
narcotic sedative narcótico sedante.
narcotize *v.* narcotizar.
nasal *adj.* nasal.
nasalis *adj.* nasal.
nasolabial *adj.* nasolabial.
nasolacrimal *adj.* nasolacrimal, nasolagrimal.
nasonnement *n.* nasalidad.
naso-oral *adj.* nasobucal, nasooral.
nasopharyngeal *adj.* nasofaríngeo,.
nasopharyngitis *n.* nasofaringitis.
nasopharynx *n.* nasofaringe.
nasus nariz, nasus.
natal *adj.* natal.
natality *n.* natalidad.
native *adj.* nativo, -va.
natremia *n.* natremia.
natriemia *n.* natremia.
natriuresis *n.* natriuresis, natruresis.
natriuretic *adj.* natriurético, -ca.
natruresis *n.* natruresis.
natruretic *adj.* natriurético, -ca.
natural *adj.* natural.
nature *n.* naturaleza.
naturopath *n.* naturópata.
naturopathic *adj.* naturopático, -ca.
naturopathy *n.* naturopatía.

nausea *n.* náusea.

  nausea gravidarum náusea gravídica.

  nausea marina náusea marítima, náusea naval.

nauseant *adj.* nauseabundo, -da, nauseante.

navel *n.* ombligo.

nebulization *n.* nebulización.

nebulize *v.* nebulizar.

nebulizer *n.* nebulizador.

necessity *n.* necesidad.

  basic human necessity necesidad básica.

neck *n.* cuello.

necrobiosis *n.* necrobiosis.

necrology *n.* necrología.

necrophile *n.* necrófilo.

necrophilia *n.* necrofilia.

necrophilous *adj.* necrófilo, -la.

necrophily *n.* necrofilia.

necrosis *n.* necrosis.

  caseation necrosis necrosis caseosa.

  caseous necrosis necrosis caseosa.

  cheesy necrosis necrosis caseosa.

  gangrenous necrosis necrosis gangrenosa.

  peripheral necrosis necrosis periférica.

  pressure necrosis necrosis por presión.

  total necrosis necrosis total.

necrotizing *adj.* necrosante, necrotizante.

need *n.* necesidad.

needle *n.* aguja.

  aspirating needle a. de aspiración, aguja aspiradora, aguja aspirante.

  aspiration needle a. de aspiración, aguja aspiradora, aguja aspirante.

  biopsy needle aguja de corte, aguja gruesa, aguja para biopsia.

  fine needle aguja fina.

  hypodermic needle aguja hipodérmica.

  intramuscular needle aguja intramuscular.

  intravenous needle aguja endovenosa, aguja intravenosa.

  knife needle aguja de bisturí, aguja-cuchilla.

  skinny needle aguja cutánea.

needle-carrier *n.* portaagujas.

needle-driver *n.* portaagujas.

needle-holder *n.* portaagujas.

negation *n.* negación.

negative *adj.* negativo, -va.

negativism *n.* negativismo.

negativity *n.* negatividad.

negligence *n.* negligencia.

neisserial *adj.* neissérico, -ca.

neoformation *n.* neoformación.

neonatal *adj.* neonatal.

neonate *n.* neonato.

  malformed neonate neonato malformado.

neonatologist *n.* neonatólogo, -ga.

neonatology *n.* neonatología.

neoplasia *n.* neoplasia.

  benign neoplasia neoplasia benigna.

  malignant neoplasia neoplasia maligna.

  mixed neoplasia neoplasia mixta.

  multiple endocrine neoplasia neoplasia endocrina múltiple.

  type I neoplasia neoplasia endocrina múltiple, tipo I.

type II neoplasia neoplasia endocrina múltiple, tipo II.

type III neoplasia neoplasia endocrina múltiple, tipo III.

neoplastic *adj.* neoplásico.

nephrectomize *v.* nefrectomizar.

nephrectomy *n.* nefrectomía.

nephric *adj.* néfrico, -ca.

nephritis *n.* nefritis, renitis.

acute interstitial nephritis nefritis intersticial aguda.

acute nephritis nefritis aguda.

acute tubulointerstitial nephritis nefritis tubulointersticial aguda.

analgesic nephritis nefritis por analgésicos.

anti-basement membrane nephritis nefritis antimembrana basal.

arteriosclerotic nephritis nefritis arteriosclerótica.

azotemic nephritis nefritis hiperazoémica.

bacterial nephritis nefritis bacteriana.

capsular nephritis nefritis capsular.

caseous nephritis nefritis caseosa.

cheesy nephritis nefritis caseosa.

chronic nephritis nefritis crónica.

congenital nephritis nefritis congénita.

focal nephritis nefritis focal.

glomerular nephritis nefritis glomerular.

glomerulocapsular nephritis nefritis glomerulocapsular.

hemorrhagic nephritis nefritis hemorrágica.

hereditary nephritis nefritis hereditaria.

immune complex nephritis nefritis por inmunocomplejos.

infective tubulointerstitial nephritis nefritis tubulointersticial infecciosa.

interstitial nephritis nefritis intersticial.

lupus nephritis nefritis del lupus, nefritis lúpica.

mesangial nephritis nefritis mesangial.

nephritis caseosa nefritis caseosa.

nephritis of pregnancy nefritis del embarazo.

parenchymatous nephritis nefritis parenquimatosa.

potassium-losing nephritis nefritis crónica por pérdida de potasio.

tubal nephritis nefritis tubular.

tubular nephritis nefritis tubular.

tubulointerstitial nephritis nefritis tubulointersticial.

nephrogenetic *adj.* nefrogenético, -ca, nefrogénico, -ca, nefrógeno, -na.

nephrolithotomy *n.* nefrolitotomía.

nephrologist *n.* nefrólogo, -ga.

nephrology *n.* nefrología.

nephron *n.* nefrón, nefrona.

nephropathia *n.* nefropatía.

nephropathy *n.* nefropatía.

analgesic nephropathy nefropatía por analgésicos.

chronic nephropathy nefropatía crónica.

hypokalemic nephropathy nefropatía hipopotasémica.

IgA nephropathy nefropatía por IgA.

IgM nephropathy nefropatía por IgM.

potassium-losing nephropathy nefropatía con pérdida de potasio.

reflux nephropathy nefropatía de reflujo, nefropatía por reflujo.

salt-losing nephropathy nefropatía con pérdida de sal.

transfusion nephropathy nefropatía postransfusional.

nephroscleria *n.* nefroesclerosis.

nephrosclerosis *n.* nefroesclerosis, nefrosclerosis.

nephrosclerotic *adj.* nefroesclerótico, -ca.

nephroscopy *n.* nefroscopia.

nephrosis *n.* nefrosis.

nephrostomy *n.* nefrostomía.

nephrotic *adj.* nefrótico, -ca.

nephrotoxic *adj.* nefrotóxico, -ca.

nephrotoxicity *n.* nefrotoxicidad.

nerve *n.* nervio.

sixth cranial nerve sexto par craneal.

nervosism *n.* nerviosismo.

nervous *adj.* nervioso, -sa.

nervousness *n.* nerviosismo.

nervus nervio, nervus.

nest *n.* nido.

net *n.* red.

nettle *n.* ortiga.

neural *adj.* neural.

neuralgia *n.* neuralgia.

cranial neuralgia neuralgia craneal.

sciatic neuralgia neuralgia ciática.

trigeminal neuralgia neuralgia del trigémino.

neuralgic *adj.* neurálgico, -ca.

neurasthenia *n.* neurastenia.

neurasthenic *adj.* neurasténico, -ca.

neurectomy *n.* neurectomía.

neurinoma *n.* neurinoma.

acoustic neurinoma neurinoma acústico.

trigeminal neurinoma neurinoma del trigémino.

neurit *n.* neurita.

neurite *n.* neurita.

neuritic *adj.* neurítico, -ca.

neuritis *n.* neuritis.

axial neuritis neuritis axial, neuritis axonal.

central neuritis neuritis central.

disseminated neuritis neuritis diseminada.

facial neuritis neuritis facial.

interstitial neuritis neuritis intersticial.

intraocular neuritis neuritis intraocular.

optic neuritis neuritis óptica.

retrobulbar neuritis neuritis retrobulbar.

neuroanastomosis *n.* neuroanastomosis.

neuroanatomy *n.* neuroanatomía.

neurobiologist *n.* neurobiólogo, -ga.

neurobiology *n.* neurobiología.

neurodermatitis *n.* neurodermatitis.

neuroectomy *n.* neurectomía, neuroectomía.

neuroglia *n.* neuroglía.

neurohormonal *adj.* neurohormonal.

neurohormone *n.* neurohormona.

neurohypophyseal *adj.* neurohipofisario, -a.

neurohypophysis *n.* neurohipófisis.

neurologic *adj.* neurológico, -ca.

neurologist *n.* neurólogo, -ga.

neurology *n.* neurología.

neuroma *n.* neuroma.

neuromuscular *adj.* neuromuscular.

neuron *n.* neurona.
 afferent neuron neurona aferente.
 efferent neuron neurona eferente.
 motor neuron neurona motora.
 postganglionic neuron neurona posganglionar.
 preganglionic neuron neurona preganglionar.
 sensory neuron neurona sensitiva, neurona sensorial.

neuronal *adj.* neuronal.

neuroncology *n.* neuroncología.

neurone *n.* neurona.

neuropathy *n.* neuropatía.
 diabetic neuropathy neuropatía diabética.

neurophysiologist *n.* neurofisiólogo, -ga.

neurophysiology *n.* neurofisiología.

neuropsychiatry *n.* neuropsiquiatría.

neuropsychology *n.* neuropsicología.

neurosciences *n.* neurociencias.

neuroscientist *n.* neurocientífico, -ca.

neurosis *n.* neurosis.

neurostimulation *n.* neuroestimulación.

neurostimulator *n.* neuroestimulador.

neurosurgeon *n.* neurocirujano.

neurosurgery *n.* neurocirugía.

neurosyphilis *n.* neurosífilis.

neurotic *adj.* neurótico, -ca.

neurotoxic *adj.* neurotóxico, -ca.

neurotoxicity *n.* neurotoxicidad.

neurotransmission *n.* neurotransmisión.

neurotransmitter *n.* neurotransmisor.

neutral *adj.* neutral, neutro, -tra.

neutralization *n.* neutralización.
 viral neutralization neutralización viral.

neutralize *v.* neutralizar.

neutropenia *n.* neutropenia.
 congenital neutropenia neutropenia congénita.
 periodic neutropenia neutropenia periódica.

neutrophil *n.* neutrófilo.
 band neutrophil neutrófilo en banda.
 hypersegmented neutrophil neutrófilo hipersegmentado.
 immature neutrophil neutrófilo inmaduro.
 mature neutrophil neutrófilo maduro.
 segmented neutrophil neutrófilo segmentado.

neutrophilia *n.* neutrofilia.

nevus *n.* naevus, nevo.
 acquired nevus nevo adquirido.
 Becker's nevus nevo de Becker.
 blue nevus nevo ampolla de forma azul, nevo azul.
 capillary nevus nevo capilar.
 congenital nevus nevo congénito.
 epidermal nevus nevo epidérmico.
 giant congenital pigmented ne

vus nevo gigante congénito pigmentado.

   pigmented nevus nevo pigmentado, nevo pigmentario, nevo pigmentoso.

   spider nevus nevo en araña.

newborn *n.* recién nacido.

nexus nexo, nexus.

nick *n.* muesca.

nicotinamide *n.* nicotinamida.

nicotine *n.* nicotina.

nidus *n.* nido.

nightmare *n.* pesadilla.

nipple *n.* pezón.

nitrogen *n.* nitrógeno.

nitrogenous *adj.* nitrogenado, -da.

nocardiosis *n.* nocardiosis.

nociception *n.* nocicepción.

nociceptive *adj.* nociceptivo, -va.

nociceptor *n.* nociceptor.

noctambulic *adj.* noctámbulo, -la.

noctambulism *n.* noctambulismo.

nocturia *n.* nicturia, nocturia.

nocturnal *adj.* nocturno, -na.

nodal *adj.* nodal.

node *n.* nódulo, nudo.

   atrioventricular node nódulo auriculoventricular.

   singer's node nódulo de cantante.

   sinoatrial node nódulo sinoauricular, nódulo sinusal.

   sinoauricular node nódulo sinoauricular, nódulo sinusal.

   syncytial node nudo sincitial.

   syphilitic node nódulo sifilítica.

nodular *adj.* nodular.

nodulate *adj.* nodulado, -da.

nodulated *adj.* nodulado, -da.

nodulation *n.* nodulación.

nodule *n.* nódulo.

nodulitis *n.* nodulitis.

nodulosis *n.* nodulosis.

nodulus nódulo, nodulus.

nodus nodus, nudo.

noise *n.* ruido.

   ambient noise ruido ambiental.

nomenclature *n.* nomenclatura.

non-adherent *adj.* no adherente.

non-antigenic *adj.* no antigénico, -ca.

non-disease *n.* no enfermedad.

non-immune *adj.* no inmune.

non-infectious *adj.* no infeccioso, -sa.

non-invasive *adj.* no invasivo, -va.

non-neoplastic *adj.* no neoplásico, -ca.

non-specific *adj.* inespecífico, -ca.

non-vascular *adj.* no vascular.

non-viable *adj.* inviable, no viable.

norma *n.* norma.

normal *adj.* normal.

normality *n.* normalidad.

normalization *n.* normalización.

normalize *v.* normalizar.

normoblast *n.* normoblasto.

normochromia *n.* normocromía.

normochromic *adj.* normocrómico.

nose *n.* nariz.

   hammer nose nariz en martillo.

   saddle nose nariz en silla de montar.

   saddle-back nose nariz en dorso de silla de montar.

   toper's nose nariz de bebedor.

   upturned nose nariz respingona.

nosebleed *n.* epistaxis.

nosocomial *adj.* nosocomial.

nosology n. nosología.
notch n. escotadura, muesca.
notochord n. notocorda, notocordio.
noxa n. noxa.
noxious adj. nocivo, -va.
nucha n. nuca.
nuchal adj. nucal.
nuclear adj. nuclear.
nucleated adj. nucleado, -da.
nucleation n. nucleación.
nucleolus n. nucléolo.
nucleotide n. nucleótido.
nucleus núcleo, nucleus.
nulligravida n. nuligrávida.
nullipara n. nulípara.
nulliparity n. nuliparidad.
number n. número.
numbness n. adormecimiento, entumecimiento.
numerical adj. numérico, -ca.
nurse n. enfermero, -ra.
nursing n. enfermería.
nutrient n. nutriente.
nutrition n. nutrición.
  adequate nutrition nutrición adecuada.
  parenteral nutrition nutrición parenteral.
  total parenteral nutrition (tpn) nutrición parenteral total (npt).
nutritional adj. nutricional.
nutritive adj. alimenticio, -cia, nutritivo, -va.
nystagmus nistagmo, nistagmus.
  central nystagmus nistagmo central.
  congenital hereditary nystagmus nistagmo congénito.

congenital nystagmus nistagmo congénito.
conjugate nystagmus nistagmo conjugado.
convergence nystagmus nistagmo convergente.
dissociated nystagmus nistagmo disociado.
lateral nystagmus nistagmo lateral.
ocular nystagmus nistagmo ocular.

O

oath n. juramento.
  hippocratic oath juramento de Hipócrates, juramento hipocrático.
  oath of Hippocrates juramento de Hipócrates, juramento hipocrático.
obese adj. obeso, -sa.
obesity n. obesidad.
  cushingoid obesity obesidad cushingoide.
  morbid obesity obesidad mórbida.
  truncal obesity obesidad troncular.
obfuscation n. obfuscación, ofuscación, ofuscamiento.
object n. objeto.
objective n. objetivo.
obligate adj. obligado, -da.
obliquity n. oblicuidad.
oblongata adj. oblongada.
observer n. observador.
obsession n. obsesión.
obsessive adj. obsesivo, -va.
obsessive-compulsive adj. obsesivo-compulsivo, -va.

obstetric *adj.* obstétrico, -ca.
obstetrical *adj.* obstétrico, -ca.
obstetrician *n.* obstetra, tocólogo, -ga.
obstetrics *n.* obstetricia.
obstruction *n.* obstrucción.
  airway obstruction obstrucción de la vía aérea.
  biliary obstruction obstrucción biliar.
  chronic airway obstruction obstrucción crónica de las vías respiratorias.
  foreign body obstruction obstrucción por cuerpo extraño.
  intestinal obstruction obstrucción intestinal.
  nasal obstruction obstrucción nasal.
  retinal central arterial obstruction obstrucción de la arteria central de la retina.
  upper airway obstruction (UAO) obstrucción de las vías respiratorias superiores (OVRS).
obstructive *adj.* obstructivo, -va.
obturation *n.* obturación.
  canal obturation obturación de un canal, obturación de un conducto.
occipital *adj.* occipital.
occipitalis *adj.* occipital, occipitalis.
occlude *v.* ocluir.
occluded *adj.* ocluido, -da.
occlusal *adj.* oclusal, oclusional.
occlusion *n.* oclusión.
  abnormal occlusion oclusión anormal.
  anatomic occlusion oclusión anatómica.

  physiologic occlusion oclusión fisiológica.
  physiological occlusion oclusión fisiológica.
occupancy *n.* ocupación.
ocellus *n.* ocelo.
ocular *adj.* ocular.
oculist *n.* oculista.
oculus oculus, ojo.
odontalgia *n.* odontalgia.
odontoid *adj.* odontoide, odontoides.
odontologist *n.* odontólogo, -ga.
odontology *n.* odontología.
odor odor, olor.
  body odor olor corporal.
  minimal identifiable odor olor mínimo identificable.
odorous *adj.* oloroso, -sa.
odynolysis *n.* odinólisis.
odynophagia *n.* odinofagia.
odynophobia *n.* odinofobia.
odynophonia *n.* odinofonía.
odynphagia *n.* odinofagia.
Oestridae Oestridae.
official *adj.* oficial.
oil *n.* aceite.
oily *adj.* oleoso, -sa.
ointment *n.* pomada, ungüento, unguentum.
  eye ointment ungüento ocular, ungüento oftálmico.
  ophthalmic ointment ungüento ocular, ungüento oftálmico.
oleaginous *adj.* oleaginoso, -sa.
olecranon *n.* olécrano, olécranon.
oleosus *adj.* oleoso, -sa.
olfact *n.* olfato.
olfactus *n.* olfato.

oligoamnios *n.* oligoamnios.

oligodendrocyte *n.* oligodendrocito.

oligonephronic *adj.* oligonefrónico, -ca.

oligophrenia *n.* oligofrenia.

oligophrenic *adj.* oligofrénico, -ca.

oligosaccharide *n.* oligosacárido.

oliguria *n.* oliguria.

oliguric *adj.* oligúrico, -ca.

omentitis *n.* omentitis.

omentum *n.* epiplón, omento.

omission *n.* omisión.

oncogene *n.* oncogén, oncogene.

oncogenesis *n.* oncogenesia, oncogénesis, oncogenia.

oncogenic *adj.* oncogénico, -ca.

oncologist *n.* oncólogo, -ga.
  radiation oncologist oncólogo radioterapeuta.

oncology *n.* oncología.
  radiation oncology oncología radioterápica.

one-armed *adj.* manco, -ca.

one-eyed *adj.* tuerto, -ta.

oneiric *adj.* onírico, -ca.

onychia *n.* oniquia.

onychomycosis *n.* onicomicosis.

oocyte *n.* oocito.
  primary oocyte oocito de primer orden, oocito primario.
  secondary oocyte oocito de segundo orden, oocito secundario.

oophorectomy *n.* ooforectomía.

oophoritis *n.* ooforitis.

opacification *n.* opacamiento, opacificación.

opacified *adj.* opacificado, -da.

opaque *adj.* opaco, -ca.

operable *adj.* operable.

operate *v.* operar.

operation *n.* operación.
  cesarean operation operación cesárea.
  Juvara's operation operación de Juvara.
  minor operation operación menor.
  open operation operación abierta.
  Trendelenburg's operation operación de Trendelenburg.

ophthalmia *n.* oftalmía.

ophthalmic *adj.* oftálmico, -ca.

ophthalmodynamometer *n.* oftalmodinamómetro.

ophthalmologic *adj.* oftalmológico, -ca.

ophthalmological *adj.* oftalmológico, -ca.

ophthalmologist *n.* oftalmólogo, -ga.

ophthalmology *n.* oftalmología.

ophthalmopathy *n.* oftalmopatía.

ophthalmoplegia *n.* oftalmoplejía.

ophthalmoplegic *adj.* oftalmopléjico, -ca.

ophthalmoscope *n.* oftalmoscopio.

ophthalmoscopy *n.* oftalmoscopia.

opiate *adj.* opiáceo, -a, opiado, -da.

opioid *n.* opioide.

opisthotonos *n.* opistótonos.

opisthotonus *n.* opistótonos.

opium opio, opium.

opponens *adj.* oponente.

opportunistic *adj.* oportunista.

opposing *adj.* oponente.

opsonin *n.* opsonina.

optic *adj.* óptico, -ca.

optical *adj.* óptico, -ca.

tician *n.* óptico, -ca.

ticist *n.* óptico, -ca.

timal *adj.* óptimo, -ma.

timism *n.* optimismo.

timum óptimo, optimum.

tist *n.* óptico, -ca.

ptometrist *n.* optometrista.

ptometry *n.* optometría.

ral *adj.* oral.

rale *n.* oral.

range *n.* naranja.

rbicular *adj.* orbicular.

rbicularis orbicular, orbicularis.

rbit *n.* órbita.

rbita *n.* órbita.

rbitalis *adj.* orbitario, -ria.

rchectomy *n.* orquectomía.

rchialgia *n.* orquialgia.

rchidectomy *n.* orquidectomía.

orchiditis *n.* orquiditis.

orchiectomy *n.* orquectomía, orquiectomía.

orchiepididymitis *n.* orquidoepididimitis, orquiepididimitis, orquioepididimitis.

orchitis *n.* orquitis.

order *n.* orden.

DNR order orden de no reanimación, orden de no resucitar.

do-not-resuscitate-without-consent order orden de no reanimación sin consentimiento.

do-not-resuscitate order orden de no reanimación, orden de no resucitar.

rdinate *n.* ordenada.

rgan *n.* órgano.

accessory organ órgano accesorio.

acoustic organ órgano acústico.

Corti's organ órgano de Corti.

digestive organ órgano digestivo.

end organ órgano final, órgano terminal.

external genital organ órgano genital externo.

extraperitoneal organ órgano extraperitoneal.

female genital organ órgano genital femenino.

female reproductive organ órgano reproductor femenino.

floating organ órgano flotante.

gustatory organ órgano del gusto, órgano gustativo, órgano gustatorio.

internal genital organ órgano genital interno.

lymphatic organ órgano linfático.

lymphoid organ órgano linfoide.

male genital organ órgano genital masculino.

male reproductive organ órgano reproductor del varón.

olfactory organ órgano del olfato, órgano olfatorio.

organ of Corti órgano de Corti.

organ of hearing órgano de la audición.

organ of smell órgano del olfato, órgano olfatorio.

organ of taste órgano del gusto, órgano gustativo, órgano gustatorio.

organ of touch órgano del tacto.

organ of vision órgano de la visión, órgano visual.

ptotic organ órgano ptótico.

reproductive organ órgano reproductor.

retroperitoneal organ órgano retroperitoneal.

sense organ órgano de los sentidos, órgano de un sentido, órgano sensorial.

sensory organ órgano de los sentidos, órgano sensorial.

target organ órgano blanco, órgano diana.

taste organ órgano del gusto, órgano gustativo, órgano gustatorio.

terminal organ órgano terminal.

touch receptor organ órgano del tacto.

urinary organ órgano urinario.

vestibular organ órgano vestibular.

vestibulocochlear organ órgano vestibulococlear.

vestigial organ órgano vestigial.

visual organ órgano de la visión, órgano visual.

wandering organ órgano errante.

organella *n.* organela, organelo.

organelle *n.* organela, organelo.

organic *adj.* orgánico, -ca.

organism *n.* organismo.

organization *n.* organización.

organizer *n.* organizador, -ra.

organogenesis *n.* organogenesia, organogénesis.

organon *n.* órgano.

organon gustus órgano del gusto, órgano gustativo, órgano gustatorio.

organon olfactus órgano del olfato, órgano olfatorio.

organotherapy *n.* organoterapia.

organ-specific *adj.* organoespecífico.

organum *n.* órgano.

organum auditus órgano auditivo.

organum extraperitoneale órgano extraperitoneal.

organum gustatorium órgano del gusto, órgano gustativo, órgano gustatorio.

organum gustus órgano del gusto, órgano gustativo, órgano gustatorio.

organum olfactorium órgano del olfato, órgano olfatorio.

organum olfactus órgano del olfato, órgano olfatorio.

organum retroperitoneale órgano retroperitoneal.

organum tactus órgano del tacto.

organum vestibulocochleare órgano vestibulococlear.

organum visuale órgano de la visión, órgano visual.

organum visus órgano de la visión, órgano visual.

orgasm *n.* orgasmo.

orgasmic *adj.* orgásmico, -ca, orgástico, -ca.

orient *v.* orientar.

orientation *n.* orientación.

sexual orientation orientación sexual.

orifice *n.* orificio.

orificium *n.* orificio.

origin *n.* origen.

ornithine *n.* ornitina.

oropharyngeal *adj.* orofaríngeo, -a.

oropharynx *n.* mesofaringe, orofaringe.

orthesis *n.* ortesis.

orthodontia *n.* ortodoncia.

orthodontics *n.* ortodoncia.

corrective orthodontics ortodoncia correctiva.

preventive orthodontics ortodoncia preventiva.

prophylactic orthodontics ortodoncia preventiva.

surgical orthodontics ortodoncia quirúrgica.

orthodontist *adj.* ortodentista, ortodontista, ortodontista.

orthognathics *n.* ortognática.

orthopedic *adj.* ortopédico, -ca.

orthopedics *n.* ortopedia.

orthopod *n.* ortopeda.

orthostatic *adj.* ortostático, -ca.

orthostatism *n.* bipedestación, ortostatismo.

os *n.* boca, hueso, os.

oscillation *n.* oscilación.

oscillatory *adj.* oscilatorio, -ria.

osmolality *n.* osmolalidad.

osmolar *adj.* osmolar.

osmolarity *n.* osmolaridad.

blood osmolarity osmolaridad sanguínea.

serum osmolarity osmolaridad del suero, osmolaridad sérica.

urine osmolarity osmolaridad de la orina, osmolaridad urinaria.

osmosis *n.* osmosis, ósmosis.

osmosity *n.* osmosidad.

ossature *n.* osamenta.

osseocartilaginous *adj.* oseocartilaginoso, -sa.

osseous *adj.* óseo, -a.

ossicle *n.* huesecillo, osículo.

ossification *n.* osificación.

ossify *v.* osificar.

ostearthritis *n.* osteartritis.

osteitis *n.* osteítis.

osteitis deformans osteítis deformante.

osteoarthritis *n.* osteoartritis.

osteoarthrosis *n.* osteoartrosis.

osteoarticular *adj.* osteoarticular.

osteoblast *n.* osteoblasto.

osteochondritis *n.* osteocondritis.

osteochondrosis *n.* osteocondrosis.

osteocyte *n.* osteocito.

osteodystrophia *n.* osteodistrofia.

osteodystrophy *n.* osteodistrofia.

osteoma *n.* osteoma.

osteomalacia *n.* osteomalacia.

osteomyelitis *n.* osteomielitis.

osteopath *n.* osteópata.

osteopathia *n.* osteopatía.

osteopathy *n.* osteopatía.

osteopenia *n.* osteopenia.

osteophyte *n.* osteófito.

osteoporosis *n.* osteoporosis.

postmenopausal osteoporosis osteoporosis posmenopáusica.

senile osteoporosis osteoporosis senil.

osteoporotic *adj.* osteoporótico, -ca.

osteosarcoma *n.* osteosarcoma.

osteosclerosis *n.* osteoesclerosis.

osteosis *n.* osteosis.

osteosynthesis *n.* osteosíntesis.

osteotomy *n.* osteotomía.

ostomate *adj.* ostomado, -da, ostomizado, -da.

ostomy *n.* ostomía.

otalgia *n.* otalgia.

otic *adj.* ótico, -ca.

otitic *adj.* otítico, -ca.

otitis *n.* otitis.

external otitis otitis externa.

otitis externa otitis externa.

otitis interna otitis interna.

otitis media otitis media.

otitis mycotica otitis micótica.

otor *adj.* ótico, -ca.

otorhinolaryngologist *n.* otorrino-laringólogo, -ga.

otorhinolaryngology *n.* otorrino-laringología.

otorrhagia *n.* otorragia.

otorrhea *n.* otorrea.

otoscope *n.* otoscopio.

outlet *n.* salida.

outlier *n.* dato aberrante.

output *n.* gasto, salidas.
  cardiac output gasto cardíaco.

oval *adj.* oval, ovalado, -da.

ovalbumin *n.* ovalbúmina.

ovarian *adj.* ovárico, -ca.

ovariectomy *n.* ovariectomía.

ovarium ovario, ovarium.

ovary *n.* ovario.
  polycystic ovary ovario poliquístico.

overdosage *n.* sobredosificación.

overdose *n.* sobredosis.

overfeeding *n.* sobrealimentación.

overlap *n.* superposición.

overlay *n.* añadido.
  functional overlay cobertura funcional.

overloading *n.* sobrecarga.

overriding *n.* cabalgamiento.

oversampling *n.* superposición.

ovicidal *adj.* ovicida.

ovicide *n.* ovicida.

ovocyte *n.* ovocito.

ovogenesis *n.* ovogenesia, ovogénesis.

ovulation *n.* ovulación.
  amenstrual ovulation ovulación amenstrual.

ovulatory *adj.* ovulativo, -va, ovulatorio, -ria.

ovule *n.* óvulo,.
  Graafian ovule óvulo de Graaf.
  primordial ovule óvulo primordial.

ovum *n.* huevo, óvulo,, ovum.
  fertilized ovum óvulo fecundado, óvulo fertilizado.
  primordial ovum óvulo primordial.
  vaginal ovum óvulo vaginal.

oxidation *n.* oxidación.
  fatty acid oxidation oxidación de ácidos grasos.

oxide *n.* óxido.

oxidized *adj.* oxidado, -da.

oxygen *n.* oxígeno.

oxygenate *v.* oxigenar.

oxygenated *adj.* oxigenado, -da.

oxygenation *n.* oxigenación.
  extracorporeal oxygenation oxigenación extracorpórea.

oxygentherapy *n.* oxigenoterapia.

oxyhemoglobin *n.* oxihemoglobina.

oxytocic *adj.* oxitócico, -ca.

oxytocin (OXT) *n.* oxitocina (OXT).

ozena *n.* ocena, ozena.

ozone *n.* ozono.

P

pacemaker *n.* marcapaso, marcapasos.
  ectopic pacemaker marcapaso ectópico.
  external pacemaker marcapaso externo.

wandering pacemaker marcapaso errante, marcapaso migratorio.

pachymeningitis *n.* paquimeningitis.

pachymeninx *n.* paquimeninge.

pack *n.* envoltura, taponamiento.

packing *n.* empacamiento, taponamiento.

nasal packing taponamiento nasal.

pad *n.* almohadilla.

buccal fat pad almohadilla grasa bucal.

fat pad almohadilla adiposa, almohadilla grasa.

kidney pad almohadilla renal.

pain *n.* algia, dolor.

abdominal pain dolor abdominal.

acute pain dolor agudo.

burning pain dolor urente.

chronic pain dolor crónico.

dull pain dolor sordo.

epigastric pain dolor epigástrico.

girdle pain dolor en cinturón.

intermenstrual pain dolor intermenstrual.

labor pain dolor de parto.

low back pain dolor de la región inferior de la espalda, lumbalgia.

referred pain dolor referido.

pairing *n.* apareamiento.

base pairing apareamiento de bases.

chromosome pairing apareamiento de los cromosomas.

random pairing apareamiento al azar.

palate *n.* paladar.

cleft palate paladar fisurado, paladar hendido.

falling palate paladar caído.

palatine *adj.* palatino, -na.

palatum paladar, palatum.

palliate *v.* paliar.

palliative *adj.* paliativo, -va.

pallor *n.* palidez.

palm *n.* palma.

palmar *adj.* palmar.

palpable *adj.* palpable.

palpation *n.* palpación.

bimanual palpation palpación bimanual.

palpebra *n.* párpado.

palpebral *adj.* palpebral.

palpebritis *n.* palpebritis.

palpitation *n.* palpitación.

paludal *adj.* palúdico, -ca.

panarteritis *n.* panarteritis.

panarthritis *n.* panartritis.

pancreas *n.* páncreas.

pancreatitis *n.* pancreatitis.

acute pancreatitis pancreatitis aguda.

pancytopenia *n.* pancitopenia.

pandemia *n.* pandemia.

pandemic *adj.* pandémico, -ca.

panencephalitis *n.* panencefalitis.

panic *n.* pánico.

panniculitis *n.* paniculitis.

pannus pannus, paño.

pant *v.* jadear.

panting *n.* jadeo.

papilla *n.* papila.

papillary *adj.* papilar.

papillate *adj.* papilar.

papilledema *n.* papiledema.

papillitis *n.* papilitis.

papilloma *n.* papiloma.

papilloma acuminatum papiloma acuminado.

papilloma venereum papiloma venéreo.

papule *n.* pápula.

paracentesis *n.* paracentesis.

abdominal paracentesis paracentesis abdominal.

paracentesis oculi paracentesis ocular.

tympanic paracentesis paracentesis timpánica.

paracusia *n.* paracusia.

paracusis *n.* paracusia, paracusis.

paradox *n.* paradoja.

paralysis *n.* parálisis.

bulbar paralysis parálisis bulbar.

central paralysis parálisis central.

centrocortical paralysis parálisis centrocortical.

cerebral paralysis parálisis cerebral.

emotional paralysis parálisis emocional.

incomplete paralysis parálisis incompleta.

infantile paralysis parálisis infantil.

obstetrical paralysis parálisis obstétrica.

ocular paralysis parálisis ocular.

paralyzant *n.* paralizador, -ra, paralizante.

parameter *n.* parámetro.

parametritis *n.* parametritis.

parametrium *n.* parametrio.

paranoia *n.* paranoia.

paranoiac *adj.* paranoico, -ca.

paranoid *adj.* paranoide.

paranormal *adj.* paranormal.

paraparesis *n.* paraparesia.

paraplectic *adj.* parapléjico, -ca.

paraplegia *n.* paraplejía.

ataxic paraplegia paraplejía atáxica.

cerebral paraplegia paraplejía cerebral.

spastic paraplegia paraplejía espástica.

paraplegic *adj.* parapléjico, -ca.

parasite *n.* parásito.

obligate parasite parásito obligado.

parasitemia *n.* parasitemia.

parasitic *adj.* parasitario, -ria, parasítico, -ca.

parasiticidal *adj.* parasiticida.

parasiticide *n.* parasiticida.

parasitologist *n.* parasitólogo, -ga.

parasitology *n.* parasitología.

parasitosis *n.* parasitosis.

parasternal *adj.* paraesternal.

parasympathetic *adj.* parasimpático, -ca.

parasympatholytic *adj.* parasimpaticolítico, -ca.

parasympathomimetic *adj.* parasimpaticomimético, -ca.

parathyroid *adj.* paratiroideo, -a, paratiroides.

paravertebral *adj.* paravertebral.

parenchyma *n.* parénquima.

parental *adj.* parental.

parenteral *adj.* parenteral, parentérico, -ca.

paresis *n.* paresia.

paresthesia *n.* parestesia.

parietal *adj.* parietal.

parity *n.* paridad.
parodontitis *n.* parodontitis.
parotid *adj.* parótida, parotídeo, -a.
parotidectomy *n.* parotidectomía.
parotiditis *n.* parotiditis.
pars *n.* pars, parte.
part *n.* parte.
particle *n.* partícula.
partition *n.* tabique.
parturient *adj.* parturienta.
partus *n.* parto.
parvule *adj.* párvulo, -la.
passage *n.* paso.
passion *n.* pasión.
passive *adj.* pasivo, -va.
paste *n.* pasta.
pasteurization *n.* pasteurización.
patch *n.* placa.
  mucous patch placa mucosa.
patella *n.* patela, rótula.
patellar *adj.* patelar.
paternalism *n.* paternalismo.
path *n.* trayecto, vía.
pathetic *adj.* patético, -ca.
pathogen *n.* patógeno.
pathogenic *adj.* patógeno, -na.
pathogenicity *n.* patogenicidad.
pathogeny *n.* patogénesis, patogenia.
pathologic *adj.* patológico, -ca.
pathological *adj.* patológico, -ca.
pathologist *n.* patólogo, -ga.
  speech-language pathologist logopeda.
pathology *n.* patología.
  cellular pathology patología celular.
  clinical pathology patología clínica.
  comparative pathology patología comparada.
  dental pathology patología dental.
  experimental pathology patología experimental.
  external pathology patología externa.
  functional pathology patología funcional.
  general pathology patología general.
  internal pathology patología interna.
  medical pathology patología médica.
  mental pathology patología mental.
  speech pathology logopedia.
  surgical pathology patología quirúrgica.
pathway *n.* vía.
  accessory pathway vía accesoria.
  alternative pathway vía alternativa.
patient *n.* paciente.
pattern *n.* patrón.
pause *n.* pausa.
pavilion *n.* pabellón.
pavor *n.* pavor.
pectoral *adj.* pectoral.
pectus *n.* pecho.
pediatric *adj.* pediátrico, -ca.
pediatrician *n.* pediatra.
pediatrics *n.* pediatría.
pedicle *n.* pedículo.
pediculate *adj.* pediculado, -da.
pediculosis *n.* pediculosis.
pediculus *n.* pedículo, pediculus, piojo.

pedophile *n.* pedófilo, -la.

pedophilia *n.* paidofilia, pedofilia.

pedophilic *adj.* pedofílico, -ca, pedófilo, -la.

peduncle *n.* pedúnculo.

pedunculated *adj.* pedunculado, -da.

pedunculus *n.* pedúnculo.

pellagra *n.* pelagra.

pellicle *n.* película.
  tear pellicle película lagrimal.

pellucid *adj.* pelúcido, -da.

pelvic *adj.* pelviano, -na, pélvico, -ca.

pelvimetry *n.* pelvimetría.

pelviography *n.* pelvigrafía, pelviografía.

pelvis *n.* pelvis.

pemphigoid *n.* penfigoide.

pemphigus *n.* pénfigo.

pendular *adj.* pendular.

penetrability *n.* penetrabilidad.

penetrance *n.* penetrancia.

penetrating *adj.* penetrante.

penetration *n.* penetración.

penis *n.* pene, verga.

pentose *n.* pentosa.

pentosuria *n.* pentosuria.

peptic *adj.* péptico, -ca.

per os *adj.* per os, peroral.

perception *n.* percepción.
  conscious perception percepción consciente.
  extrasensory perception (ESP) percepción extrasensorial (PES).

perceptive *adj.* perceptivo, -va.

percussion *n.* percusión.
  bimanual percussion percusión bimanual.
  deep percussion percusión profunda.
  direct percussion percusión directa.
  finger percussion percusión digital.

perennial *adj.* perenne.

perfectionism *n.* perfeccionismo.

perforans *adj.* perforante.

perforated *adj.* perforado, -da.

perforation *n.* perforación.

perfusate *adj.* perfundido, -da.

perfuse *v.* perfundir.

perfusion *n.* perfusión.

perianal *adj.* perianal.

periapical *adj.* periapical.

pericardiac *adj.* pericardíaco, -ca, pericárdico, -ca.

pericardial *adj.* pericardíaco, -ca, pericárdico, -ca.

pericarditis *n.* pericarditis.

pericardium *n.* pericardio.

perichondritis *n.* pericondritis.

peridural *adj.* peridural.

perifolliculitis *n.* perifoliculitis.

perimeter *n.* perímetro.

perimetric *adj.* perimetral, perimétrico, -ca.

perinatal *adj.* perinatal.

perinatology *n.* perinatología.

perineal *adj.* perineal.

perineum *n.* periné, perineo.

period *n.* período, regla.
  fertile period período fértil.
  incubative period período de incubación.
  menstrual period período menstrual.
  puerperal period período puerperal.

periodic *adj.* periódico, -ca.

periodicity *n.* periodicidad.

periodontal *adj.* periodontal.
periodontics *n.* periodoncia.
periodontist *n.* periodoncista.
periodontitis *n.* periodontitis.
periorbital *adj.* periorbitario, -ria.
periosteum *n.* periostio.
periostitis *n.* periostitis.
peripheral *adj.* periférico, -ca.
periphery *n.* periferia.
peristalsis *n.* peristaltismo.
peristaltic *adj.* peristáltico, -ca.
peritoneal *adj.* peritoneal.
peritoneum *n.* peritoneo.
peritonitis *n.* peritonitis.
periumbilical *adj.* periumbilical.
perivascular *adj.* perivascular.
perivertebral *adj.* perivertebral.
permeability *n.* permeabilidad.
permeable *adj.* permeable.
pernicious *adj.* pernicioso, -sa.
peroneal *adj.* peroneo, -a.
persistence *n.* persistencia.
persona *n.* persona.
personality *n.* personalidad.
  split personality personalidad escindida.
persuasion *n.* persuasión.
perversion *n.* perversión.
  sexual perversion perversión sexual.
perverted *adj.* pervertido, -da.
pes pes, pie.
  pes cavus pes cavus, pie cavo.
  pes equinovalgus pes equinovalgus, pie equinovalgo.
  pes equinovarus pes equinovarus, pie equinovaro.
  pes equinus pie equino.
  pes planus pes planus, pie plano.

pes valgus pes valgus, pie valgo.
pes varus pes varus, pie varo.
pessary *n.* pesario.
pessimism *n.* pesimismo.
pestilence *n.* pestilencia.
pestilential *adj.* pestilente.
pestis *n.* peste.
petechia *n.* petequia.
petechial *adj.* petequial.
petrolatum *n.* vaselina.
petrous *adj.* pétreo, -a.
phacoemulsification *n.* facoemulsificación, facoemulsión.
phagocyte *n.* fagocito.
phalanx *n.* falange.
pharmaceutic *adj.* farmacéutico, -ca.
pharmaceutical *adj.* farmacéutico, -ca.
pharmaceutics *n.* farmacia.
pharmaceutist *n.* farmacéutico, -ca.
pharmacist *n.* farmacéutico, -ca.
pharmacokinetic *adj.* farmacocinético, -ca.
pharmacokinetics *n.* farmacocinética.
pharmacologic *adj.* farmacológico, -ca.
pharmacological *adj.* farmacológico, -ca.
pharmacology *n.* farmacología.
pharmacotherapy *n.* farmacoterapia.
pharmacy *n.* farmacia.
pharyngitis *n.* faringitis.
pharynx *n.* faringe.
phase *n.* fase.
phenomenon *n.* fenómeno.
phenotype *n.* fenotipo.

phenotypic *adj.* fenotípico, -ca.

phenylketonuria (FKU) *n.* fenilcetonuria (FCU).

pheromone *n.* feromonas.

phimosis *n.* fimosis.

phlebectomy *n.* flebectomía.

phlebitic *adj.* flebítico, -ca.

phlebitis *n.* flebitis.

phlebography *n.* flebografía.

phlebotomy *n.* flebotomía.

phlegm *n.* flema.

phlegmon *n.* flemón.

phobia *n.* fobia.

phocomelia *n.* focomelia.

phonation *n.* fonación.

phonendoscope *n.* fonendoscopio.

phosphatemia *n.* fosfatemia.

phospholipid *n.* fosfolípido.

photophobia *n.* fotofobia.

photosensitization *n.* fotosensibilización.

phrenic *adj.* frénico, -ca.

phthiriasis *n.* ftiriasis, ptiriasis.

phthisic *adj.* tísico, -ca.

phthisis *n.* tisis.

physician *n.* médico, -ca.
  emergency physician médico de urgencia.
  family physician médico de familia.
  osteopathic physician médico osteópata.
  primary care physician médico de atención primaria.
  resident physician médico residente.

physiologic *adj.* fisiológico, -ca.

physiological *adj.* fisiológico, -ca.

physiology *n.* fisiología.

physiopathologic *adj.* fisiopatológico, -ca.

physiopathology *n.* fisiopatología.

physiotherapeutist *n.* fisioterapeuta.

physiotherapist *n.* fisioterapeuta.

physiotherapy *n.* fisioterapia.

phytotherapy *n.* fitoterapia.

pica *n.* pica.

piece *n.* pieza.

piedra *n.* piedra.

pigment *n.* pigmento.
  bile pigment pigmento biliar.
  visual pigment pigmento visual.

pigmentation *n.* pigmentación.

pigmented *adj.* pigmentado, -da.

pile *n.* almorrana.

pill *n.* píldora.

piloerection *n.* piloerección.

pilose *adj.* piloso, -sa.

pilosebaceous *adj.* pilosebáceo, -a.

pilus *n.* cabello, capillus.

pineal *adj.* pineal.

pinealocyte *n.* pinealocito.

piorrea *n.* piorrea.

pipet *n.* pipeta.

pipette *n.* pipeta.

pituitarism *n.* pituitarismo.

pituitarium *n.* pituitaria.

pituitary *adj.* pituitario, -ria.

pityriasis *n.* pitiriasis.
  pityriasis capitis pitiriasis capitis.
  pityriasis rosea pitiriasis rosácea, pitiriasis rosada.
  pityriasis versicolor pitiriasis versicolor.

placebo *n.* placebo.

placement *n.* colocación.

placenta *n.* placenta.

fetal placenta placenta fetal.

maternal placenta placenta materna.

placenta fetalis placenta fetal.

placenta previa placenta previa.

plague *n.* peste.

   ...ague peste negra.

   bubonic plague peste bubónica.

plane *n.* plano.

planing *n.* aplanamiento.

plantar *adj.* plantar.

planum *n.* plano, planum.

plaque *n.* placa.

   bacterial plaque placa bacteriana.

   dental plaque placa dentaria.

   senile plaque placa senil.

plasma *n.* plasma.

   blood plasma plasma sanguíneo.

plasmapheresis *n.* plasmaféresis.

plasmid *n.* plásmido.

plaster *n.* emplasto, yeso.

plastic *adj.* plástico, -ca.

plasty *n.* plástia.

plate *n.* placa.

   bone plate placa ósea.

   neural plate placa neural.

plateau *n.* meseta.

platelet *n.* plaqueta.

plateletpheresis *n.* plaquetaféresis.

pleasure *n.* placer.

pledge *n.* juramento.

pleura *n.* pleura.

pleurisy *n.* pleuresía.

pleuritis *n.* pleuritis.

pleurodynia *n.* pleurodinia.

plexus *n.* plexo.

plug *n.* tapón.

   cerumen plug tapón de cerumen.

pluripotential *adj.* pluripotencial.

pneumarthrosis *n.* neumartrosis, neumoartrosis.

pneumocyte *n.* neumocito.

pneumology *n.* neumología.

pneumonia *n.* neumonía.

   acute pneumonia neumonía aguda.

   aspiration pneumonia neumonía por aspiración.

   atypical pneumonia neumonía atípica, neumonía atípica primaria.

   bacterial pneumonia neumonía bacteriana.

   caseous pneumonia neumonía caseosa.

   cheesy pneumonia neumonía caseosa.

   congenital aspiration pneumonia neumonía congénita, neumonía congénita por aspiración, neumonía por aspiración congénita.

   extrinsic allergic pneumonia neumonía alérgica extrínseca.

   influenza virus pneumonia neumonía por virus de la gripe.

   influenzal pneumonia neumonía por virus de la gripe.

   inhalation pneumonia neumonía por inhalación.

   interstitial pneumonia neumonía intersticial.

   metastatic pneumonia neumonía metastásica.

   parenchymatous pneumonia neumonía parenquimatosa.

   primary atypical pneumonia neumonía atípica, neumonía atípica primaria, neumonía primaria atípica.

secondary pneumonia neumonía secundaria.

septic pneumonia neumonía séptica.

staphylococcal pneumonia neumonía estafilocócica.

streptococcal pneumonia neumonía estreptocócica.

terminal pneumonia neumonía terminal.

tuberculous pneumonia neumonía tuberculosa.

unresolved pneumonia neumonía no resuelta.

varicella pneumonia neumonía por varicela.

viral pneumonia neumonía viral, neumonía vírica.

pneumonitis *n.* neumonitis.
pneumopathy *n.* neumopatía.
pneumopericardium *n.* neumopericardio.
pneumoperitoneal *adj.* neumoperitoneal.
pneumotherapy *n.* neumoterapia.
pneumothorax *n.* neumotórax.

pressure pneumothorax neumotórax a presión.

spontaneous pneumothorax neumotórax espontáneo.

tension pneumothorax neumotórax a tensión, neumotórax hiperbárico.

valvular pneumothorax neumotórax valvular.

pocket *n.* bolsa.

gingival pocket bolsa gingival.

podagra *n.* podagra, podagrismo.
podalic *adj.* podálico, -ca.

podologist *n.* podólogo, -ga.
podology *n.* podología.
point *n.* punta, punto.

painful point punto doloroso.

point dolorosum punto doloro

point of ossification punto ficación.

pressure point punto de presi

poison *n.* veneno.
poisoning *n.* envenenamiento, intoxicación.

ergot poisoning intoxicación por cornezuelo del centeno.

food poisoning intoxicación alimentaria, intoxicación alimenticia.

mushroom poisoning intoxicación por setas.

polar *n.* polar.
polarity *n.* polaridad.
polarization *n.* polarización.
pole *n.* polo.
polio *n.* polio.
poliomyelitis *n.* poliomielitis.
poliomyeloencephalitis *n.* poliomieloencefalitis.
polishing *n.* pulido.
pollakiuria *n.* polaquiuria.
polyadenitis *n.* poliadenia, poliadenitis.
polyarthritis *n.* poliartritis.
polyarticular *adj.* poliarticular.
polyclinic *n.* policlínica.
polycythemia *n.* policitemia, poliglobulia.

polycythemia vera policitemia vera, policitemia verdadera.

polydactylia *n.* polidactilia.
polydactyly *n.* polidactilia.
polydipsia *n.* polidipsia.

polymer *n.* polímero.

polyneuritis *n.* polineuritis.

polynuclear *adj.* polinuclear.

polynucleate *adj.* polinucleado, -da.

polynucleated *adj.* polinucleado, -da.

polyopia *n.* poliopía.

polyp *n.* pólipo.

  bronchial polyp pólipo bronquial.

  fibrous polyp pólipo fibroso.

  juvenile polyp pólipo juvenil.

  laryngeal polyp pólipo laríngeo.

  nasal polyp pólipo nasal.

  vascular polyp pólipo vascular.

polypeptide *n.* polipéptido.

polypharmacy *n.* polifármacia.

polysaccharide *n.* polihósido, polisacárido.

polyvalent *adj.* polivalente.

ponderable *adj.* ponderable.

ponderal *adj.* ponderal.

pons *n.* puente.

pontocerebellar *adj.* pontocerebeloso, -sa.

popliteal *adj.* poplíteo, -a.

pore *n.* poro.

porphobilinogen *n.* porfobilinógeno.

porphyria *n.* porfiria.

porta *n.* porta.

portion *n.* porción.

position *n.* posición.

  anatomical position posición anatómica.

  dorsal position posición dorsal.

  dorsal recumbent position posición de decúbito dorsal, posición de decúbito supino.

  fetal position posición fetal.

  frontotransverse position posición frontal transversa, posición frontotransversa.

  lateral recumbent position posición de decúbito lateral, posición lateroabdominal.

  lithotomy position posición de litotomía.

  obstetric position posición obstétrica.

  prone position posición de decúbito prono, posición prona.

  supine position posición supina.

  Trendelenburg's position posición de Trendelenburg.

positive *adj.* positivo, -va.

posology *n.* posología.

posterior *adj.* posterior, -ra.

posteroanterior *adj.* posteroanterior.

posteroinferior *adj.* posteroinferior.

posterointernal *adj.* posterointerno, -na.

posterolateral *adj.* posterolateral.

posteromedian *adj.* posteromediano, -na.

posteroparietal *adj.* posteroparietal.

posterosuperior *adj.* posterosuperior, -ra.

posthumous *adj.* póstumo, -ma.

postmenopausal *adj.* posmenopáusico, -ca.

postnatal *adj.* posnatal.

postoperative *adj.* posoperatorio, -ria.

postprandial *adj.* posprandial.

post-traumatic *adj.* postraumáti-co, -ca.

postulate *n.* postulado.

postural *adj.* postural.

posture *n.* postura.

potable *adj.* potable.

potassemia *n.* potasemia.

potassium *n.* potasio.

potency *n.* potencia.

potential *n.* potencial.

potentiation *n.* potenciación.

pouch *n.* bolsa.

  pouch of Douglas bolsa de Dou-glas.

power *n.* poder.

practice *n.* práctica.

prandial *adj.* prandial.

praxis *n.* praxis.

precancerous *adj.* precanceroso, -sa.

precipitate *n.* precipitado.

precipitation *n.* precipitación.

preclinical *adj.* preclínico, -ca.

precocious *adj.* precoz.

precocity *n.* precocidad.

precursor *adj.* precursor, -ra.

pre-eclampsia *n.* preeclampsia.

pregnancy *n.* embarazo.

  ectopic pregnancy embarazo ectó-pico.

  extrauterine pregnancy embarazo extrauterino.

  molar pregnancy embarazo afetal, embarazo molar.

  multiple pregnancy embarazo múl-tiple.

  ovarian pregnancy embarazo ová-rico.

  tubal pregnancy embarazo tubárico.

  twin pregnancy embarazo gemelar.

  uterine pregnancy embarazo eutó-pico, embarazo uterino.

pregnant *adj.* embarazada.

prehension *n.* prensión.

premalignant *adj.* premaligno, -na.

premature *n.* prematuro, -ra.

premenstrual *adj.* premenstrual.

prenatal *adj.* prenatal.

preneoplastic *adj.* preneoplásico, -ca.

preoptic *adj.* preóptico, -ca.

preparation *n.* preparación.

preperforative *adj.* preperforati-vo, -va.

preputium *n.* prepucio.

presbyacusia *n.* presbiacusia, pres-biacusis.

presbyopia *n.* presbicia, presbiopía, presbitismo.

prescription *n.* prescripción, receta.

presenile *adj.* presenil.

presentation *n.* presentación.

  anterior presentation presenta-ción mentoanterior.

  breech complete presentation presentación de nalgas completa.

  breech presentation presentación de nalgas.

  brow presentation presentación de frente.

  cephalic presentation presenta-ción cefálica.

  double breech presentation pre-sentación doble de nalgas.

  face presentation presentación de cara, presentación facial.

  footing presentation presentación podálica.

  knee presentation presentación de rodillas.

oblique presentation presentación oblicua.

pelvic presentation presentación pelviana, presentación pélvica.

placental presentation presentación de la placenta.

posterior presentation presentación mentoposterior.

shoulder presentation presentación de hombros.

transverse presentation presentación transversa.

trunk presentation presentación de tronco.

vertex presentation presentación de vértice.

preservation *n.* conservación.

cold preservation conservación en frío.

preservative *n.* conservante.

pressor *adj.* presor, -ra.

pressure *n.* presión.

atmospheric pressure presión atmosférica.

back pressure presión de fondo, presión retrógrada.

blood pressure presión arterial.

capillary pressure presión capilar.

central venous pressure (CVP) presión venosa central (PVC).

cerebral perfusion pressure (CPP) presión de perfusión cerebral (PPC).

cerebrospinal pressure presión cefalorraquídea.

critical pressure presión crítica.

diastolic blood pressure presión arterial diastólica.

filling pressure presión de llenado.

high blood pressure hipertensión.

hydrostatic pressure presión hidrostática.

intra-abdominal pressure presión intraabdominal.

intracranial pressure presión intracraneal.

intraocular pressure presión intraocular.

intraventricular pressure presión intraventricular.

negative pressure presión negativa.

osmotic pressure presión osmótica.

pleural pressure presión pleural.

positive pressure presión positive.

pulmonary pressure presión pulmonar.

pulse pressure presión del pulso.

static pressure presión estática.

systolic pressure presión sistólica.

venous pressure presión venosa.

wedge pressure presión de enclavamiento.

presynaptic *n.* presináptico.

presystole *n.* presístole.

prevalence *n.* prevalencia.

prevention *n.* prevención.

primary prevention prevención primaria.

secondary prevention prevención secundaria.

tertiary prevention prevención terciaria.

preventive *adj.* preventivo, -va.

previous *adj.* previo, -via.

priapism *n.* priapismo.

primary *adj.* primario, -ria.

primigravida *n.* primigrávida.

primipara *n.* primípara.

primitive *adj.* primitivo, -va.

primordial *adj.* primordial.

principle *n.* principio.

abstinence principle principio de abstinencia.

active principle principio activo.

prion *n.* prión.

probiotic *adj.* probiótico, -ca.

procedure *n.* intervención, procedimiento.

invasive procedure procedimiento invasivo.

process *n.* proceso.

procreate *n.* procrear.

proctologist *n.* proctólogo, -ga.

proctology *n.* proctología.

prodomous *adj.* prodrómico, -ca.

prodrome *n.* pródromo.

prodromic *adj.* prodrómico, -ca.

product *n.* producto.

productive *adj.* productivo, -va.

proenzyme *n.* proenzima.

profile *n.* perfil.

antigenic profile perfil antigénico.

biochemical profile perfil bioquímico.

personality profile perfil de la personalidad.

test profile perfil de pruebas.

progenitor *n.* progenitor, -ra.

progeny *n.* progenie.

progeria *n.* progeria.

progestational *adj.* progestacional.

progesterone *n.* progesterona.

progestogen *n.* progestágeno, progestógeno.

prognathism *n.* prognatismo.

progress *n.* progreso.

progression *n.* progresión.

progressive *adj.* progresivo, -va.

prohormone *n.* prohormona.

projection *n.* proyección.

visual projection proyección visual.

prokaryote *n.* procariota.

prolactin *n.* prolactina.

prolapse *n.* prolapso.

mitral valve prolapse prolapso de la válvula mitral.

prolapse of the umbilical cord prolapso del cordón umbilical.

proliferation *n.* proliferación.

proliferative *adj.* proliferativo, -va.

prolongation *n.* prolongación.

prominence *n.* prominencia.

prominent *adj.* prominente.

prominentia *n.* prominencia.

pronation *n.* pronación.

pronation of the foot pronación del pie.

pronation of the forearm pronación del antebrazo.

pronator *adj.* pronador, -ra.

prone *n.* prono.

propagate *v.* propagar.

propagation *n.* propagación.

prophase *n.* profase.

prophylactic *adj.* diafiláctico, -ca, profiláctico, -ca.

prophylaxis *n.* profilaxis.

active prophylaxis profilaxis activa.

chemical prophylaxis profilaxis química.

passive prophylaxis profilaxis pasiva.

propioception *n.* propiocepción.
propositus *n.* propósito.
propulsion *n.* propulsión.
prostate *n.* próstata.
prostatectomy *n.* prostatectomía.
prostatic *adj.* prostático, -ca.
prostatitis *n.* prostatitis.
prosthesis *n.* prótesis.
  cardiac valve prosthesis prótesis de válvula cardíaca.
  cochlear prosthesis prótesis coclear.
  dental prosthesis dentaria, prótesis dental.
  fixed partial prosthesis prótesis parcial fija.
  full prosthesis prótesis total.
  implant prosthesis prótesis de implante.
  ocular prosthesis prótesis ocular.
  overlay prosthesis prótesis superpuesta.
  partial prosthesis prótesis parcial.
  provisional prosthesis prótesis provisional.
  removable partial prosthesis prótesis parcial removible.
  temporary prosthesis prótesis temporal.
  transitional prosthesis prótesis transitoria.
  trial prosthesis prótesis de prueba.
prosthetic *adj.* prostético, -ca, protésico, -ca.
protamine *n.* protamina.
protean *adj.* proteico, -ca.
protein *n.* proteína.
proteinaceous *adj.* proteináceo, -a.
proteinogram *n.* proteinograma.

proteinuria *n.* proteinuria, proteuria.
  gestational proteinuria proteinuria gestacional.
  transient proteinuria proteinuria transitoria.
  true proteinuria proteinuria verdadera.
prototype *n.* prototipo.
protozoal *adj.* protozoario, -ria.
protozoon *n.* protozoo.
protrusion *n.* protrusión.
protuberance *n.* protuberancia.
proximal *adj.* proximal.
pruriginous *adj.* prurígeno, -na, pruriginoso, -sa.
prurigo *n.* prurigo.
pruritus *n.* prurito.
  essential pruritus prurito esencial, prurito generalizado, prurito idiopático.
  pruritus ani prurito anal, prurito ani.
  pruritus vulvae prurito vulvar.
pseudarthrosis *n.* seudoartrosis.
pseudoarthrosis *n.* seudoartrosis.
pseudopregnancy *n.* seudoembarazo.
psoriasis *n.* psoriasis.
psyche *n.* psique.
psychiatrist *n.* psiquiatra.
psychiatry *n.* psiquiatría.
psychic *adj.* psíquico, -ca.
psycho-analysis *n.* psicoanálisis.
psychoanalyst *n.* psicoanalista.
psychologist *n.* psicólogo, -ga.
psychology *n.* psicología.
  educational psychology psicología de la educación, psicología educacional.

psychopath *n.* psicópata.

psychopathology *n.* psicopatología.

psychopathy *n.* psicopatía.

psychopharmaceutical *n.* psicofármaco.

psychosis *n.* psicosis.

psychosocial *adj.* psicosocial.

psychosomatic *adj.* psicosomático, -ca.

psychostimulant *n.* psicoestimulante.

psychotherapist *n.* psicoterapeuta.

psychotherapy *n.* psicoterapia.

psychotic *adj.* psicótico, -ca.

ptosis *n.* ptosis.

pubarche *n.* pubarquia.

puberty *n.* pubertad.

  precocious puberty pubertad precoz.

pubis *n.* pubis.

puericulture *n.* puericultura.

puerperal *adj.* puerperal.

puerperium *n.* puerperio.

pulmonitis *n.* pulmonía.

pulp *n.* pulpa.

  dental pulp pulpa dental.

  devitalized pulp pulpa desvitalizada.

  digital pulp pulpa del dedo, pulpa digital.

  non-vital pulp pulpa no vital.

  pulp of the finger pulpa del dedo, pulpa digital.

  radicular pulp pulpa radicular.

pulpa *n.* pulpa.

pulpalgia *n.* pulpalgia.

pulpectomy *n.* pulpectomía.

pulpitis *n.* pulpitis.

pulsatile *adj.* pulsátil.

pulsation *n.* pulsación.

pulsator *n.* pulsador.

pulse *n.* pulso.

  abdominal pulse pulso abdominal.

  anacrotic pulse pulso anacrótico, pulso anacroto.

  bigeminal pulse pulso bigémino.

  celer pulse pulso celer.

  filiform pulse pulso filiforme.

  intermittent pulse pulso intermitente.

  irregular pulse pulso irregular.

  jugular pulse pulso yugular.

  Kussmaul's paradoxical pulse pulso paradójico, pulso paradójico de Kussmaul.

  paradoxical pulse pulso paradójico, pulso paradójico de Kussmaul.

  peripheral pulse pulso periférico.

  popliteal pulse pulso poplíteo.

  rapid pulse pulso rápido.

  undulating pulse pulso ondulante.

pulsion *n.* pulsión.

pulsus *n.* pulso.

  pulsus alternans pulso alternante.

  pulsus celer pulso acelerado.

  pulsus inaequalis pulso desigual.

pulverization *n.* pulverización.

pulverize *v.* pulverizar.

pump *n.* bomba, bombear.

  breast pump bomba mamaria, bomba para mamas, bomba sacaleches.

  constant infusion pump bomba para infusión constante.

  infusion pump bomba de infusión.

  infusion-withdrawal pump bomba de infusión y extracción.

insulin infusion pump bomba de infusión de insulina.

insulin pump bomba de insulina.

peristaltic pump bomba peristáltica.

proton pump bomba de protones.

sodium pump bomba de sodio.

sodium-potassium pump bomba de Na y K, bomba de sodio-potasio.

stomach pump bomba del estómago, bomba estomacal, bomba gástrica.

punctiform *adj.* puntiforme.

puncture *n.* punción.

lumbar puncture (LP) punción lumbar (PL).

pupil *n.* pupila.

fixed pupil pupila fija.

pinhole pupil pupila puntiforme.

tonic pupil pupila tónica.

pupilla *n.* pupila.

purgative *adj.* purgante.

purple púrpura.

purpura *n.* púrpura.

allergic purpura púrpura alérgica.

hemorrhagic purpura púrpura hemorrágica.

Henoch-Schönlein purpura púrpura de Henoch-Schönlein.

thrombocytopenic purpura púrpura trombocitopénica.

purulent *adj.* purulento, -ta.

pus *n.* pus.

pustular *adj.* pustular, pustuloso, -sa.

pustule *n.* pústula.

pustulosis *n.* pustulosis.

putrefaction *n.* putrefacción, putrescencia.

putrid *adj.* pútrido, -da.

pyelitis *n.* pielitis.

pyelography *n.* pielografía.

pyelonephritis *n.* pielonefritis.

pyelonephrosis *n.* pielonefrosis.

pyeloplasty *n.* pieloplastia.

pyloritis *n.* piloritis.

pyloroplasty *n.* piloroplastia.

pylorospasm *n.* piloroespasmo.

pylorus *n.* píloro.

pyogen *n.* piógeno.

pyogenic *adj.* piogénico, -ca.

pyramid *n.* pirámide.

pyramidal *adj.* piramidal.

pyrectic *adj.* pirético, -ca.

pyretic *adj.* pirético, -ca.

pyrogen *n.* pirógeno.

pyrosis *n.* pirosis.

pyuria *n.* piuria.

Q

quadrant *n.* cuadrante.

quadriceps *adj.* cuádriceps.

quarantine *n.* cuarentena.

quiescent *adj.* quiescente.

quintipara *n.* quintípara.

quintuplet *adj.* quintillizo, -za, quíntuplo, -pla.

R

rabies *n.* rabia.

race *n.* raza.

rachialgia *n.* raquialgia.

rachianalgesia *n.* raquianalgesia.

rachianesthesia *n.* raquianestesia.

rachidial *adj.* raquídeo, -a.

rachitic *adj.* raquítico, -ca.

rachitis *n.* raquitis, raquitismo.
 resistant rachitis raquitismo vitaminorresistente.

racial *adj.* racial.

radiate *v.* irradiar, radiado, -da, radiar.

radiation *n.* radiación.
 ultraviolet radiation radiación ultravioleta.
 X-radiation radiación X.

radiato *n.* radiación.

radicular *adj.* radicular.

radiculitis *n.* radiculitis.

radiculopathy *n.* radiculopatía.

radioactive *adj.* radiactivo, -va, radioactivo, -va.

radioactivity *n.* radiactividad, radioactividad.

radiogram *n.* radiografía, radiograma.
 panoramic radiogram radiografía panorámica.

radiography *n.* radiografía.
 digital radiography radiografía digital.

radioimmunoassay (RIA) *n.* radioinmunoanálisis (RIA).

radiologist *n.* radiólogo, -ga.

radiology *n.* radiología.

radiopaque *adj.* radioopaco, -ca, radiopaco, -ca.

radiosensibility *n.* radiosensibilidad.

radiosensible *adj.* radiosensible.

radiosensitive *adj.* radiolábil, radiosensible.

radiosensitiveness *n.* radiosensibilidad.

radiosensitivity *n.* radiosensibilidad.

radiotherapy *n.* radioterapia.
 intracavitary radiotherapy radioterapia intracavitaria.

radium *n.* radio, radium.

radius radio, radius.

radix radix, raíz.

rage *n.* ira.

rales *n.* sibilancia.
 sibilant rales sibilancia.
 whistling rales sibilancia.

ramification *n.* ramificación.

ramified *adj.* ramificado, -da.

ramify *v.* ramificar.

ramus *n.* rama, ramo, ramus.

range *n.* gama, rango.
 range of motion rango de movimiento.

rape *n.* violación.
 acquaintaince rape violación por conocido.
 date rape violación por conocido.
 marital rape violación marital.
 statutory rape violación de menores.

raptus *n.* rapto.

rash *n.* exantema, rash.
 butterfly rash exantema en alas de mariposa, exantema en mariposa, rash en mariposa.
 caterpillar rash rash por orugas.
 diaper rash exantema del pañal, rash del pañal.
 nettle rash exantema por ortigas, rash por ortigas.
 summer rash rash de verano.
 wildfire rash rash de erisipela.

rat *n.* rata.

rate *n.* índice, tasa, velocidad.

death rate índice de muertes, tasa de mortalidad.

glomerular filtration rate (GFR) índice de filtración glomerular (GFR), tasa de filtración glomerular (TFG).

metabolic rate índice metabólico.

morbidity rate índice de morbilidad, tasa de morbidad.

mortality rate índice de mortalidad.

sedimentation rate velocidad de sedimentación.

raticide *n.* raticida.

ratio *n.* proporción, razón.

rational *adj.* racional.

rattle *n.* estertor.

crepitant rattle estertor crepitante.

rattus *n.* rata.

ray *n.* rayo.

ultraviolet ray rayo ultravioleta.

reabsorb *v.* reabsorber.

reabsorbable *adj.* reabsorbible.

reabsorption *n.* reabsorción.

bone reabsorption reabsorción ósea.

gingival reabsorption reabsorción gingival.

tubular reabsorption reabsorción tubular.

react *v.* reaccionar.

reaction *n.* reacción.

reactivation *n.* reactivación.

reading *n.* lectura.

lip reading lectura de labios, lectura del habla.

speech reading lectura de labios, lectura del habla.

reagent *n.* reactivo.

real *adj.* real.

reality *n.* realidad.

reamputation *n.* reamputación.

rebound *n.* rechazo.

recalcification *n.* recalcificación.

recall *n.* recuerdo.

recanalization *n.* recanalización.

recanalize *v.* recanalizar.

receptor *n.* receptor, -ra.

alpha-adrenergic receptor receptor alfa-adrenérgico.

beta-adrenergic receptor receptor beta-adrenérgico.

chemical receptor receptor químico.

cholinergic receptor receptor colinérgico.

dopamine receptor receptor de dopamina.

estrogen receptor receptor de estrógenos.

hormone receptor receptor hormonal.

insulin receptor receptor de insulina.

LDL receptor receptor de lipoproteínas de baja densidad (LDL).

opiate receptor receptor para opiáceo.

pain receptor receptor de dolor.

pressure receptor receptor de presión.

progesterone receptor receptor de progesterona.

sensory receptor receptor sensitivo.

touch receptor receptor táctiles.

volume receptor receptor de volumen.

recession *n.* recesión.

recessive *adj.* recesivo, -va.

recidivation *n.* recidiva.

recipe *n.* receta.

recognition *n.* reconocimiento.

recombinant *adj.* recombinante.

recombination *n.* recombinación.

reconstitution *n.* reconstitución.

reconstruction *n.* reconstrucción.

record *n.* registro.

  electrocardiographic record registro electrocardiografico.

  electroencefalographic record registro electroencefalografico.

  hospital record registro hospitalario.

  medical record registro médico.

  patient's hospital record registro hospitalario de pacientes.

recovery *n.* recuperación, restablecimiento.

  postoperatory recovery recuperación posoperatoria.

  spontaneous recovery recuperación espontánea.

recrudescence *n.* recrudecimiento, recrudescencia.

recruitment *n.* reclutamiento.

rectal *adj.* rectal.

rectalgia *n.* rectalgia.

rectification *n.* rectificación.

rectify *v.* rectificar.

rectitis *n.* rectitis.

rectoabdominal *adj.* rectoabdominal.

rectovaginal *adj.* rectovaginal, vaginorrectal.

rectovesical *adj.* rectovesical.

rectovulvar *adj.* rectovulvar.

rectum *n.* recto.

recuperate *v.* recuperarse.

recuperation *n.* recuperación.

recurrence *n.* recurrencia.

recurrent *adj.* recurrente.

red *n.* rojo, rojo, -ja.

red-haired *adj.* pelirrojo, -ja, taheño, -ña, tajeño, -ña.

red-headed *adj.* pelirrojo, -ja, taheño, -ña, tajeño, -ña.

redness *n.* rubor.

redressement *n.* enderezamiento.

reduce *v.* reducir.

reducible *adj.* reducible.

reductant *n.* reductor.

reduction *n.* reducción.

  breast reduction reducción de la mama, reducción mamaria.

  closed reduction reducción cerrada.

  closed reduction of fracture reducción cerrada de fractura.

  mammaplasty reduction reducción de la mama, reducción mamaria.

  open reduction reducción abierta.

  open reduction of fracture reducción abierta de fractura.

  reduction of fracture reducción de fractura.

  weight reduction reducción de peso.

reference *n.* referencia.

referral *n.* derivación.

refine *v.* refinar.

reflect *v.* reflejar, reflexionar.

reflected *adj.* reflejado, -da.

reflex *n.* reflejo, -ja.

  accommodation reflex reflejo de acomodación.

Achilles tendon reflex reflejo del tendón de Aquiles, reflejo tendinoso de Aquiles.

acquired reflex reflejo adquirido.

anal reflex reflejo anal.

attention reflex of the pupil reflejo de atención de la pupila.

conditional reflex reflejo condicionado.

conditioned reflex reflejo condicionado.

cry reflex reflejo del llanto.

defense reflex reflejo de defensa.

eye reflex reflejo ocular.

Guillain-Barré reflex reflejo de Guillain-Barré, reflejo plantar en hiperflexión.

knee reflex reflejo de la rodilla.

knee-jerk reflex reflejo de la sacudida de la rodilla, reflejo patelar.

muscular reflex reflejo motor muscular, reflejo muscular.

patellar reflex reflejo rotuliano.

patellar tendon reflex reflejo del tendón rotuliano.

pathologic reflex reflejo patológico.

plantar reflex reflejo plantar.

postural reflex reflejo postural.

pupillary reflex reflejo pupilar.

sole reflex reflejo plantar.

static reflex reflejo estático, reflejo estatocinético.

statokinetic reflex reflejo estático, reflejo estatocinético.

tendon reflex reflejo tendinoso.

trained reflex reflejo condicionado.

reflux *n.* reflujo.

gastroesophageal reflux reflujo gastroesofágico.

refraction *n.* refracción.

refresh *v.* refrescar.

refrigeration *n.* refrigeración.

refringent *adj.* refringente.

regenerate *v.* regenerar.

regeneration *n.* regeneración.

regimen *n.* régimen.

region *n.* región.

regression *n.* regresión.

regular *adj.* regular.

regularity *n.* regularidad.

regulation *n.* regulación.

regulatory *adj.* regulador, -ra.

regurgitant *adj.* regurgitante.

regurgitate *v.* regurgitar.

regurgitation *n.* regurgitación.

valvular regurgitation regurgitación valvular.

rehospitalize *v.* rehospitalizar.

rehydratation *n.* rehidratación.

rehydrate *v.* rehidratar.

reimplantation *n.* reimplantación.

reinforcement *n.* reforzamiento, refuerzo.

positive reinforcement refuerzo positivo.

reintubation *n.* reintubación.

rejection *n.* rechazo, reyección.

acute rejection rechazo agudo.

humoral rejection rechazo humoral.

organ rejection rechazo de órgano.

rejuvenescence *n.* rejuvenecimiento.

relapse *n.* recaída, recidiva.

tumor relapse recidiva de los tumores.

relapsing adj. recurrente.

relation n. relación.

relationship n. relación.

relative adj. relativo, -va.

relax v. relajar.

relaxant n. relajante.

  muscular relaxant relajante muscular.

relaxation n. relajación, relajamiento.

reliability n. fiabilidad.

relief n. alivio.

remanent n. remanente.

remedy n. remedio.

remineralization n. remineralización.

remission n. remisión.

  spontaneous remission remisión espontánea.

remit v. remitir.

renal adj. renal.

repair n. reparación.

reparation n. reparación.

reparative adj. reparador, -ra, reparativo, -va.

repellent adj. repelente.

replacement n. sustitución.

  hip replacement sustitución de cadera.

  knee replacement sustitución de rodilla.

  total hip replacement sustitución total de la cadera.

replant n. reimplante.

replication n. replicación.

repolarization n. repolarización.

report n. informe.

repositioning n. reposición.

reproduction n. reproducción.

  sexual reproduction reproducción sexual.

reproductive adj. reproductivo, -va, reproductor, -ra.

request n. demanda.

research n. investigación.

  clinical research investigación clínica.

resect v. resecar.

resectable adj. resecable.

resection n. resección.

reserve n. reserva.

reservoir n. reservorio.

  reservoir of infection reservorio de infección.

residual adj. residual.

residue n. residuo, resto.

  embryonic residue resto embrionario.

resilience n. elasticidad, resiliencia.

resistance n. resistencia.

  insulin resistance resistencia a la insulina.

resolve v. resolver.

resonance n. resonancia.

respirable adj. respirable.

respiration n. respiración.

  abdominal respiration respiración abdominal.

  aerobic respiration respiración aeróbica.

  anaerobic respiration respiración anaeróbica.

  artificial respiration respiración artificial.

  assisted respiration respiración asistida.

  costal respiration respiración costal.

cutaneous respiration respiración cutánea.

diaphragmatic respiration respiración diafragmática.

interrupted respiration respiración entrecortada, respiración interrumpida.

mouth-to-mouth respiration respiración boca a boca.

paradoxical respiration respiración paradójica.

stertorous respiration respiración estertorosa.

thoracic respiration respiración torácica.

respirator *n.* respirador.

respiratory *adj.* respiratorio, -ria.

respire *v.* respirar.

response *n.* respuesta.

immune response respuesta inmune.

no response (NR) no respuesta (NR).

rest *n.* apoyo, descanso, reposo, soporte.

incisal rest apoyo incisal.

occlusal rest apoyo oclusal.

restoration *n.* restauración.

restorative *adj.* reconstituyente, reparativo, va, restaurativo, -va.

restraint *n.* restricción, sujeción.

result *n.* resultado.

resuscitation *n.* reanimación, resucitación, resurrección.

cardiopulmonary resuscitation reanimación cardiopulmonar.

do not attempt resuscitation (DNAR) no intentar la reanimación (NIR).

mouth-to-mouth resuscitation reanimación boca a boca.

resuscitator *n.* resucitador.

retardate *adj.* retardado, retrasado, -da.

retardation *n.* retraso.

mental retardation retraso mental.

mild mental retardation retraso mental leve.

moderate mental retardation retraso mental moderado.

profound mental retardation retraso mental profundo.

psychomotor retardation retraso psicomotor.

severe mental retardation retraso mental grave.

rete *n.* red, rete.

retention *n.* retención.

denture retention retención protésica.

retention of placental fragments retención placentaria.

retention of urine retención de orina.

urine retention retención de orina.

reticulated *adj.* reticulado, -da.

reticulosis *n.* reticulosis, retoteliosis.

reticulum *n.* retículo.

retina *n.* retina.

detached retina retina desprendida.

retinal *adj.* retinal, retiniano, -na.

retinitis *n.* dictitis, retinitis.

retinoblastoma *n.* retinoblastoma.

retinochoroiditis *n.* retinocoroiditis.

retinopapillitis *n.* retinopapilitis.

retinopathy *n.* retinopatía.

hypertensive retinopathy retinopatía hipertensiva.

macular retinopathy retinopatía macular.

proliferative retinopathy retinopatía proliferativa.

retinopathy of prematurity retinopatía de los prematuros.

retinoscope *n.* retinoscopio.

retinoscopy *n.* retinoscopia.

retinosis *n.* retinosis.

retractile *adj.* retráctil.

retraction *n.* retracción.

uterine muscle retraction retracción del útero.

retractor *n.* retractor, separador.

retrocession *n.* retrocesión, retroceso.

retrognathia *n.* retrognatia.

retroperitoneal *adj.* retroperitoneal.

retroperitonitis *n.* retroperitonitis.

retroplacental *adj.* retroplacentario, -ria.

retrorectal *adj.* retrorrectal.

retrospection *n.* retrospección.

retrospective *adj.* retrospectivo, -va.

retrosternal *adj.* retroesternal, retrosternal.

retroversion *n.* retroversión.

retrovirus *n.* retrovirus.

return *n.* retorno.

venous return retorno venoso.

revaccination *n.* revacunación.

revascularization *n.* revascularización.

reversible *adj.* reversible.

reversion *n.* reversión.

revulsion *n.* derivación, revulsión.

reward *n.* recompensa.

rheum *n.* legaña, reuma, reúma.

rheuma *n.* reuma, reúma.

rheumatic *adj.* reumático, -ca.

rheumatism *n.* reumatismo.

rheumatismal *adj.* reumático, -ca.

rheumatologist *n.* reumatólogo, -ga.

rheumatology *n.* reumatología.

rhexis *n.* rotura.

rhinitis *n.* rinitis.

allergic rhinitis rinitis alérgica.

anaphylactic rhinitis rinitis analfiláctica.

rhinolaryngitis *n.* rinolaringitis.

rhinopharyngeal *adj.* rinofaríngeo, -a.

rhinopharyngitis *n.* rinofaringitis.

rhinopharynx *n.* rinofaringe.

rhinoplasty *n.* rinoplastia.

rhinorrhea *n.* rinorrea.

rhinovirus *n.* rinovirus.

rhythm *n.* ritmo.

atrioventricular nodal rhythm ritmo nodal auriculoventricular.

cantering rhythm ritmo de galope.

coronary sinus rhythm ritmo sinusal coronario.

fast rhythm ritmo rápido.

fetal rhythm ritmo fetal.

nodal rhythm ritmo nodal.

sinus rhythm ritmo sinusal.

ventricular rhythm ritmo ventricular.

rhythmical *adj.* rítmico, -ca.

rib *n.* costa, costilla.

ribbon *n.* cinta.

ribonucleotide *n.* ribonucleótido.

ribosome *n.* ribosoma.

rickets *n.* raquitismo.

rickety *adj.* raquítico, -ca.

rictus *n.* rictus.

rigidity *n.* rigidez.

cadaveric rigidity rigidez cadavérica.

catatonic rigidity rigidez catatónica.

cogwheel rigidity rigidez en rueda dentada.

postmortem rigidity rigidez post mortem.

rigor *n.* rigor.

rigor mortis rigor mortis.

rim *n.* borde.

occlusal rim borde de oclusión.

occlusion rim borde de oclusión.

ring *n.* anillo.

neck ring anillo cervical.

umbilical ring anillo umbilical.

vascular ring anillo vascular.

ringworm *n.* tiña, tinea.

ringworm of the scalp tiña del cuero cabelludo.

risk *n.* riesgo.

risus *n.* risa.

ritual *n.* ritual.

rod *n.* bastoncillo.

retinal rod bastoncillo retiniano.

role *n.* rol.

room *n.* sala.

delivery room paritorio, sala de partos.

emergency room (ER) sala de urgencias (SU).

intensive therapy room sala de cuidados intensivos.

operating room (OR) sala de operaciones (SO).

postdelivery room sala posparto.

recovery room sala de recuperación.

recovery room (RR) sala de reanimación.

root *n.* raíz.

rosacea *n.* rosácea.

rose *n.* rosa.

roseola *n.* roséola.

rotation *n.* rotación.

intestinal rotation rotación intestinal.

rotator *adj.* rotador, rotatorio, -ria.

rotula *n.* rótula.

round *n.* sesión.

teaching round sesión docente.

route *n.* vía.

route of administration vía de administración.

rubbing *n.* roce.

pericardial rubbing roce pericárdico.

pleuritic rubbing roce pleurítico.

rubefacient *adj.* rubefaciente.

rubefaction *n.* rubefacción.

rubella *n.* rubella, rubéola.

rubeola *n.* rubella, rubéola.

rubor *n.* rubor.

ructus *n.* eructo, ructus.

rudimentary *adj.* rudimental, rudimentario, -ria.

ruga arruga, ruga.

rugose *adj.* rugoso, -sa.

rugosity *n.* rugosidad.

rugous *adj.* rugoso, -sa.

rule *n.* norma, regla.

rupture *n.* rotura, ruptura.

rutin *n.* rutina.

S

sac *n.* bolsa, saccus, saco.

amniotic sac bolsa amniótica.

saccade *n.* sacudida.

saccate *adj.* enquistado, -da.

saccharin *n.* sacarina.

saccular *adj.* sacular.

sacculocochlear *adj.* saculococlear.

saccus *n.* saccus, saco.

sacral *adj.* sacral.

sacrococcygeal *adj.* sacrococcígeo, -a.

sacrococcyx *n.* sacrocóccix.

sacrum *n.* sacro.

sadism *n.* sadismo.

sadist *n.* sádico, -ca.

sadness *n.* tristeza.

sadomasochism *n.* sadomasoquismo.

sadomasochistic *adj.* sadomasoquista.

sagittal *adj.* sagital.

sal *n.* sal.

saline *adj.* salino, -na.

saliva *n.* saliva.

salivary *adj.* salival.

salivation *n.* salivación.

salpingectomy *n.* salpingectomía.

salpingitis *n.* salpingitis.

salt *n.* sal.

salubrious *adj.* salubre.

salubrity *n.* salubridad.

salutary *adj.* saludable, salutífero, -ra.

sample *n.* muestra.
   biased sample muestra sesgada.
   random sample muestra al azar.

sampling *n.* muestreo, toma.
   random sampling muestreo aleatorio.

sanatorium *n.* sanatorio.

sane *n.* cuerdo, -da.

sanguine *adj.* sanguíneo, -a.

sanguineous *adj.* sanguíneo, -a.

sanguinolent *adj.* sanguinolento, -ta.

sanitary *adj.* sanitario, -ria.

sanitation *n.* saneamiento, sanidad.

sanitize *v.* sanear.

sanity *n.* cordura, sanidad.

sapo *n.* jabón.

sarcoidosis *n.* sarcoidosis.

sarcoma *n.* sarcoma.

sarcomere *n.* sarcómera, sarcómero.

satellite *n.* satélite.

saturated *adj.* saturado, -da.

saturation *n.* saturación.
   hemoglobin oxygen saturation saturación de oxígeno en la hemoglobina.
   oxygen saturation saturación de oxígeno.

saturnism *n.* saturnismo.

saucerization *n.* aplanamiento, saucerización.

saw *n.* sierra.

scabies *n.* escabiasis, sarna.

scabietic *adj.* escabético, -ca, escabiético, -ca, escabioso, -sa, sarnoso, -sa.

scala *n.* rampa.

scale *n.* descamar, escala, escama, gama.

scaling *n.* escarificación.

scalp cuero cabelludo.

scalprum *n.* escalpro.

scaly *adj.* escamoso, -sa.

scan *n.* rastreo, scan.
   isotopic scan rastreo isotópico.

scanner *n.* escáner.

scanning *n.* barrido.

scaphoid *adj.* escafoide, escafoideo, -a, escafoides.

scapula *n.* escápula.

scar *n.* cicatriz.

scarification *n.* escarificación.

scarlatina *n.* escarlatina.

scatologia *n.* escatología.

scatology *n.* escatología.

scatoma *n.* escatoma.

schema *n.* esquema.

scheme *n.* esquema.

schistocyte *n.* esquistocito.

schistosome *n.* esquistosoma, tecosoma.

schistosomiasis *n.* esquistosomiasis.

schizophrenia *n.* esquizofrenia.

schizophrenic *adj.* esquizofrénico, -ca.

sciatica *n.* ciática.

scissors *n.* tijeras.

sclera *n.* esclera.

scleritis *n.* escleritis.

scleroderma *n.* escirrosarca, escleremia, esclerodermia.

sclerosant *adj.* esclerosante.

sclerosed *adj.* esclerosado, -da.

sclerosing *adj.* esclerosante.

sclerosis *n.* esclerismo, escleropatía, esclerosis.

  amyotrophic lateral sclerosis (ALS) esclerosis lateral amiotrófica (ELA).

sclerotica *n.* esclerótica.

scoliosis *n.* escoliosis.

scopophilia *n.* escopofilia, voyeurismo.

scotoma *n.* escotoma.

screen *n.* pantalla.

screening *n.* detección, screening.

  genetic screening detección selectiva genética.

scrotum *n.* escroto.

scurvy *n.* escorbuto.

searching *n.* investigación.

sebaceous *adj.* sebáceo, -a.

sebaceus *adj.* sebáceo, -a.

seborrhea *n.* seborragia, seborrea.

seborrheic *adj.* seborreico, -ca.

sebum *n.* sebo, sebum.

secondary *n.* secundario, -ria.

secrete *v.* secretar, segregar.

secretion *n.* secreción.

  apocrine secretion secreción apocrina.

  autocrine secretion secreción autocrina.

  bronchial secretion secreción bronquial.

  external secretion secreción externa.

  holocrine secretion secreción holocrina.

  internal secretion secreción interna.

  merocrine secretion secreción merocrina.

  paracrine secretion secreción paracrina.

  paralytic secretion secreción paralítica.

secretory *adj.* secretor, -ra.

sectarian *adj.* sectario, -ria.

sectio *n.* sección.

  sectio alta sección alta, sección hipogástrica, sección suprapúbica.

  sectio lateralis sección lateral.

  sectio mediana sección mediana.

section *n.* corte, sección.

  abdominal section sección abdominal.

  cesarean section sección cesárea.

frontal section corte frontal, sección frontal.

perineal section sección perineal.

sagittal section sección sagital.

sector *n.* sector.

secundipara *n.* secundípara.

secundiparity *n.* secundiparidad.

sedation *n.* sedación.

sedative *n.* sedante, sedativo, -va.

nervous sedative sedante nervioso.

respiratory sedative sedante respiratorio.

sedativus *n.* sedante, sedativo, -va.

sedentary *adj.* sedentario, -ria.

sediment *n.* sedimento.

segment *n.* segmento.

segmental *adj.* segmentario, -ria.

segmentation *n.* segmentación.

segmentum *n.* segmento.

segregation *n.* segregación.

seizure *n.* acceso, convulsión, crisis.

absence seizure crisis de ausencia.

atonic seizure crisis atónica.

clonic seizure convulsión clónica.

convulsive seizure crisis convulsiva.

epileptic seizure crisis epiléptica.

febrile seizure convulsión febril.

focal seizure convulsión focal.

generalized seizure crisis generalizada.

generalized tonic-clonic seizure convulsión tónico-clónica generalizada.

grand mal seizure crisis de gran mal.

hysterical seizure convulsión histérica, convulsión histeroide.

Jacksonian seizure crisis jacksoniana.

motor seizure crisis motora.

myoclonic seizure crisis mioclónica.

neonatal seizure convulsión neonatal.

partial complex seizure crisis parcial compleja.

partial seizure convulsión parcial, crisis parcial.

partial simple seizure crisis parcial simple.

petit mal seizure crisis de pequeño mal.

secondarily generalized seizure crisis generalizada secundaria.

tonic seizure convulsión tónica.

tonic-clonic seizure crisis generalizada tónico-clónica.

selection *n.* selección.

multiple selection selección múltiple.

natural selection selección natural.

random selection selección aleatoria.

truncate selection selección sesgada, selección truncada.

selective *adj.* selectivo, -va.

selectivity *n.* selectividad.

self *n.* sí mismo.

sella *n.* sella, silla.

semen *n.* semen.

seminal *adj.* seminal.

seminoma *n.* seminoma.

senile *adj.* senil.

senility *n.* senilidad.

senium *n.* senectud.

senography *n.* senografía.

sensation *n.* sensación.
 dermal sensation sensación dérmica.
 sensation of warmth sensación de calor.
 skin sensation sensación cutánea.
sense *n.* sentido.
 sense of equilibrium sentido del equilibrio.
sensibility *n.* sensibilidad.
sensitive *adj.* sensible.
sensitivity *n.* sensibilidad.
 contrast sensitivity sensibilidad de contraste.
 cross sensitivity sensibilidad cruzada.
 phototoxic sensitivity sensibilidad fototóxica.
sensitization *n.* sensibilización.
 cross sensitization sensibilización cruzada.
 Rh sensitization sensibilización Rh.
sensitized *adj.* sensibilizado, -da.
sensor *n.* sensor, -ra.
sensorial *adj.* sensorial.
sensorimotor *adj.* sensitivomotor, -ra, sensoriomotor, -triz.
sensory *adj.* sensitivo, -va.
sensual *adj.* sensual.
sensualism *n.* sensualidad, sensualismo.
sentiment *n.* sentimiento.
separation *n.* separación.
separator *n.* separador.
sepsis *n.* sepsis.
 puerperal sepsis sepsis puerperal.
septate *adj.* septado, -da, tabicado, -da.
septic *adj.* séptico, -ca.

septicemia *n.* septicemia.
septicemic *adj.* septicémico, -ca.
septum *n.* septo, septum, tabique.
sequela *n.* secuela.
sequence *n.* secuencia.
sequester *v.* secuestrar.
sequestration *n.* secuestro.
sequestrum *n.* secuestro.
seralbumin *n.* seroalbúmina.
serial *adj.* seriado, -da, serial.
series *n.* serie.
 leukocytic series serie leucocítica.
seroconversion *n.* seroconversión.
seroconvert *v.* seroconvertir.
seroculture *n.* serocultivo.
serogroup *n.* serogrupo.
serologic *adj.* serológico, -ca.
serological *adj.* serológico, -ca.
serology *n.* serología.
 diagnostic serology serología diagnóstica.
seroma *n.* seroma.
seronegative *adj.* seronegativo, -va.
seronegativity *n.* seronegatividad.
seropositive *adj.* seropositivo, -va.
serotonin *n.* serotonina.
serotoninergic *adj.* serotoninérgico, -ca.
serpiginous *adj.* serpiginoso, -sa.
serrated *adj.* serrado, -da, serratus.
serratus *adj.* serrado, -da, serrato, -ta, serratus.
serum *n.* serum, suero.
serumal *adj.* sérico, -ca.
service *n.* servicio.
 basic health service servicio básico de salud.
 day health care service servicio de hospital de día.

detoxification service servicio de toxicología.

environmental service servicio interno.

maternal and child (MCH) service servicio de salud maternoinfantil.

psychiatric emergency service servicio de urgencias de psiquiatría.

sesamoid *adj.* sesamoide, sesamoideo, -a.

sesamoiditis *n.* sesamoiditis.

sex *v.* sexar, sexo.

chromosomal sex sexo cromosómico.

endocrinologic sex sexo endocrinológico.

genetic sex sexo genético.

gonadal sex sexo gonadal.

morphological sex sexo morfológico.

nuclear sex sexo nuclear.

psychological sex sexo psicológico.

safe sex sexo seguro.

social sex sexo social.

sexology *n.* sexología.

sexopathy *n.* sexopatía.

sextigravida *n.* sextigrávida.

sextipara *n.* sextípara.

sextuplet *adj.* sextillizo, -za, sextúpleto, -ta.

sexual *adj.* sexual.

sexuality *n.* sexualidad.

infantile sexuality sexualidad infantil.

shadow *n.* sombra.

acoustic shadow sombra acústica.

shakes *n.* sacudidas.

sheath *n.* vaina.

shift *n.* desplazamiento, desviación.

axis shift desplazamiento axial, desviación axial.

chemical shift desviación química.

Doppler shift desplazamiento de Doppler.

luteoplacental shift desviación luteoplacentaria.

regenerative blood shift desviación sanguínea regenerativa.

shift to the left desplazamiento hacia la izquierda, desviación hacia la izquierda.

shift to the right desplazamiento hacia la derecha, desviación hacia la derecha.

threshold shift desplazamiento del umbral.

shin *n.* espinilla.

shock *n.* choque, shock.

anaphylactic shock choque anafiláctico.

anaphylactoid shock choque anafilactoide.

anesthetic shock choque anestésico, choque por anestesia.

bacteriemic shock choque bacteriémico.

cardiogenic shock choque cardiogénico.

chronic shock choque crónico.

cultural shock choque cultural, shock cultural.

declamping shock choque por descompresión.

delirious shock choque delirante.

electric shock choque eléctrico.

endotoxic shock choque endotóxico.

endotoxin shock choque por endotoxinas.

hemorrhagic shock choque hemorrágico.

histamine shock choque histamínico.

hypovolemic shock choque hipovolémico.

insulin shock choque insulínico.

irreversible shock choque irreversible.

reversible shock choque reversible.

septic shock choque séptico.

serum shock choque sérico.

spinal shock choque espinal, choque medular.

surgical shock choque quirúrgico.

traumatic shock choque traumático.

shoe *n.* zapato.

cast shoe zapato para escayola.

normal last shoe zapato de horma normal.

orthopedic Oxford shoe zapato ortopédico de tacón bajo.

shoulder *n.* hombro.

shunt *n.* derivación, shunt.

arteriovenous (A-V) shunt derivación arteriovenosa (AV).

sialorrhea *n.* sialorrea.

sibilant *adj.* sibilante.

sibling *n.* mellizo.

sibship *n.* consanguinidad.

sick *adj.* enfermo, -ma, mareado, -da, nauseado, -da.

sicklemia *n.* drepanocitemia.

sickness *n.* enfermedad.

morning sickness enfermedad matinal.

mountain sickness enfermedad de la montaña.

sleeping sickness enfermedad del sueño.

side *n.* lado.

sideroblast *n.* sideroblasto.

siderocyte *n.* siderocito.

siderosis *n.* siderosis.

sigh *n.* suspiro.

sight *n.* visión, vista.

day sight visión diurna, vista diurna.

far sight visión de lejos.

long sight visión de lejos, vista larga, vista lejana.

near sight visión de cerca.

night sight vista nocturna.

short sight visión corta, vista cercana, vista corta.

sigmoid *adj.* sigmoide, sigmoideo, -a, sigmoides.

sigmoidectomy *n.* sigmoidectomía.

sign *n.* signo.

meningeal sign signo meníngeo.

physical sign signo físico.

positive sign of pregnancy signo positivo de embarazo.

presumptive sign signo de presunción.

prodromic sign signo prodrómico.

soft neurologic sign signo neurológico leve.

visual sign signo visual.

vital sign signo vital.

signal *n.* señal.

significance *n.* significación.

statistical significance significación estadística.

silence *n.* silencio.

silent *adj.* silencioso, -sa, silente.

silhouette *n.* silueta.

cardiac silhouette silueta cardíaca.

silicone *n.* silicona.

injectable silicone silicona inyectable.

silicosis *n.* silicosis.

silk *n.* seda.

surgical silk seda quirúrgica.

simple *adj.* simple.

simulation *n.* simulación.

simulator *adj.* simulador, simulador, -ra.

simultaneous *adj.* simultáneo, -a.

sinew *n.* tendón.

sinistrality *n.* sinistralidad.

sinus seno, sinus.

sinusitis *n.* sinuitis, sinusitis.

site lugar, sitio, situs, zona.

situation *n.* situación.

skeletal *adj.* esquelético, -ca.

skeleton *n.* esqueleto.

skill *n.* destreza, habilidad.

skin *n.* piel.

bronzed skin piel bronceada.

loose skin piel laxa.

skull *n.* cráneo.

slant *n.* inclinación, pendiente.

slaver *n.* baba.

sleep somnus, sueño.

deep sleep sueño profundo.

fast sleep sueño rápido.

light sleep sueño ligero, sueño liviano.

NREM sleep sueño NREM.

rapid eye movement sleep sueño de movimientos oculares rápidos (MOR).

REM sleep sueño de movimientos oculares rápidos (MOR), sueño REM.

sleepwalker *n.* sonámbulo, -la.

sleepwalking *n.* sonambulismo.

sling *n.* cabestrillo, fronda.

smallpox *n.* viruela.

smear *n.* frotis.

blood smear frotis sanguíneo.

cervical smear frotis cervical.

Pap smear frotis de Pap, frotis de Papanicolaou.

smegma *n.* esmegma.

smell *v.* oler.

snake *n.* serpiente.

sneeze *n.* estornudo.

snore *n.* ronquido.

snuffbox *n.* tabaquera.

anatomic snuffbox tabaquera anatómica.

anatomical snuffbox tabaquera anatómica.

anatomist's snuffbox tabaquera anatómica.

snuffling *n.* nasalización.

soap *n.* jabón.

socket *n.* alveolo, alvéolo.

sodium *n.* sodio.

softening *n.* reblandecimiento.

sol *n.* sol.

solid *adj.* sólido, -da.

solitary *adj.* solitario, -ria.

solubility *n.* solubilidad.

soluble *adj.* soluble.

solum solum, suelo.

solutio *n.* solución, solutio.

solution solución, solutio.

somatic *adj.* somático, -ca.

somatization *n.* somatización.

somnambulance *n.* sonambulismo.

somnambulism *n.* sonambulismo.

somnambulist *n.* sonámbulo, -la.

spine

somniferous *adj.* somnífero, -ra.

somnific *adj.* somnífero, -ra.

somnolence *n.* somnolencia.

somnolency *n.* somnolencia.

somnolent *adj.* somnoliento, -ta.

somnolentia *n.* somnolencia.

sonitus ruido, sonido, sonitus.

sopor *n.* sopor.

soporiferous *adj.* soporífero, -ra.

sore , llaga, ulcus.

 pressure sore llaga por presión.

souffle *n.* soplo.

 cardiac souffle soplo cardíaco.

sound *n.* ruido, sonda sonido.

 auscultatory sound ruido auscultatorio, sonido auscultatorio.

 bowel sound ruido intestinal.

 cardiac sound ruido cardíaco.

 esophageal sound sonda esofágica.

 heart sound ruido del corazón, sonido cardíaco.

 Korotkoff sound sonido de Korotkoff, ruido de Korotkoff.

 respiratory sound ruido respiratorio, sonido respiratorio.

 vesicular breath sound ruido respiratorio vesicular, sonido respiratorio vesicular.

space *n.* espacio.

spasm *n.* espasmo.

spasmolytic *adj.* espasmolítico, -ca.

spasmus espasmo, spasmus.

spastic *adj.* espástico, -ca.

spasticity *n.* espasticidad.

spatium *n.* espacio.

spatula *n.* espátula.

spay *v.* castrar.

specialist *n.* especialista.

specific *adj.* específico, -ca.

specificity *n.* especificidad.

specimen *n.* espécimen, muestra.

 clean-catch specimen muestra no contaminada.

 cytologic specimen muestra citológica.

 midstream-catch urine specimen muestra de orina de mitad de micción.

 random voided specimen muestra miccional aleatoria.

 sputum specimen muestra de esputo.

spectacles *n.* anteojos, gafas.

 bifocal spectacles anteojos bifocales.

 trifocal spectacles anteojos trifocales.

speculum *n.* espéculo.

speech *n.* habla, lenguaje.

 jumbled speech habla confusa.

speed *n.* velocidad.

spermatogenesis *n.* espermatogénesis.

spermatozoid *n.* espermatozoide.

spermicide *n.* espermicida.

sphenoid *adj.* esfenoideo, -a, esfenoides.

sphincter *n.* esfínter.

sphygmomanometer *n.* esfigmomanómetro.

spider *n.* araña.

 arterial spider araña arterial.

 vascular spider araña vascular.

spill *n.* derramamiento.

spina *n.* espina.

spindle *n.* huso.

spine *n.* espina.

spirometer *n.* espirómetro.
spirometry *n.* espirometría.
spleen *n.* bazo.
 accessory spleen bazo accesorio.
 cyanotic spleen bazo cianótico.
 enlarged spleen bazo aumentado de tamaño.
 floating spleen bazo flotante.
 movable spleen bazo movible, bazo móvil.
 speckled spleen bazo moteado.
 wandering spleen bazo errante.
 waxy spleen bazo céreo.
splen *n.* bazo.
splenectomy *n.* esplenectomía.
splenomegaly *n.* esplenomegalia.
splint *n.* férula.
 abutment splint férula de lindero, férula de sostén.
 plaster splint férula de yeso.
 surgical splint férula quirúrgica.
splinting *n.* entablillado, ferulización.
splitting *n.* desdiferenciación, desdoblamiento, escisión.
spondylarthrosis *n.* espondilartrosis.
spondylitis *n.* espondilitis.
spondylopathy *n.* espondilopatía.
sponge *n.* esponja, tampón.
 menstrual sponge tampón menstrual.
spot *n.* mancha.
 café au lait spot mancha de café con leche.
 cherry-red spot mancha de color rojo de cereza, mancha rojo cereza.
 corneal spot mancha corneana, mancha de la córnea.

Fuchs' spot mancha de Fuchs.
Mongolian spot mancha de Baelz, mancha mongólica.
Port wine spot mancha en vino de Oporto.
spotting *n.* manchado.
sprain *n.* esguince, torcedura.
 sprain of the ankle or foot esguince de tobillo o de pie.
spray *n.* nebulización.
spreader *n.* distribuidor, espaciador, untador.
sprue *n.* bebedero de molde, esprue.
sputum *n.* esputo.
squama *n.* escama.
squamate *adj.* escamado, -da, escamoso, -sa.
squame *n.* escama.
squamous *adj.* escamoso, -sa.
squatting *n.* cuclillas.
squint *v.* bizquear, bizqueo, bizquera.
 accommodative squint bizqueo de la acomodación.
 comitant squint bizqueo concomitante.
 concomitant squint bizqueo concomitante.
 convergent squint bizqueo convergente.
 divergent squint bizqueo divergente.
 upward and downward squint bizqueo hacia arriba y hacia abajo.
stabile *adj.* estable.
stabilization *n.* estabilización.
stable *adj.* estable.
stage *n.* estadio, etapa, fase, platina.
 resting stage fase de descanso.

tumor stage estadio tumoral.
stagnation *n.* estancamiento.
stain *v.* colorante, teñir.
staining *adj.* coloración, colorante.
stalk *n.* tallo.
  body stalk tallo corporal.
  optic stalk tallo óptico.
standard *n.* estándar.
stapes *n.* estribo.
starch *n.* almidón.
starvation *n.* inanición.
stasis *n.* estasia, estasis.
state *n.* estado.
  vegetative state estado vegetativo.
statistics *n.* estadística.
stature *n.* estatura, talla.
  short stature baja estatura, talla baja.
status *n.* estado, status.
  mental status estado mental.
steatorrhea *n.* esteatorrea.
steatosis *n.* esteatosis.
stenosis *n.* estenosis.
  aortic stenosis estenosis aórtica.
  valvular stenosis estenosis valvular.
step *n.* paso.
sterile *adj.* estéril.
sterilitas *n.* esterilidad.
sterility *n.* esterilidad.
sterilization *n.* esterilización, uperisación.
sterilizer *n.* esterilizador.
sternoclavicular *adj.* esternoclavicular.
sternocleidal *adj.* esternocleidal, esternocleido, -da.
sternum esternón, sternum.
sternutatio *n.* estornudo.

sternutation *n.* estornudo.
stertor *n.* estertor.
stethoscope *n.* estetoscopio.
stigma *n.* estigma.
stillborn *adj.* mortinato, -ta.
stimulant *n.* estimulante.
  central nervous system stimulant estimulante del sistema nervioso central, neuroestimulante.
stimulation *n.* estimulación.
stimulus *n.* estímulo.
sting *n.* picadura.
stippling *n.* punteado.
stoma *n.* estoma.
stomach *n.* estómago.
stomatitis *n.* estomatitis.
stool *n.* deposición, excremento, heces.
  fatty stool heces grasas.
strabismal *adj.* estrábico, -ca.
strabismus *n.* estrabismo.
straight *adj.* recto, -ta.
strain *n.* cepa, distensión, esfuerzo, estirpe.
  wild type strain cepa tipo salvaje.
straining *n.* tenesmo.
strait *n.* estrecho.
strand *n.* hebra.
strangle *n.* estrangulación.
strangulated *adj.* estrangulado, -da.
strangulation *n.* estrangulación.
strapping *n.* strapping, vendaje.
streak *n.* estría, raya.
strength *n.* fuerza, intensidad.
streptococcus *n.* estreptococito, estreptococo.
stress *n.* estrés, tensión.
stretching *n.* estiramiento.
stria *n.* estría, stria.

stricture n. estrechez.

stridor n. estridor.

stripe n. banda.

stroke n. ataque.

   heat stroke ataque de calor.

structure n. estructura.

struma n. estruma.

study n. estudio.

   cross sectional study estudio transversal.

   cross-selectional study estudio transversal.

   prospective study estudio prospectivo.

   retrospective study estudio retrospectivo.

   single-blind study estudio simple ciego.

stump n. muñón.

   conical stump muñón cónico.

   duodenal stump muñón duodenal.

   gastric stump muñón gástrico.

   rectal stump muñón rectal.

stupefacient adj. estupefaciente.

stupefactive adj. estupefaciente.

stuttering n. tartamudez.

sty n. orzuelo.

   external sty orzuelo externo.

   internal sty orzuelo interno.

stye n. orzuelo.

succedaneous adj. sucedáneo, -a.

succus jugo, succus.

   succus entericus jugo intestinal.

   succus gastricus jugo gástrico.

   succus pancreaticus jugo pancreático.

   succus prostaticus jugo prostático.

suckle v. amamantar.

sucrose n. sacarosa.

suction n. succión.

sudor n. sudor.

sudoriparous adj. sudoríparo, -ra.

suffering n. sufrimiento.

suffocation n. ahogamiento, opresión.

sugar n. azúcar.

suggestion n. sugestión.

suicidal adj. suicida.

suicide n. suicida, suicidio.

sulcus n. sulcus, surco.

sulfonamide n. sulfamida.

superacid adj. superácido, -da.

superacidity n. superacidez.

superactivity n. sobreactividad, superactividad.

superacute adj. sobreagudo, -da, superagudo, -da.

superalimentation n. sobrealimentación, superalimentación.

superficial adj. superficial.

superficialis adj. superficial.

superinfection n. superinfección.

supernumerary adj. supernumerario, -ria.

superposition n. superposición.

supersensitivity n. supersensibilidad.

supinate v. supinar.

supination n. supinación.

   supination of the foot supinación del pie.

   supination of the forearm supinación del antebrazo.

supinator n. supinador.

supine adj. supino, -na.

supplemental adj. suplementario, -ria.

support n. apoyo, soporte.

life support soporte vital.

midstance support apoyo medio.

suppressant *n.* supresor, -ra.

suppression *n.* supresión.

suppurate *v.* supurar.

suppuration *n.* supuración.

suppurative *adj.* supurativo, -va.

suprapubic *adj.* suprapúbico, -ca.

suprarenal *adj.* suprarrenal.

supraspinous *adj.* supraespinoso, -sa, supraspinoso, -sa.

surdimute *adj.* sordomudo, -da.

surdimutitas *n.* sordomudez.

surface *n.* superficie.

surgeon *n.* cirujano, -na.

surgery *n.* cirugía.

abdominal surgery cirugía abdominal.

ambulatory surgery cirugía ambulatoria.

antiseptic surgery cirugía antiséptica.

aseptic surgery cirugía aséptica.

aural surgery cirugía ótica, cirugía otológica.

cardiac surgery cirugía cardíaca.

closed surgery cirugía cerrada.

conservative surgery cirugía conservadora.

cosmetic surgery cirugía cosmética.

dental surgery cirugía dental.

esthetic surgery cirugía estética.

general surgery cirugía general.

major surgery cirugía mayor.

minor surgery cirugía menor.

operative surgery cirugía operatoria.

oral surgery cirugía bucal, cirugía oral.

orthopedic surgery cirugía ortopédica.

plastic surgery cirugía plástica.

radical surgery cirugía radical.

reconstructive surgery cirugía reconstructiva, cirugía reconstructora.

transsexual surgery cirugía transexual.

surgical *adj.* quirúrgico, -ca.

surrogate *n.* suplente.

surveillance *n.* vigilancia.

inmune surveillance vigilancia inmune, vigilancia inmunológica.

inmunological surveillance vigilancia inmune, vigilancia inmunológica.

survey *n.* vigilancia.

metastatic survey vigilancia metastática.

susceptibility *n.* susceptibilidad.

genetic susceptibility susceptibilidad genética.

susceptible *adj.* susceptible.

suspension *n.* suspensión.

sustentaculum soporte, sustentáculo, sustentaculum.

susurrus *n.* susurro.

susurrus aurium susurro auricular.

sutura *n.* sutura.

suture *n.* sutura.

absorbable surgical suture sutura absorbible.

absorbable suture sutura absorbible.

anatomical suture sutura anatómica.

non-absorbable surgical suture sutura no absorbible, sutura quirúrgica no absorbible.

swallow *v.* deglutir.

swayback *n.* caída de espaldas.

swoon *n.* vahído.

sycosis *n.* sicosis.

  sycosis barbae sicosis de la barba.

symbiosis *n.* simbiosis.

symbol *n.* símbolo.

symmetric *adj.* simétrico, -ca.

symmetrical *adj.* simétrico, -ca.

symmetry *n.* simetría.

sympathectomy *n.* simpatectomía.

sympathetic *n.* simpático.

sympathic *n.* simpático.

sympathy *n.* simpatía.

symphysis *n.* sínfisis.

symptom *n.* síntoma.

  abstinence symptom síntoma de abstinencia.

  concomitant symptom síntoma concomitante.

  delayed symptom síntoma aplazado, síntoma diferido, síntoma retrasado.

  presenting symptom síntoma de presentación.

  prodromal symptom síntoma prodrómico.

  target symptom síntoma diana.

symptomatic *adj.* sintomático, -ca.

synapse *n.* sinapsis.

synapsis *n.* sinapsis.

synaptic *adj.* sináptico, -ca.

synchronism *n.* sincronismo.

synchronous *adj.* sincrónico, -ca.

syncopal *adj.* sincopal.

syncope *n.* síncope.

  cardiac syncope síncope cardíaco.

  syncope anginosa síncope anginoso.

syndactylia *n.* sindactilia.

syndactyly *n.* palmidactilia, sindactilia.

syndrome *n.* síndrome.

  abstinence syndrome síndrome de abstinencia.

  abused-child syndrome síndrome de abuso del niño.

  acquired immunodeficiency syndrome (AIDS) síndrome de inmunodeficiencia adquirida (SIDA).

  adult respiratory distress syndrome (ARDS) síndrome de dificultad respiratoria del adulto (SDRA), síndrome de distrés respiratorio del adulto (SDRA), síndrome de insuficiencia respiratoria del adulto.

  anginal syndrome síndrome anginoso.

  anginose syndrome síndrome anginoso.

  anxiety syndrome síndrome de ansiedad.

  compartmental syndrome síndrome compartimental.

  fetal alcohol syndrome síndrome alcohólico fetal, síndrome de alcoholismo fetal.

  fetal aspiration syndrome síndrome de aspiración fetal.

  Henoch-Schönlein syndrome síndrome de Henoch-Schönlein.

  irritable bowel syndrome síndrome del intestino irritable.

  malabsortion syndrome síndrome de mala absorción, síndrome de malabsorción.

  respiratory distress syndrome of the newborn síndrome de dificultad respiratoria del recién nacido.

  runting syndrome síndrome de injerto contra huésped.

sleep apnea syndrome síndrome de apnea del sueño.

stroke syndrome síndrome de accidente vascular.

withdrawal syndrome síndrome de abstinencia.

withdrawal syndrome for alcohol síndrome de abstinencia del alcohol.

withdrawal syndrome for sedatives síndrome de abstinencia de sedantes.

syndromic *adj.* sindrómico, -ca.

synechia *n.* sinequia.

synergia *n.* sinergia.

synergic *adj.* sinérgico, -ca.

synergism *n.* sinergismo.

synergy *n.* sinergia.

synoscheos *n.* sinósqueo.

synovitis *n.* sinovitis.

synthesis *n.* síntesis.

syphilis *n.* sífilis.

syphilitic *adj.* sifilítico, -ca.

syringe *n.* jeringa, jeringuilla.

air syringe jeringa de aire.

aspiration syringe jeringa de aspiración.

hypodermic syringe jeringa hipodérmica.

water syringe jeringa de agua.

syrup *n.* jarabe.

system *n.* sistema.

autonomic nervous system sistema nervioso autónomo.

blood group system sistema de grupos sanguíneos.

central nervous system sistema nervioso central.

digestive system sistema digestivo.

endocrine system sistema endocrino.

genital system sistema genital.

glandular system sistema glandular.

Haversian system sistema de Havers, sistema haversiano.

hematopoietic system sistema hematopoyético, sistema hemopoyético.

immune system sistema inmunitario, sistema inmunológico.

international system of units sistema internacional de unidades (SI).

locomotor system sistema locomotor.

lymphatic system sistema linfático.

mononuclear phagocyte system sistema mononuclear fagocítico.

mononuclear phagocyte system (MPS) sistema fagocítico mononuclear (SFM).

muscular system sistema muscular.

nervous system sistema nervioso.

neuromuscular system sistema neuromuscular.

parasympathetic nervous system sistema nervioso parasimpático.

reproductive system sistema reproductor.

skeletal system sistema esquelético.

sympathetic nervous system sistema nervioso del tronco simpático, sistema nervioso simpático.

system respiratorium sistema respiratorio.

urinary system sistema urinario.

urogenital system sistema urogenital.

vegetative nervous system sistema nervioso vegetativo.

visceral nervous system sistema nervioso visceral.

systematized *adj.* sistematizado, -da.

systemic *adj.* sistémico, -ca.

systole *n.* sístole.

T

tabacism *n.* tabaquismo.

tabacosis *n.* tabacosis.

tabagism *n.* tabaquismo.

tabes *n.* tabefacción, tabes.

table *n.* mesa, tabla.

examining table mesa de examen.

operating table mesa de operaciones.

tilt table mesa basculante, mesa inclinada.

tablet *n.* comprimido, tableta.

buccal tablet tableta bucal.

compressed tablet tableta comprimida.

enteric coated tablet tableta con cubierta entérica.

tabula *n.* tabla, tabula.

tabular *adj.* tabular.

tache *n.* mancha.

tachyarrhythmia *n.* taquiarritmia.

tachycardia *n.* taquicardia.

atrial tachycardia taquicardia auricular.

atrioventricular tachycardia taquicardia auriculoventricular.

auriculoventricular tachycardia taquicardia auriculoventricular.

fetal tachycardia taquicardia fetal.

sinus tachycardia taquicardia sinusal.

supraventricular tachycardia (SVT) taquicardia supraventricular (TSV).

tachycardiac *adj.* taquicárdico, -ca.

tachycardic *adj.* taquicárdico, -ca.

tachypnea *n.* taquipnea.

tactile *adj.* táctil.

tactual *adj.* táctil.

tactus *n.* tacto.

taenia *n.* taenia, tenia.

taeniasis *n.* teniasis.

tail *n.* cola.

talalgia *n.* talalgia.

talus talón, talus.

tamponade *n.* taponamiento.

cardiac tamponade taponamiento cardíaco, taponamiento de Rose.

pericardial tamponade taponamiento pericárdico.

tantrum *n.* berrinche, rabieta.

tape *n.* cinta.

adhesive tape cinta adhesiva, esparadrapo.

dental tape cinta dental.

tapeworm *n.* tenia.

tara *n.* tara.

tardive *adj.* tardío, -a.

tardy *adj.* tardío, -a.

tare *n.* tara.

target *n.* blanco.

tarsal *adj.* tarsal, tarsiano, -na.

tarsalgia *n.* tarsalgia.

tarsus *n.* tarso, tarsus.

tartar *n.* sarro.

taste *n.* gusto.

tattoo *n.* taraceo, tatuaje.

tattooing *n.* tatuaje.

taxonomy *n.* taxonomía.

tear¹ *n.* desgarramiento, desgarro.
  ligamental tear desgarro ligamentoso.
  vaginal tear desgarro vaginal.

tear² *n.* lágrima.
  artificial tear lágrima artificial.

tearing *n.* lagrimeo.

technique *n.* técnica.
  assisted reproduction technique técnica de reproducción asistida.
  relaxation technique técnica de relajación.

teething *n.* dentición.

telangiectasia *n.* telangiectasia.

telediastolic *adj.* telediastólico, -ca.

telepathy *n.* telepatía.

telomere *n.* telómero.

telophase *n.* telofase.

temperament *n.* temperamento.
  choleric temperament temperamento bilioso, temperamento colérico.

temperature *n.* temperatura.
  ambient temperature temperatura ambiental.
  axillary temperature temperatura axilar.
  basal temperature temperatura basal.
  body temperature temperatura corporal.
  room temperature temperatura ambiental.
  temperature of infant temperatura del lactante.

template *n.* plantilla, templado.

temple *n.* sien.

temporal *adj.* temporal.

temporalis *adj.* temporal.

tendinitis *n.* tendinitis.

tendinous *adj.* tendinoso, -sa.

tendo *n.* tendo, tendón.
  tendo Achillis tendón de Aquiles.

tendon *n.* tendón.
  Achilles' tendon tendón de Aquiles.
  pulled tendon tendón desgarrado.

tendonitis *n.* tendinitis, tendonitis.

tendosynovitis *n.* tendosinovitis.

tenesmus *n.* tenesmo.
  rectal tenesmus tenesmo rectal.
  vesical tenesmus tenesmo vesical.

tenia *n.* tenia.

teniasis *n.* teniasis.

tense *adj.* tenso, -sa.

tensiometer *n.* tensiómetro.

tension *n.* tensión.
  arterial tension tensión arterial.
  fatigue tension tensión de fatiga.
  muscular tension tensión muscular.
  oxygen tension tensión de oxígeno.

tepid *adj.* tibio, -bia.

teratogen *n.* teratógeno.

teratogenesis *n.* teratogénesis, teratogenia.

teratogenous *adj.* teratógeno.

teratoma *n.* teratoide, teratoma.

term *n.* término.

terminal *n.* terminal.

terminatio *n.* terminación.

termination *n.* terminación.

terminology *n.* terminología.

terminus *n.* término, terminus.

terror *n.* terror.
  night terror terror nocturno.

tertian *n.* terciano, -na.

test *n.* prueba, test.

   intelligence test test de inteligencia.

   intradermal skin test test intracutáneo.

   personality test test de personalidad.

   test tube probeta.

testicle *n.* testículo.

   ectopic testicle testículo ectópico.

   undescended testicle testículo no descendido.

testicular *adj.* testicular.

testing *n.* valoración.

testis testículo, testis.

testosterone *n.* testosterona.

tetanization *adj.* tetanización.

tetanize *v.* tetanizar.

tetanus *n.* tétanos.

tetany *n.* tetania.

   hypocalcemic tetany tetania hipocalcémica.

   neonatal tetany tetania del recién nacido, tetania neonatal.

tetralogy *n.* tetralogía.

   Fallot's tetralogy tetralogía de Fallot.

   tetralogy of Fallot tetralogía de Fallot.

tetraplegia *n.* tetraplejía.

tetraplegic *adj.* tetrapléjico, -ca.

tetrasomy *n.* tetrasomía.

tetter *n.* sarpullido.

   crusted tetter sarpullido costroso.

   prickly heat tetter sarpullido por calor.

textus tejido, textus.

thalamic *adj.* talámico, -ca.

thalamus *n.* tálamo.

thalassemia *n.* talasemia.

thanatos *n.* tánatos.

theca *n.* teca.

theorem *n.* teorema.

theoretical *adj.* teórico, -ca.

theorist *n.* teórico, -ca.

theory *n.* teoría.

   Baeyer's theory teoría de Baeyer.

theque *n.* teca.

therapeutic *adj.* terapéutico, -ca.

therapeutics terapéutica.

therapia *n.* terapia.

therapist *n.* terapeuta.

   occupation therapist terapeuta ocupacional.

   physical therapist terapeuta físico.

   sexual therapist terapeuta sexual.

   speech therapist terapeuta del lenguaje.

therapy *n.* terapia.

   adjuvant therapy terapia adyuvante.

   anticoagulant therapy terapia anticoagulante.

   biological therapy terapia biológica.

   combined therapy terapia combinada.

   electroconvulsive therapy terapia electroconvulsiva (TEC).

   hyperbaric oxygen therapy terapia con oxígeno hiperbárico.

   immunesuppresive therapy terapia inmunosupresora.

   immunization therapy terapia de inmunización.

   inhalation therapy terapia de inhalación.

   intravenous therapy terapia intravenosa.

oxygen therapy terapia con oxígeno.

play therapy terapia de juego, terapia lúdica.

radiation therapy terapia con radiación, terapia con radio.

relaxation therapy terapia de relajación.

sexual therapy terapia sexual.

shock therapy terapia de choque, terapia de shock.

vaccine therapy terapia con vacunas.

thermal *adj.* termal, térmico, -ca.

thermic *adj.* térmico, -ca.

thermolabile *adj.* termolábil.

thermometer *n.* termómetro.

Celsius thermometer termómetro centígrado, termómetro de Celsius.

electronic thermometer termómetro electrónico.

Fahrenheit thermometer termómetro de Fahrenheit.

fever thermometer termómetro para la fiebre.

mercury thermometer termómetro de mercurio.

rectal thermometer termómetro rectal.

thermoreceptor *n.* termorreceptor.

thermoregulation *n.* termorregulación.

thermostabile *adj.* termoestable, termostábil, termostable.

thermostable *adj.* termoestable.

thermostat *n.* termostato, termóstato.

hypothalamic thermostat termostato hipotalámico.

thiazide *n.* tiacida, tiazida.

thigh *n.* muslo.

thinking *n.* pensamiento.

abstract thinking pensamiento abstracto.

autistic thinking pensamiento autista.

creative thinking pensamiento creativo.

thinness *n.* delgadez.

thioflavine *n.* tioflavina.

thirst *n.* sed.

thoracentesis *n.* toracentesis.

thoracic *adj.* torácico, -ca.

thorax *n.* tórax.

thought *n.* pensamiento.

threshold *n.* umbral.

throat *n.* garganta.

thrombectomy *n.* trombectomía.

thrombin *n.* trombina.

thrombocythemia *n.* trombocitemia.

essential thrombocythemia trombocitemia esencial.

thrombocytosis *n.* trombocitosis.

thromboembolism *n.* tromboembolia, tromboembolismo.

thrombolytic *adj.* trombolítico, -ca.

thrombopenia *n.* trombopenia.

thrombopeny *n.* trombopenia.

thrombophilia *n.* trombofilia.

thrombophlebitis *n.* tromboflebitis.

thrombosed *adj.* trombosado, -da.

thrombosis *n.* trombosis.

venous thrombosis trombosis venosa.

thrombotic *adj.* trombótico, -ca.

thrombus *n.* trombo.

thrush *n.* algodoncillo, muguet.

thumb *n.* pulgar.

thymus *n.* timo.

thyroid *adj.* tiroideo, -a.

thyroidectomize *v.* tiroidectomiza-do, -da, tiroidectomizar.

thyroidectomy *n.* tiroidectomía.

thyroidism *n.* tiroidismo.

thyroiditis *n.* tiroiditis.

thyrotoxicosis *n.* tirotoxicosis.

tibia *n.* tibia.

  tibia valga tibia valga.

  tibia vara tibia vara.

tibial *adj.* tibial, tibialis.

tibialis *adj.* tibial, tibialis.

tic *n.* tic.

  chronic tic tic crónico.

  convulsive tic tic convulsivo.

  diaphragmatic tic tic diafragmáti-co, tic respiratorio.

  local tic tic local.

  spasmodic tic tic espasmódico.

  tic douloureux tic doloroso, tic do-loroso de la cara.

  tic facial tic facial.

tide *n.* marea.

timbre *n.* timbre.

time *n.* tiempo.

  activated partial thromboplastin time (APTT) tiempo de trombo-plastina parcial activada (TTPa).

  clotting time tiempo de coagula-ción, tiempo de formación del coá-gulo.

  partial thromboplastin time (PTT) tiempo de tromboplastina parcial (TTP).

  prothrombin time tiempo de pro-trombina.

  reaction time tiempo de reacción.

  relaxation time tiempo de relaja-ción.

  sedimentation time tiempo de se-dimentación.

tinction *n.* tinción.

tinea *n.* tiña, tinea.

  tinea corporis tiña corporal, tiña del cuerpo.

tinnitus *n.* acúfeno, tinnitus, zum-bido.

  vibratory tinnitus zumbido vibra-torio.

tissue *n.* tejido.

  adipose tissue tejido adiposo.

  bone tissue tejido óseo.

  cancellous tissue tejido esponjoso, tejido poroso.

  cartilaginous tissue tejido cartila-ginoso.

  cicatricial tissue tejido cicatricial.

  connective tissue tejido conectivo, tejido conjuntivo.

  elastic tissue tejido elástico, tejido elástico amarillo.

  embryonic tissue tejido embriona-rio, tejido primario.

  fibroelastic tissue tejido fibroelás-tico.

  loose connective tissue tejido con-juntivo laxo.

  lymphatic tissue tejido linfático.

  lymphoid tissue tejido linfoide, te-jido linfoideo.

  muscular tissue tejido muscular.

  nervous tissue tejido nervioso.

  osseous tissue tejido óseo.

  scar tissue tejido cicatricial.

  skeletal tissue tejido esquelético.

tissular *adj.* tisular.

titer *n.* título.

titrate *v.* titular.

titration *n.* titulación, valoración.

titubation *n.* titubeo.

tobacco *n.* tabaco.

tocology *n.* tocología.

toe *n.* dedo.

tennis toe dedo del pie de tenista.

toenail *n.* uña.

tolerance *n.* tolerancia.

drug tolerance tolerancia a los fármacos, tolerancia farmacológica.

exercise tolerance tolerancia al ejercicio.

immunologic tolerance tolerancia inmunológica.

tolerance pain tolerancia al dolor.

toll *n.* mortandad.

tomography *n.* tomografía.

computed tomography (CT) tomografía computadorizada (TC).

computer axial tomography (CAT) tomografía axial computadorizada (TAC).

emission computed tomography (ECT) tomografía computadorizada por emisión (TCE).

positron emission tomography (PET) tomografía por emisión de positrones (PET).

single-photon emission computed tomography (SPECT) tomografía computadorizada por emisión de fotón único (SPECT).

tone *n.* tono.

affective tone tono afectivo.

fetal heart tone (FHT) tono cardíaco fetal (TCF).

heart tone tono cardíaco.

muscular tone tono muscular.

vagal tone tono vagal.

tongue *n.* lengua.

fissured tongue lengua arrugada, lengua fisurada, lingua fissurata.

furred tongue lengua saburral.

tonic *n.* tónico, -ca.

tonicity *n.* tonicidad.

tonoclonic *adj.* tonoclónico, -ca.

tonsil *n.* amígdala.

tonsillar *adj.* tonsilar.

tonsillary *adj.* tonsilar.

tonsillectomy *n.* tonsilectomía.

tonsillitis *n.* amigdalitis, tonsilitis.

acute tonsillitis amigdalitis aguda.

diphtheritic tonsillitis amigdalitis diftérica.

herpetic tonsillitis amigdalitis herpética.

mycotic tonsillitis amigdalitis micótica.

preglottic tonsillitis amigdalitis preglótica.

streptococcal tonsillitis amigdalitis estreptocócica.

superficial tonsillitis amigdalitis superficial, tonsilitis superficial.

supurative tonsillitis amigdalitis supurativa.

Vincent's tonsillitis amigdalitis de Vincent.

tonsilloadenoidectomy *n.* adenoamigdalectomía.

tonus *n.* tonicidad, tono, tonus.

tooth *n.* diente, muela.

acrylic resin tooth diente de acrílico, diente de resina acrílica.

anatomic tooth diente anatómico.

artificial tooth diente artificial.

buck tooth diente prominente, diente salido.

crossbite tooth diente en mordida cruzada.

dead tooth diente muerto.

deciduous tooth diente decidual.

devitalized tooth diente desvitalizado.

fused tooth diente fusionado.

impacted tooth diente impactado.

malposed tooth diente en malposición.

migrating tooth diente migratorio.

milk tooth diente de leche.

mottled tooth diente manchado.

natal tooth diente natal.

neonatal tooth diente neonatal.

non-anatomic tooth diente no anatómico.

non-vital tooth diente no vital.

normally posed tooth diente en posición normal.

permanent tooth diente permanente.

premature tooth diente prematuro.

primary tooth diente primario.

protruding tooth diente protruido.

second tooth diente secundario.

vital tooth diente vital.

wandering of a tooth diente errante.

wisdom tooth muela del juicio.

tophus *n.* tofo.

topical *adj.* tópico, -ca.

topicum *n.* tópico.

torcula *n.* prensa, tórcula.

torpid *adj.* tórpido, -da.

torsion *n.* torsión.

torsion of the testis torsión del cordón espermático, torsión del testículo, torsión testicular.

torso *n.* torso.

torticollis *n.* torticolis, tortícolis.

tortuous *adj.* tortuoso, -sa.

totipotential *adj.* totipotencial.

touch *n.* tacto.

rectal touch tacto rectal.

vaginal touch tacto vaginal.

tour *n.* vuelta.

tourniquet *n.* torniquete.

toxemia *n.* toxemia.

toxemia of pregnancy toxemia del embarazo, toxemia gravídica.

toxic *adj.* tóxico, -ca.

toxicity *n.* toxicidad.

acute toxicity toxicidad aguda.

toxicolgy *n.* toxicología.

toxicologic *adj.* toxicológico, -ca.

toxicosis *n.* toxicosis.

toxin *n.* tóxico, toxina.

toxoplasmosis *n.* toxoplasmosis.

trabecula *n.* trabécula.

trabecular *adj.* trabecular.

trabeculate *adj.* trabeculado, -da.

tracer *n.* trazador.

trachea *n.* tráquea.

tracheal *adj.* traqueal.

tracheitis *n.* traqueítis.

tracheostomize *v.* traqueostomizar.

tracheostomy *n.* traqueostomía.

tracheotomy *n.* traqueotomía.

trachitis *n.* traqueítis, traquitis.

trachoma *n.* tracoma.

tracing *n.* trazado, trazo.

tract *n.* haz, tracto.

uveal tract úvea.

traction *n.* tracción.

tractus haz, tracto, tractus.

training *n.* adiestramiento, entrenamiento.

trait *n.* rasgo.

acquired trait rasgo adquirido.

character trait rasgo caracterial, rasgo del carácter.

chromosomal trait rasgo cromosómico.

codominant trait rasgo codominante.

dependent trait rasgo dependiente.

dominant trait rasgo dominante.

hereditary trait rasgo hereditario.

intermediate trait rasgo intermedio.

non-penetrant trait rasgo no penetrante.

personality trait rasgo de la personalidad.

sex-conditioned trait rasgo condicionado por el sexo.

sex-influenced trait rasgo influido por el sexo.

sex-limited trait rasgo limitado por el sexo.

sex-linked trait rasgo ligado al sexo.

trance *n.* trance.

tranquilizer *n.* tranquilizante.

major tranquilizer tranquilizante mayor.

minor tranquilizer tranquilizante menor.

transaminasemia *n.* transaminasemia.

transcutaneous *adj.* transcutáneo, -a.

transdermal *adj.* transdérmico, -ca.

transduction *n.* transducción.

transfer *n.* transferencia, traslado.

transference *n.* transferencia.

negative transference transferencia negativa.

positive transference transferencia positiva.

transformation *n.* transformación.

transfuse *v.* transfundir.

transfusion *n.* transfusión.

arterial transfusion transfusión arterial.

blood transfusion transfusión de sangre.

drip transfusion transfusión por goteo.

fetomaternal transfusion transfusión fetomaterna.

twin-to-twin transfusion transfusión gemelo-gemelar.

transgenic *adj.* transgénico, -ca.

transient *adj.* transitorio, -a.

transit *n.* tránsito.

intestinal transit tránsito intestinal.

translocation *n.* translocación, traslocación.

balanced translocation translocación balanceada, translocación equilibrada.

transmembrane *n.* transmembrana.

transmigration *n.* transmigración.

transmissible *adj.* transmisible.

transmission *n.* transmisión.

synaptic transmission transmisión sináptica.

transmural *adj.* transmural.

transparent *adj.* transparente.

transpirable *adj.* transpirable.

transpiration *n.* transpiración.

transplacental *adj.* transplacentario, -a.

transplant *n.* trasplantar, trasplante.

  bone marrow transplant trasplante de médula ósea.

  corneal transplant trasplante corneal, trasplante de córnea.

  fetal tissue transplant trasplante de tejido fetal.

  heart transplant trasplante cardíaco, trasplante de corazón.

  HLA-identical transplant trasplante HLA idéntico.

  liver transplant trasplante hepático.

  pancreatic transplant trasplante pancreático.

  renal transplant trasplante renal.

  tendon transplant trasplante del tendón, trasplante tendinosos.

transplantation *n.* trasplante.

transport *n.* transporte.

transsexual *adj.* transexual.

transsexualism *n.* transexualismo.

transudation *n.* transudación, trasudación.

transvestism *n.* travestismo.

transvestite *n.* travestido, -da.

trapezium *n.* trapecio.

trascendence *n.* trascendencia.

trascendent *adj.* trascendental, trascendente.

traslation *n.* traslación.

trasplantar *adj.* trasplantar.

trauma *n.* trauma.

  acoustic trauma trauma acústico.

  birth trauma trauma del nacimiento.

  cranioencephalic trauma trauma craneoencefálico.

  missile wound trauma trauma por herida de bala.

  psychic trauma trauma psíquico.

traumatic *adj.* traumático, -ca.

traumatism *n.* traumatismo.

traumatologist *n.* traumatólogo, -ga.

traumatology *n.* traumatología.

tray *n.* bandeja.

treat *v.* tratar.

treatment *n.* tratamiento.

  active treatment tratamiento activo.

  adjuvant treatment tratamiento adyuvante.

  causal treatment tratamiento causal.

  coadjuvant treatment tratamiento coadyuvante.

  combined modality treatment tratamiento combinado.

  conservative treatment tratamiento conservador.

  curative treatment tratamiento curativo.

  diabetic treatment tratamiento de la diabetes.

  dietetic treatment tratamiento dietético.

  empiric treatment tratamiento empírico.

  hygienic treatment tratamiento higiénico.

  immunosuppressive treatment tratamiento inmunosupresor.

organ treatment tratamiento orgánico.

palliative treatment tratamiento paliativo.

preventive treatment tratamiento preventivo.

prophylactic treatment tratamiento profiláctico.

radical treatment tratamiento radical.

specific treatment tratamiento específico.

stepped treatment tratamiento escalonado.

surgical treatment tratamiento quirúrgico.

symptomatic treatment tratamiento sintomático.

tremor *n.* temblor, tremor.

benign essential tremor temblor esencial, temblor esencial benigno, temblor esencial hereditario.

essential tremor temblor esencial, temblor esencial benigno, temblor esencial hereditario.

familial tremor temblor familiar.

hereditary essential tremor temblor esencial, temblor esencial benigno, temblor esencial hereditario.

physiologic tremor temblor fisiológico.

postural tremor temblor postural.

rest tremor temblor de reposo.

resting tremor temblor de reposo.

senile tremor temblor senil.

tremulous *adj.* tembloroso, -sa, trémulo, -la.

trend *n.* tendencia.

trepan *n.* trépano.

trepanation *n.* trepanación.

trepanner *n.* trepanador, -ra.

triad *n.* tríada.

trial *n.* ensayo.

triangle *n.* triángulo.

triangulum triángulo, triangulum.

trichinosis *n.* triquinosis.

trichosis *n.* tricosis.

tricipital *adj.* tricipital, tricípite.

tricuspid *adj.* tricúspide.

tricuspidal *adj.* tricúspide.

tricuspidate *adj.* tricúspide.

tricyclic *adj.* tricíclico, -ca.

trigeminus *n.* trigémino.

trigger *n.* desencadenante, gatillo.

triglyceride *n.* triglicérido.

trigone *n.* trígono.

trigonitis *n.* trigonitis.

trigonum trígono, trigonum.

trilaminar *adj.* trilaminar.

trilateral *adj.* trilateral.

trilogy *n.* trilogía.

trimensual *adj.* trimensual, trimestral.

trimester *n.* trimestre.

tripara *n.* trípara.

triphasic *adj.* trifásico, -ca.

triplet *n.* triplete.

triplets *adj.* trillizo, -za.

triplex *adj.* triple, triplex.

trisomia *n.* trisomía.

trisomy *n.* trisomía.

triturate *v.* triturar.

trocar *n.* trócar.

trochanter *n.* trocánter.

trochiter *n.* troquíter.

trophic *adj.* trófico, -ca.

trophism *n.* trofismo.

trophoblast *n.* trofoblasto.

trophology *n.* trofología.

tropism *n.* tactismo, tropismo.

true *adj.* real.

truncate *v.* truncado, -da, truncar.

truncatus *adj.* truncado, -da.

truncus *n.* tronco.

trunk *n.* tronco.

truss *n.* braguero.

trypanosome *n.* tripanosoma.

trypanosomiasis *n.* tripanosomiasis, tripnosomiosis.

trypsinogen *n.* tripsinógeno.

tryptic *adj.* tríptico, -ca.

tuba *n.* trompa.

tubal *adj.* tubárico, -ca, tubario, -ria.

tube *n.* sonda, trompa, tubo.
 drainage tube sonda de drenaje, tubo de drenaje.
 esophageal tube sonda esofágica.
 feeding tube sonda de alimentación, tubo de alimentación.
 nasogastric tube sonda nasogástrica.
 nasotracheal tube sonda nasotraqueal.
 nephrostomy tube sonda de nefrostomía.
 stomach tube sonda gástrica.
 test tube tubo de ensayo.
 X-ray tube tubo de rayos X.

tuberculin *n.* tuberculina.

tuberculocidal *adj.* tuberculocida.

tuberculocide *n.* tuberculocida.

tuberculosis *n.* tuberculosis.
 pulmonar tuberculosis tuberculosis pulmonar.

tuberculostatic *adj.* tuberculostático, -ca.

tuberculous *adj.* tuberculoso, -sa.

tuberositas tuberosidad, tuberositas.

tuberosity *n.* tuberosidad.

tubular *adj.* tubular.

tubule *n.* túbulo.

tubulus *n.* túbulo.

tubus tubo, tubus.

tugging *n.* tiro.

tularemia *n.* tularemia.

tumefacient *adj.* tumefaciente.

tumefaction *n.* tumefacción.

tumor *n.* tumor.
 benign tumor tumor benigno.
 malignant tumor tumor maligno.

tunic *n.* túnica.

tunica *n.* túnica.

tunnel *n.* túnel.

turbid *adj.* túrbido, -da, turbio, -bia.

turbidity *n.* enturbiamiento, turbiedad.

tussal *adj.* tusivo, -va.

tussis tos, tussis.

tussive *adj.* tusivo, -va.

twin *n.* gemelo, -la.
 identical twin gemelo idéntico.

twinge *n.* punzada.

twitch *n.* contracción.

tyloma *n.* tiloma.

tympanum *n.* tímpano.

type *n.* tipo.
 constitutional type tipo constitucional.

typhus *n.* tifo, tifus.

typing *n.* tipificación.
 blood typing tipificación de la sangre, tipificación de los grupos sanguíneos.
 HLA typing tipificación de los HLA.

typology *n.* tipología.

tyrotoxicosis *n.* tirotoxicosis.
tyroxine *n.* tiroxina.

U

ulcer *n.* llaga, úlcera, ulcus.
  gastric ulcer ulcus gástrico.
ulcerate *v.* ulcerar.
ulcerated *adj.* ulcerado, -da.
ulceration *n.* ulceración.
ulcus *n.* ulcus.
ulna *n.* cúbito, cubitus, ulna.
ultrasonic *adj.* ultrasónico, -ca.
ultrasonography *n.* ultrasonografía.
ultraviolet *adj.* ultravioleta.
umbilical *adj.* umbilical.
umbilicate *adj.* umbilicado, -da.
umbilicated *adj.* umbilicado, -da.
umbilication *n.* umbilicación.
umbilicus *n.* ombligo.
unconscious *n.* inconsciente.
unconsciousness *n.* inconsciencia.
unction *n.* unción.
underweight *n.* bajo peso.
ungual *adj.* ungueal, ungular.
unguent *n.* ungüento, unguentum.
unguis *n.* uña, unguis.
  unguis aduncus uña encarnada, uña incardinada, uñero.
  unguis incarnatus uña encarnada, uña incardinada, uñero.
unicellular *adj.* unicelular.
unigravida *adj.* unigrávida.
union *n.* reunión, unión.
unipotent *adj.* unipotente.
unit *n.* unidad.

  clinical unit unidad clínica.
  intensive care unit (ICU) unidad de cuidados intensivos (UCI).
  international unit unidad internacional.
  neonatal intensive care unit (NICU) unidad de cuidados intensivos neonatales (UCIN).
universal *adj.* universal.
univitelline *adj.* univitelino, -na.
unphysiologic *adj.* no fisiológico, -ca.
unsaturated *adj.* insaturado, -da.
urea *n.* urea.
uremia *n.* uremia, uroemia.
uremic *adj.* urémico, -ca.
ureter *n.* uréter.
urethra *n.* uretra.
  membranous urethra uretra membranosa.
  penile urethra uretra peneana.
  prostatic urethra uretra prostática.
  urethra masculina uretra masculina.
urethral *adj.* uretral.
urethritis *n.* uretritis.
urgency *n.* urgencia.
  motor urgency urgencia motora.
  sensory urgency urgencia sensorial.
uric *adj.* úrico, -ca.
uricemia *n.* uricemia.
uricosuria *n.* uricosuria.
urina *n.* orina.
urinal *n.* orinal.
urinalysis *n.* urinálisis.
urinary *adj.* urinario, -ria.
urinate *v.* orinar.
urination *n.* micción, urinación.

precipitant urination micción precipitante.

stuttering urination micción tartamuda, micción tartamudeante.

urine *n.* orina, urina.

cloudy urine orina turbia.

maple syrup urine orina en jarabe de arce.

urogenital *adj.* urogenital.

urography *n.* urografía.

urologic *adj.* urológico, -ca.

urologist *n.* urólogo, -ga.

urology *n.* urología.

urothelium *n.* urotelio.

urticant *adj.* urticante.

urticaria *n.* urticaria.

uterine *adj.* uterino, -na.

uterus *n.* útero, uterus.

gravid uterus útero grávido.

utricle *n.* utrículo.

utriculus *n.* utrículo.

uvea *n.* úvea.

uveitis *n.* uveítis.

uvula *n.* úvula.

uvulitis *n.* uvulitis.

V

vaccinal *adj.* vaccinal, vacunal.

vaccination *n.* vacunación.

vaccine *n.* vacuna.

antirabic vaccine vacuna antirrábica.

attenuated vaccine vacuna atenuada.

bacterial vaccine vacuna bacteriana, vacuna bactérica.

combined vaccine vacuna polivalente.

diphtheria vaccine vacuna antidiftérica, vacuna de la difteria.

hepatitis B vaccine vacuna contra la hepatitis B, vacuna de la hepatitis B.

human diploid cell rabies vaccine (HDRV) vacuna antirrábica preparada de células diploides humanas, vacuna antirrábica preparada en células diploides humanas (HDRV).

inactivated poliovirus vaccine (IPV) vacuna antipoliomielítica inactivada (IPV).

inactivated vaccine vacuna de virus inactivados, vacuna inactivada.

influenza virus vaccine vacuna antigripal, vacuna de virus de influenza, vacuna de virus de la influenza.

killed vaccine vacuna de organismos muertos.

live rubella virus vaccine vacuna antirrubeólica de virus vivos, vacuna de virus de la rubéola vivos, vacuna de virus de rubéola vivos.

measles vaccine vacuna antisarampión, vacuna antisarampionosa, vacuna del sarampión.

measles virus vaccine vacuna antisarampión, vacuna antisarampionosa, vacuna de virus sarampionoso, vacuna del sarampión.

meningococcal polysaccharide vaccine vacuna antimeningocócica de polisacáridos.

mumps virus vaccine vacuna antiparotidítica, vacuna antiparotiditis, vacuna de virus de las paperas.

oral poliovirus vaccine (OPV) vacuna antipoliomielítica oral (OPV).

pertussis vaccine vacuna anticoqueluchosa, vacuna antipertussis, vacuna antitosferinosa, vacuna contra la tos ferina, vacuna de la tos ferina.

pneumococcal vaccine vacuna antineumocócica.

poliovirus vaccine vacuna antipoliomielítica, vacuna antipoliomielitis, vacuna de la poliomielitis, vacuna de poliovirus.

polyvalent vaccine vacuna polivalente.

rabies vaccine vacuna de la rabia.

recombinant hepatitis B vaccine vacuna recombinante de la hepatitis B.

rubella virus vaccine vacuna antirrubéola, vacuna antirrubeólica.

Sabin's oral vaccine vacuna antipoliomielítica de Sabin, vacuna de Sabin bucal.

Salk vaccine vacuna antipoliomielítica de Salk, vacuna de Salk.

smallpox vaccine vacuna antivariólica, vacuna de la viruela.

staphylococcus vaccine vacuna de estafilococo, vacuna estafilocócica.

streptococcic vaccine vacuna de estreptococos, vacuna estreptocócica.

tetanus vaccine vacuna antitetánica.

triple vaccine vacuna triple, vacuna triple vírica.

trivalent vaccine vacuna triple, vacuna triple vírica.

tuberculosis vaccine vacuna antituberculosa, vacuna de la tuberculosis.

whooping cough vaccine vacuna contra la tos ferina, vacuna de la tos ferina.

yellow fever vaccine vacuna antia-marílica, vacuna anti-fiebre amarilla, vacuna de Aragão, vacuna de la fiebre amarilla.

vaccinum vaccinum.

vacuole n. vacuola.

vacuum n. vacío, vacuum.

vagal adj. vagal.

vagina n. vagina, vaina.

  septate vagina vagina septada, vagina tabicada.

vaginal adj. vaginal.

vaginismus n. vaginismo.

vaginosis n. vaginosis.

vagotomy n. vagotomía.

vagus n. vago.

valgus adj. valgo, -ga, valgus.

valid adj. válido, -da.

validation n. validación.

validity n. validez.

valley n. valle.

value n. valor.

  mean value valor medio.

  normal value valor normal.

  threshold value valor umbral.

valva n. válvula.

valve n. valva, válvula.

  prosthetic heart valve válvula cardíaca protésica.

valvotomy n. valvotomía.

valvular adj. valvular.

valvule n. válvula.

valvulitis n. valvulitis.

vapor n. vapor.

vaporization n. vaporización.

vaporizer n. vaporizador.

variability n. variabilidad.

  baseline variability of fetal heart rate variabilidad basal de la frecuencia cardíaca fetal.

variable n. variable.

variance n. varianza.

variant n. variante.

variation n. variación.

varicella n. varicela.

varicocele n. varicocele.

varicose adj. varicoso, -sa.

varicosity n. varicosidad.

variety n. variedad.

variola n. variola, viruela.

varus varo, -ra, varus.

vas vas, vaso.

vascular adj. vascular.

vascularity n. vascularidad.

vascularization n. vascularización.

vascularized adj. vascularizado, -da.

vasculitis n. vasculitis.

vasculopathy n. vasculopatía.

vasectomized adj. vasectomizado, -da.

vasectomy n. vasectomía.

vasoconstriction n. vasoconstricción.

vasoconstrictive adj. vasoconstrictivo, -va, vasoconstrictor, -ra.

vasoconstrictor adj. vasoconstrictor, -ra.

vasodilatation n. vasodilatación.

vasodilative adj. vasodilatador, -ra, vasodilatativo, -va.

vasodilator adj. vasodilatador, -ra.

vasomotive adj. vasomotor, -ra.

vasopressin (VP) n. vasopresina (VP).

vasospasm n. vasoespasmo, vasospasmo.

vasovagal adj. vasovagal.

vault n. bóveda.

vector n. vector.

biological vector vector biológico.

veganism n. veganismo.

vegetarian n. vegetariano, -na.

vegetarianism n. vegetarianismo, vegetarismo.

vegetation n. vegetación.

adenoid vegetation vegetación adenoide.

bacterial vegetation vegetación bacteriana.

vegetative adj. vegetante, vegetativo, -va.

veil n. velo, velum.

vein n. vena.

vellus n. vello.

velocity n. velocidad.

sedimentation velocity velocidad de sedimentación.

velum n. velo, velum.

vena n. vena.

venepuncture n. venopunción.

venereal adj. venéreo, -a.

venereology n. venereología.

venipuncture n. venepunción, venepuntura, venipuntura.

venography n. venografía.

venom n. veneno.

snake venom veneno de las serpientes.

viper venom veneno de víbora.

venose adj. venoso, -sa.

venous adj. venoso, -sa.

venter n. venter, vientre.

ventilate v. ventilar.

ventilation n. ventilación.

artificial ventilation ventilación artificial.

assisted ventilation ventilación asistida.

ventilator *n.* ventilador.

ventral *adj.* ventral.

ventralis *adj.* ventral.

ventricle *n.* ventrículo, ventriculus.

ventricular *adj.* ventricular.

ventriculus *n.* ventrículo, ventriculus.

venula *adj.* vénula, venular.

venule *n.* vénula.

verbiage *n.* verborrea.

vermis vermes, vermis.

verruca *n.* verruca, verruga.

 verruca vulgaris verruga vulgar.

verruga *n.* verruca, verruga.

version *n.* versión.

vertebra *n.* vértebra.

vertebral *adj.* vertebral.

vertebrated *adj.* vertebrado, -da.

vertex vertex, vértice.

vertical *adj.* vertical.

verticalis *adj.* vertical.

vertiginous *adj.* vertiginoso, -sa.

vertigo *n.* vértigo.

 central vertigo vértigo central.

 disabling positional vertigo vérti-go posicional incapacitante.

 height vertigo vértigo de altura.

 labyrinthine vertigo vértigo labe-ríntico.

 peripheral vertigo vértigo periférico.

 positional vertigo vértigo de posi-ción, vértigo posicional.

 postural vertigo vértigo postural.

 rotary vertigo vértigo rotatorio.

 rotatory vertigo vértigo rotatorio.

vesica *n.* vejiga, vesica.

 vesica biliaris vejiga biliar.

 vesica urinaria vejiga urinaria, vesi-ca urinalis, vesica urinaria.

vesical *adj.* vesical.

vesicle *n.* vesícula.

 seminal vesicle vesícula seminal.

vesicula *n.* vesícula.

 vesicula bilis vesícula biliar.

 vesicula fellea vesícula biliar, vesí-cula fellea, vesícula fellis.

 vesicula seminalis vesícula semi-nal.

vesicular *adj.* vesicular.

vessel *n.* vaso.

vestibular *adj.* vestibular.

vestibule *n.* vestíbulo.

vestibulum *n.* vestíbulo.

vestige *n.* vestigio.

vestigium *n.* vestigio.

via *n.* vía.

viability *n.* viabilidad.

viable *adj.* viable.

vial *n.* vial.

vibration *n.* vibración.

vibrative *adj.* vibrante, vibrativo, -va.

vibrator *n.* vibrador.

vibrio *n.* vibrión.

vice *n.* vicio.

vicious *adj.* vicioso, -sa.

view *n.* vista.

vigilance *n.* vigilia.

vigor *n.* vigor.

villose *adj.* velloso, -sa, velludo, -da.

villous *adj.* velloso, -sa.

villus *n.* vellosidad, villus.

 amniotic villus vellosidad amnióti-ca.

vinculum *n.* vínculo, vinculum.

violaceous *adj.* violáceo, -a.

violation *n.* violación.

violet *adj.* violeta.

viral *adj.* viral, vírico, -ca, virósico, -ca, viroso, -sa.

viremia *n.* viremia.

virgin *adj.* virgen.

virginity *n.* virginidad.

viricidal *adj.* viricida, virucida, virulicida.

virile *adj.* viril.

virility *n.* virilidad.

virilization *n.* virilización.

virilizing *adj.* virilizador, -ra, virilizante.

virion *n.* virión.

virosis *n.* virosis.

virtual *adj.* virtual.

virulent *adj.* virulento, -ta.

virus *n.* virus.

virustatic *adj.* virustático, -ca.

viscera *n.* víscera.

visceral *adj.* visceral.

visceralgia *n.* visceralgia.

viscoelasticity *n.* viscoelasticidad.

viscosity *n.* viscosidad.

viscus víscera, viscus.

visibility *n.* visibilidad.

visible *adj.* visible.

vision *n.* visión.
  central vision visión central.
  color vision visión de color.
  double vision visión doble.
  low vision visión baja.
  monocular vision visión monocular.
  night vision visión nocturna.
  scotopic vision visión escotópica.
  stereoscopic vision visión estereoscópica.

visit *n.* visita.

visual *adj.* visual.

visualization *n.* visualización.

visualize *v.* visualizar.

vital *adj.* vital.

vitality *n.* vitalidad.

vitalize *v.* vitalizar.

vitamin *n.* vitamina, vitazima.

vitelline *adj.* vitelina, vitelino, -na.

vitiligo *n.* vitíligo.

vitium vicio, vitium.

vitrectomy *n.* vitrectomía.

viviparous *adj.* vivíparo, -ra.

vivisection *n.* vivisección.

vocal *adj.* vocal.

voice *n.* voz.
  cavernous voice voz cavernosa.
  eunuchoid voice voz de falsete, voz eunucoide.
  whispered voice voz susurrada.

voix *n.* voz.

volatile *adj.* volátil.

volume *n.* volumen.
  blood volume volumen sanguíneo.
  mean corpuscular volume (MCV) volumen corpuscular medio VMC.

voluntary *adj.* voluntario, -ria.

volvulus *n.* vólvulo.

vomer *n.* vómer.

vomit *n.* vómito.
  bilious vomit vómito bilioso.
  black vomit vómito negro.
  coffee-ground vomit vómito de borra de café, vómito en posos de café.

vomiting *n.* vomición, vómito.
  incoercible vomiting vómito incoercible.
  morning vomiting vómito matinal.
  periodic vomiting vómito periódico.
  projectile vomiting vómito en escopetazo.

recurrent vomiting vómito recurrente.

vomiting of pregnancy vómito del embarazo.

vomitive *adj.* vomitivo, -va.

vomitory *n.* vomitivo, vomitorio.

vomitus vómito, vomitus.

vomitus niger vómito negro.

vortex vortex, vórtice.

vox vox, voz.

voyeurism *n.* voyeurismo.

vulgaris *adj.* vulgar.

vulnerability *n.* vulnerabilidad.

vulnerable *adj.* vulnerable.

vulva *n.* vulva.

vulval *adj.* vulvar.

vulvar *adj.* vulvar.

vulvitis *n.* vulvitis.

W

waist *n.* cintura, talle.

wakefulness *n.* vigilia.

walk *n.* marcha.

wall *n.* pared.

cell wall pared celular.

warblefly *n.* tábano.

ward *n.* sala.

warm *adj.* templado, -da.

wart *n.* verruca, verruga.

watershed *n.* cuenca, divisoria de aguas.

wave *n.* onda.

electroencephalographic wave onda electroencefalográfica.

P wave onda P.

pulse wave onda del pulso.

Q wave onda Q.

R wave onda R.

S wave onda S.

T wave onda T.

way *n.* vía.

weakening *n.* debilitación, depauperación.

weakness *n.* debilidad.

wean *v.* destetar.

weaning *n.* destete.

weanling *n.* destetado, -da.

wear *n.* desgaste.

weather *n.* clima.

webbed *adj.* membranoso, -sa.

wedge *n.* cuña.

weightlessness *n.* ingravidez.

well-being *n.* bienestar.

well-being of the patient bienestar del enfermo.

wellness *n.* bienestar.

high-level wellness bienestar de alto nivel.

wheal *n.* roncha.

wheel *n.* rueda.

wheeze *n.* jadeo, sibilancia.

whey *n.* suero.

whim *n.* antojo.

whiplash *n.* latigazo.

whisper *n.* cuchicheo.

whistle *n.* silbato, silbido.

white *n.* blanco, -ca.

white of the eye blanco del ojo.

will *n.* voluntad.

window *n.* ventana.

wire *n.* alambre.

orthodontic wire alambre de ortodoncia.

separating wire alambre de separación, alambre separador.

wiring *n.* alambrado.

work *n.* trabajo.

   work of mourning trabajo del duelo.

worm *n.* gusano.

wound *n.* herida, herir.

   non-penetrating wound herida no penetrante.

   open wound herida abierta.

   penetrating wound herida penetrante.

   septic wound herida séptica.

wrinkle *n.* arruga.

wrinkled *adj.* rugoso, -sa.

wrist *n.* muñeca.

   tennis wrist muñeca de tenis.

X-Y-Z

xanthelasma *n.* xantelasma.

xanthelasmatosis *n.* xantelasmatosis.

xanthin *n.* xantina.

xanthine *n.* xantina.

xanthogranuloma *n.* xantogranuloma.

xanthogranulomatosis *n.* xantogranulomatosis.

xanthoma *n.* xantoma.

xanthomatosis *n.* xantomatosis.

xanthosis *n.* xantosis.

xenograft *n.* xenograft, xenoinjerto.

xenophobia *n.* xenofobia.

xerosis *n.* xerosis.

xerostomia *n.* xerostomía.

xiphoid *adj.* xifoide, xifoides.

xiphoiditis *n.* xifoiditis.

xylose *n.* xilosa.

yeast *n.* levadura.

yellow *n.* amarillo.

zona *n.* zona.

zone *n.* zona.

   epileptogenic zone zona epileptógena.

   epileptogenous zone zona epileptógena.

   erogenous zone zona erógena, zona erotógena.

   erotogenic zone zona erógena, zona erotógena.

   trigger zone zona desencadenante, zona gatillo.

   visual zone zona visual.

zoology *n.* zoología.

zoom *n.* zoom.

zoonosis *n.* zoonosis.

zoophilia *n.* zoofilia.

zoospermia *n.* zoospermia.

zoster *n.* zoster.

   ophthalmic zoster zoster oftálmico.

zygoma *n.* cigoma, zigoma.

zygomatic *adj.* cigomático, -ca.

zygote *n.* cigoto.

zymogenic *adj.* cimogénico, -ca, zimógeno, -na.

zymogenous *adj.* zimógeno, -na.

zymogic *adj.* zimógeno, -na.

Español - Inglés
Spanish - English

A

abacteriano, -na *adj.* abacterial.
abandono *m.* abandonment.
  abandono infantil child neglect.
abasia *f.* abasia.
abdomen *m.* abdomen.
  abdomen agudo acute abdomen.
  abdomen quirúrgico surgical abdomen.
  abdomen en tabla abdominal splinting, wooden belly.
abdominal *adj.* abdominal.
abdominalgia *f.* abdominalgia.
abducción *f.* abduction.
abductor *adj.* abductor.
aberración *f.* aberration, aberratio.
  aberración cromosómica chromosomal aberration, chromosome aberration.
aberrante *adj.* aberrant.
abetalipoproteinemia *f.* abetalipoproteinemia.
ablación *f.* ablatio.
  ablación placentaria ablatio placentae.
  ablación retiniana ablatio retinae.
ablefaria *f.* ablephary.
abordaje *m.* approach.
abortante *adj.* abortient, abortigenic.
abortar *v.* abort.
abortivo, -va *adj.* abortive.
aborto *m.* abortion, abortus.
  aborto accidental accidental abortion.
  aborto en curso abortion in progress.

aborto diferido missed abortion.
aborto electivo elective abortion.
aborto espontáneo spontaneous abortion.
aborto ilegal illegal abortion.
aborto inevitable inevitable abortion.
aborto provocado induced abortion.
aborto retenido missed abortion.
aborto terapéutico therapeutic abortion.
abrasión *f.* abrasion, grinding, abrasio.
  abrasión corneal corneal abrasion, abrasio corneae.
  abrasión dental, abrasión dentaria tooth abrasion, abrasion of the teeth, abrasio dentium.
abrazadera *f.* brace.
absceso *m.* abscess.
  absceso abdominal abdominal abscess.
  absceso agudo acute abscess.
  absceso alveolar alveolar abscess.
  absceso amigdalino tonsillar abscess.
  absceso anorrectal anorectal abscess.
  absceso biliar biliary abscess.
  absceso cerebral brain abscess, cerebral abscess.
  absceso dental, absceso dentoalveolar dental abscess, dentoalveolar abscess.
  absceso orbitario orbital abscess.
  absceso peridental, absceso periodontal, absceso periodóntico peridental, periodontal abscess.
  absceso pulmonar pulmonary abscess.

absceso renal renal abscess.
absorción *f.* absorption.
absorción cutánea cutaneous absorption.
absorción de fármaco drug absorption.
absorción intestinal intestinal absorption.
absorción parenteral parenteral absorption.
absorción patológica pathologic absorption, pathological absorption.
absorción percutánea percutaneous absorption.
abstinencia *f.* abstinence.
abstinencia alimentaria alimentary abstinence.
abstinencia de sustancias substance abstinence.
abstracto *m.* abstract.
abulia *f.* abulia.
abúlico, -ca *adj.* abulic.
abuso *m.* abuse.
abuso de medicamentos drug abuse.
abuso de sustancias, abuso de sustancias psicoactivas substance abuse, psychoactive substance abuse.
abuso sexual del adulto sexual abuse of an adult.
abuso sexual del niño sexual child abuse.
acalasia *f.* acalasia.
acantosis *f.* acanthosis.
acariasis *f.* acariasis.
ácaro *m.* mite.
acaudado, -da *adj.* acaudate.
acceso[1] *m.* access.
acceso[2] *m.* attack, crisis, seizure.

accesorio *m.* accessorius.
accesorio, -ria *adj.* accessory.
accidental *adj.* accidental.
accidente *m.* accident.
accidente cerebrovascular (ACV) cerebrovascular accident (CVA).
accidente laboral occupational accident, professional accident.
acción *f.* action.
acción farmacológica drug action.
acción refleja reflex action.
acefalia *f.* acephalia, acephaly.
acéfalo *m.* acephalus.
aceite *m.* oil.
acelerador *m.* accelerator.
acelular *adj.* acellular.
aceptación *f.* acceptance.
acetábulo *m.* acetabulum.
acético, -ca *adj.* acetic.
acetona *f.* acetone.
acetonemia *f.* acetonemia.
acetonuria *f.* acetonuria.
acidez *f.* acidity.
acidez del estómago acidity of the stomach.
acídico, -ca *adj.* acidic.
acidificación *f.* acidification.
acidificar *v.* acidify.
ácido *m.* acid, acidum.
acidosis *f.* acidosis.
acidosis compensada compensated acidosis.
acidosis descompensada uncompensated acidosis.
acidosis diabética diabetic acidosis.
acidosis láctica lactic acidosis.
acidosis metabólica metabolic acidosis.

acidosis renal renal acidosis.

acidosis respiratoria respiratory acidosis.

aciduria *f.* aciduria.

acinesia *f.* akinesia.

Acinetobacter Acinetobacter.

acínico, -ca *adj.* acinic.

ácino *m.* acinus.

aclaramiento *m.* clearance.

aclaramiento de fármaco drug clearance.

aclaramiento de creatinina creatinine clearance.

aclorhidria *f.* achlorhydria.

acné, acne *f.* acne.

acné común common acne.

acné conglobata conglobate acne, acne conglobata.

acné infantil infantile acne.

acné rosácea acne rosacea.

acné sebácea acne sebacea.

acné vulgar acne vulgaris.

acolia *f.* acholia.

acoluria *f.* acholuria.

acolúrico, -ca *adj.* acholuric.

acomodación *f.* accommodation.

acomodación del ojo accommodation of the eye.

acondroplasia *f.* achondroplasia, chondroplasty.

acoso sexual *m.* sexual harassment.

acrocianosis *f.* acrocyanosis.

acromegalia *f.* acromegalia, acromegaly.

acromegálico, -ca *adj.* acromegalic.

acromion *m.* acromion.

Actinobacillus Actinobacillus.

actinomicosis *f.* actinomycosis.

Actinomyces Actinomyces.

actitud *f.* attitude.

actividad *f.* activity.

actividad biológica biological activity.

actividad colinérgica cholinergic activity.

actividad enzimática enzyme activity.

activo, -va *adj.* active.

acto *m.* act.

acto compulsivo compulsive act.

acto impulsivo impulsive act.

acto reflejo reflex act.

acto voluntario voluntary act.

acúfeno *m.* tinnitus.

acupuntor, -ra *m., f.* acupuncturist.

acupuntura *f.* acupuncture.

acusia *f.* acusis.

adaptable *adj.* adaptive.

adaptación *f.* adaptation.

adaptación a la oscuridad dark adaptation.

adaptador *m.* adapter, adaptor.

addisoniano, -na *adj.* Addisonian.

adducción *f.* adduction.

adducir *v.* adduct.

adductor, -ra *adj.* adductor.

adenitis *f.* adenitis.

adenoamigdalectomía *f.* adenotonsillectomy, tonsilloadenoidectomy.

adenocarcinoma *m.* adenocarcinoma.

adenohipófisis *f.* adenohypophysis.

adenoides *f.* adenoids.

adenoidectomía *f.* adenoidectomy.

adenoiditis *f.* adenoiditis.

adenoma *m.* adenoma.

adenoma adrenal adrenal adenoma.

adenoma bronquial bronchial adenoma.

adenoma renal adenoma of the kidney.

adenoma tóxico toxic adenoma.

adenosis *f.* adenosis.

adherencia *f.* adherence, adhesion.

adherencia abdominal abdominal adhesion.

adherencia amniótica amniotic adhesion.

adherencia traumática uterina traumatic uterine adhesion.

adherente *adj.* adherent.

adherir *v.* adhere.

adhesión *f.* adhesion, adhesio.

adhesivo, -va *adj.* adhesive.

adicción *f.* addiction.

adipocito *m.* adipocyte.

adipogénesis *f.* adipogenesis.

adiposidad *f.* adiposity, adipositas.

aditivo, -va *adj.* additive.

aditivo alimentario food additive.

administración *f.* administration.

administración bucal de la medicación buccal administration of medication.

administración de fármacos drug administration.

administración de líquidos parenterales administration of parenteral fluids.

administración de medicación mediante inhalación inhalation administration of medication.

administración oftálmica de medicamentos ophthalmic administration of medication.

adolescencia *f.* adolescence.

adolescente *m., f. y adj.* adolescent.

adquirido, -da *adj.* acquired.

adrenal *adj.* adrenal.

adrenalectomía *f.* adrenalectomy.

adrenalina *f.* adrenaline.

adrenérgico, -ca *adj.* adrenergic.

aducción *f.* adduction.

aductor, -ra *adj.* adductor.

adulteración *f.* adulteration.

adultez *f.* adulthood.

adulto, -ta *m., f. y adj.* adult.

adyacente *adj.* adjacent.

adyuvante *m. y adj.* adjuvant.

aéreo, -a *adj.* aerial.

aeróbico, -ca *adj.* aerobic.

aerobio, -bia *adj.* aerobe.

aerodinámica *f.* aerodynamics.

aerofagia *f.* aerophagia, aerophagy air swallowing.

aerosol *m.* aerosol.

aeroterapia *f.* aerotherapeutics, aerotherapy.

afagia *f.* aphagia.

afasia *f.* aphasia.

afasia anósmica anosmic aphasia.

afasia auditiva auditory aphasia.

afasia de Broca Broca's aphasia.

afasia central central aphasia.

afasia completa complete aphasia.

afasia global global aphasia.

afasia gráfica, afasia grafomotora graphic, graphomotor aphasia.

afasia infantil childhood aphasia.

afasia motora motor aphasia.

afasia óptica optic aphasia.

afasia verbal verbal aphasia.

afasia visual visual aphasia.

afasia de Wernicke Wernicke's aphasia.

afásico, -ca *m., f.* aphasiac.

afebril *adj.* afebrile.

afección *f.* affection.

afectado, -da *adj.* affected.

afectividad *f.* affectivity.

afirmación *f.* affirmation.

afonía *f.* aphonia.

afónico, -ca *adj.* aphonic.

afrodisíaco, -ca *adj.* aphrodisiac.

afta *f.* aphtha.

aftoide *adj.* aphthoid.

agalactia *f.* agalactia.

agalactorrea *f.* agalactorrhea.

agammaglobulinemia *f.* agamma-globulinemia.

agenesia *f.* agenesia, agenesis.

  agenesia cortical agenesia cortica-lis.

  agenesia del cuerpo calloso agenesia of the corpus callosum.

  agenesia gonadal gonadal agenesia.

  agenesia ovárica ovarian agenesia.

  agenesia renal renal agenesia.

  agenesia tímica thymic agenesia.

  agenesia vaginal vaginal agenesia.

agente *m.* agent.

  agente activador activating agent.

  agente alquilante alkylating agent.

  agente ansiolítico, agente antiansiedad antianxiety agent.

  agente antipsicótico antipsychotic agent.

  agente bloqueador, agente bloqueante blocking agent.

  agente bloqueador de los canales del calcio calcium channel blocking agent.

  agente bloqueador de los recep- **tores beta-adrenérgicos** beta-adrenergic receptor blocking agent.

  agente bloqueador neuromuscular neuromuscular blocking agent.

  agente de cambio change agent.

  agente diluyente diluting agent.

  agente dispersante dispersing agent.

  agente embolizador embolization agent.

  agente enmascarador masking agent.

  agente farmacológico pharmacological agent.

  agente fijadores fixing agent.

  agente midriático y ciclopéjico mydriatic and cycloplegic agent.

  agente oxidante oxidizing agent.

  agente progestacional progestational agent.

  agente quelante chelating agent.

  agente químico chemical agent.

  agente quimioterápico chemotherapeutic agent.

  agente reductor reducing agent.

  agente sinérgico synergistic agent.

  agente tensioactivo surfactant agent.

  agente teratógeno teratogenic agent.

agitación *f.* agitation.

  agitación psicomotriz pyschomotor agitation.

agitado, -da *adj.* agitated.

aglosia *f.* aglossia.

aglutinable *adj.* agglutinable.

aglutinación *f.* agglutination.

  aglutinación plaquetaria platelet agglutination.

aglutinante *adj.* agglutinant.

aglutinina *f.* agglutinin.

 aglutinina anti-RH anti-RH agglutinin.

 aglutinina inmune immune agglutinin.

agnosia *f.* agnosia.

 agnosia auditiva acoustic agnosia, auditory agnosia.

 agnosia de la imagen corporal body-image agnosia.

 agnosia óptica optic agnosia.

 agnosia táctil tactile agnosia.

 agnosia visual visual agnosia.

 agnosia visuoespacial visual-spatial agnosia, visuospatial agnosia.

agonadal *adj.* agonadal.

agonía *f.* agony.

agónico, -ca *adj.* agonal.

agonista *adj.* agonist.

agotamiento *m.* exhaustion.

 agotamiento nervioso nervous exhaustion.

 agotamiento por calor heat exhaustion.

agotar *v.* deplete.

agrafia *f.* agraphia.

 agrafia literal literal agraphia.

 agrafia mental mental agraphia.

 agrafia verbal verbal agraphia.

agráfico, -ca *adj.* agraphic.

agranulocitosis *f.* agranulocytosis.

agregación *f.* aggregation.

 agregación de hematíes red cell aggregation.

 agregación familiar familial aggregation.

 agregación plaquetaria platelet aggregation.

agregado, -da *adj.* aggregated.

agresión *f.* aggression.

 agresión autodestructiva inward aggression.

 agresión destructiva destructive aggression.

 agresión sexual sexual assault.

agresivo, -va *adj.* aggressive.

agrupación *f.* assortment.

agrupamiento *m.* grouping.

 agrupamiento sanguíneo blood grouping.

agudeza *f.* acuity.

 agudeza visual visual acuity.

aguja *f.* needle.

 aguja aspiradora, aguja aspirante, aguja de aspiración aspirating needle, aspiration needle.

 aguja-cuchilla knife needle.

 aguja cutánea skinny needle.

 aguja endovenosa intravenous needle.

 aguja fina fine needle.

 aguja gruesa biopsy needle.

 aguja hipodérmica hypodermic needle.

 aguja intramuscular intramuscular needle.

 aguja intravenosa intravenous needle.

agujetas *f.* stitch.

ahogamiento *m.* drowning.

 ahogamiento incompleto near drowning.

 ahogamiento secundario secondary drowning.

ahogo *m.* choke.

aire *m.* air.

 aire alveolar alveolar air.

aire de reserva reserve air.

airear *v.* aerate.

aislado, -da *adj.* isolated.

aislamiento[1] *m.* insulation.

aislamiento[2] *m.* isolation.

aislamiento genético genetic isolate.

aislamiento infeccioso infectious isolation.

aislamiento social social isolation.

aislante *m.* insulator, isolator.

aislante quirúrgico surgical isolator.

ajuste *m.* adjustment.

alalia *f.* alalia.

alambrado *m.* wiring.

alambre *m.* wire.

alambre de ortodoncia orthodontic wire.

alambre de separación, alambre separador separating wire.

alanina *f.* alanine.

alantoide *adj.* allantoid.

alantoides *f.* allantois.

albinismo *m.* albinism.

albinismo oculocutáneo oculocutaneous albinism.

albino, -na *adj.* albino.

albugínea *f.* albuginea.

albuginitis *f.* albuginitis.

albúmina *f.* albumin.

albúmina circulante circulating albumin.

albúmina normal del suero humano normal human serum albumin.

albúmina sérica serum albumin.

albuminemia *f.* albuminemia.

albuminuria *f.* albuminuria.

albuminuria cardíaca cardiac albuminuria.

albuminuria falsa false albuminuria.

albuminuria fisiológica physiologic albuminuria, physiological albuminuria.

albuminuria sérica serous albuminuria.

albuminuria transitoria transient albuminuria.

albuminuria verdadera true albuminuria.

alcalinidad *f.* alkalinity.

alcalosis *f.* alkalosis.

alcalosis compensada compensated alkalosis.

alcalosis descompensada decompensated alkalosis.

alcalosis metabólica metabolic alkalosis.

alcalosis respiratoria respiratory alkalosis.

alcaptonuria *f.* alkaptonuria.

alcohol *m.* alcohol.

alcoholemia *f.* alcoholemia.

alcohólico, -ca *adj.* alcoholic.

alcoholismo *m.* alcoholism.

alcoholismo agudo acute alcoholism.

alcoholización *f.* alcoholization.

aldosterona *f.* aldosterone.

aldosteronismo *m.* aldosteronism.

aldosteronismo idiopático idiopathic.

aldosteronismo primario primary aldosteronism.

aldosteronismo secundario secondary aldosteronism.

alélico, -ca *adj.* allelic.

alelo *m.* allele.

  alelo codominante codominant allele.

  alelo dominante dominant allele.

  alelo múltiple multiple allele.

  alelo recesivo recessive allele.

  alelo silencioso silent allele.

alergénico, -ca *adj.* allergenic.

alergeno *m.* allergen.

alergia *f.* allergy.

  alergia alimentaria food allergy.

  alergia a fármacos drug allergy.

  alergia al frío cold allergy.

  alergia al polen pollen allergy.

  alergia provocada induced allergy.

  alergia retardada delayed allergy.

alérgico, -ca *adj.* allergic.

alergología *f.* allergology.

aleta *f.* flange.

  aleta bucal buccal flange.

  aleta labial labial flange.

  aleta lingual lingual flange.

aleteo *m.* flutter.

  aleteo auricular auricular flutter.

  aleteo nasal nasal flaring, flaring of the nostrils.

  aleteo ocular ocular flutter.

alexia *f.* alexia.

  alexia motora motor alexia.

  alexia musical musical alexia.

alfa1-antitripsina *f.* alpha1-antitrypsin.

alfa-beta-bloqueante *f.* alpha-beta-blocker.

alfa-fetoproteína (AFP) *f.* alpha-fetoprotein (AFP).

alfa-globulina *f.* alpha-globulin.

alfa-lipoproteína *f.* alpha-lipoprotein.

alfa2-macroglobulina *f.* alpha2-macroblogulin.

algia *f.* pain.

álgido, -da *adj.* algid.

algodón *m.* cotton.

algodoncillo *m.* thrush.

alianza *f.* alliance.

  alianza terapéutica therapeutic alliance.

aliento *m.* breath.

  aliento fétido bad breath.

  aliento hepático liver breath.

  mal aliento bad breath.

  aliento urémico uremic breath.

alimentación *f.* alimentation, feeding.

  alimentación al pecho breast feeding.

  alimentación artificial artificial alimentation, artificial feeding.

  alimentación con biberón bottle feeding.

  alimentación forzada forced alimentation, forcible feeding, forced feeding.

  alimentación gástrica gastric feeding.

  alimentación mediante gastrostomía gastrostomy feeding.

  alimentación nasogástrica nasogastric feeding.

  alimentación parenteral parenteral alimentation.

  alimentación parenteral total total parenteral alimentation.

alimentario, -ria *adj.* alimentary.

alimenticio, -cia *adj.* nutritive.

alimento *m.* food.
  alimento dietético dietetic food.
alineación *f.* alignment.
alineamiento *m.* alignment.
alivio *m.* relief.
almidón *m.* starch.
almohadilla *f.* pad.
  almohadilla adiposa fat pad.
  almohadilla grasa fat pad.
  almohadilla renal kidney pad.
almorrana *f.* pile.
aloanticuerpo *m.* alloantibody.
aloantígeno *m.* alloantigen.
alodinia *f.* allodynia.
alogrupo *m.* allogroup.
aloinjerto *m.* allograft.
aloinmune *adj.* alloimmune.
alopecia *f.* alopecia.
  alopecia androgénica androgenetic alopecia, androgenic alopecia, alopecia androgenetica.
  alopecia areata alopecia areata.
  alopecia cicatricial, alopecia cicatrisata cicatricial alopecia.
  alopecia circunscrita alopecia circumscripta.
  alopecia por compresión pressure alopecia.
  alopecia congénita congenital alopecia, alopecia congenitalis.
  alopecia de distribución masculina male pattern alopecia.
  alopecia de estrés stress alopecia.
  alopecia generalizada alopecia generalisata.
  alopecia hereditaria alopecia hereditaria.
  alopecia orbicular alopecia orbicularis.

  alopecia posparto postpartum alopecia.
  alopecia prematura premature alopecia, alopecia prematura.
  alopecia por presión pressure alopecia.
  alopecia psicógena psychogenic alopecia.
  alopecia por radiación radiation alopecia.
  alopecia por rayos X X-ray alopecia.
  alopecia seborreica alopecia seborrheica.
  alopecia senil senile alopecia, alopecia senilis.
  alopecia total alopecia totalis.
  alopecia tóxica alopecia toxica.
  alopecia universal alopecia universalis.
alopécico, -ca *adj.* alopecic.
alosensibilización *f.* allosensitization.
alotipia *f.* allotypy.
alotipo *m.* allotype.
alta *f.* discharge.
  alta definitiva absolute discharge.
  alta involuntaria involuntary discharge.
  alta sin permiso (ASP) absent without leave (AWOL).
alteración *f.* alteration.
  alteración cualitativa qualitative alteration.
  alteración cuantitativa quantitative alteration.
  alteración nerviosa nervous breakdown.
  alteración del nivel de conscien-

cia (ANC) altered state of consciousness (ASC).

alternación *f.* alternation.

alternancia *f.* alternans.

altruismo *m.* altruism.

altura *f.* height.

alucinación *f.* hallucination.

alucinación alcohólica alcoholic hallucination.

alucinación auditiva auditory hallucination.

alucinación consciente hallucinosis.

alucinación olfatoria olfactory hallucination.

alucinación somática somatic hallucination.

alucinación táctil tactile hallucination.

alucinación visual visual hallucination.

alucinógeno *m.* hallucinogen.

alucinosis *f.* hallucinosis.

alumbramiento *m.* accouchement.

aluminosis *f.* aluminosis.

alveobronquiolitis *f.* alveobronchiolitis.

alveolitis *f.* alveolitis.

alveolitis alérgica, alveolitis alérgica extrínseca allergic alveolitis, extrinsic allergic alveolitis.

alvéolo, alveolo *m.* socket, alveolus.

amalgama *f.* amalgam.

amalgama dental, amalgama dentaria dental amalgam.

amamantar *v.* suckle.

amargo, -ga *adj.* bitter.

amarillo *m.* yellow.

amaurosis *f.* amaurosis.

amaurosis congénita congenital amaurosis, amaurosis congenita.

amaurosis diabética diabetic amaurosis.

amaurosis fugaz amaurosis fugax.

ambidextro, -tra *adj.* ambidexter.

ambiente *m.* environment.

ambisexual *adj.* ambisexual.

ambivalencia *f.* ambivalence.

ambliopía *f.* amblyopia.

ambliopía estrabísmica strabismic amblyopia.

ambliopiatría *f.* amblyopiatrics.

ambiópico, -ca *f.* amblyopic.

ambliocospio *m.* amblyoscope.

Amblyomma Amblyomma.

ambo *m.* ambo.

ambomaleal *adj.* ambomalleal.

ambón *m.* ambo.

ambulancia *f.* ambulance.

ambulatorio, -a *adj.* ambulatory.

amebiasis *f.* amebiasis.

amebiasis hepática hepatic amebiasis.

amebiasis intestinal intestinal amebiasis.

amebicida *adj.* amebicidal.

amenorrea *f.* amenorrhea.

amenorrea emocional emotional amenorrhea.

amenorrea por estrés stress amenorrhea.

amenorrea fisiológica physiologic amenorrhea.

amenorrea hipofisaria hypophyseal amenorrhea.

amenorrea hipotalámica hypothalamic amenorrhea.

amenorrea nutricional nutritional amenorrhea.

amenorrea ovárica ovarian amenorrhea.

amenorrea patológica pathologic amenorrhea.

amenorrea posparto amenorrhea postpartum.

amenorrea pospíldora postpill amenorrhea.

amenorrea premenopáusica premenopausal amenorrhea.

amenorrea secundaria secondary amenorrhea.

amenorrea traumática traumatic amenorrhea.

amenorreico, -ca *adj.* amenorrheic.

ametropía *f.* ametropia.

amielínico, -ca *adj.* amyelinic.

amígdala *f.* amygdala, tonsil.

amigdalectomía *f.* amygdalectomy.

amigdalitis *f.* tonsillitis.

amigdalitis aguda acute tonsillitis.

amigdalitis diftérica diphtheritic tonsillitis.

amigdalitis estreptocócica streptococcal tonsillitis.

amigdalitis herpética herpetic tonsillitis.

amigdalitis micótica mycotic tonsillitis.

amigdalitis preglótica preglottic tonsillitis.

amigdalitis superficial superficial tonsillitis.

amigdalitis supurativa supurative tonsillitis.

amigdalitis de Vincent Vincent's tonsillitis.

amiloide *m.* amyloid.

amiloidosis *f.* amyloidosis.

amiloidosis cutánea, amiloidosis cutis cutaneous amyloidosis, amyloidosis cutis.

amiloidosis familiar familial amyloidosis.

amiloidosis hereditaria, amiloidosis heredofamiliar hereditary amyloidosis, heredofamilial amyloidosis.

amiloidosis idiopática idiopathic amyloidosis.

amiloidosis nodular nodular amyloidosis.

amiloidosis primaria primary amyloidosis.

amiloidosis secundaria secondary amyloidosis.

amiloidosis senil senile amyloidosis.

aminoácido *m.* aminoacid.

aminoácido esencial essential aminoacid.

aminoácido no esencial non-essential aminoacid.

aminoacidopatía *f.* aminoacidopathy.

aminoaciduria *f.* aminoaciduria.

amiotrofia *f.* amyotrophy.

amnesia *f.* amnesia.

amnesia anterógrada anterograde amnesia.

amnesia auditiva auditory amnesia.

amnesia continua continuous amnesia.

amnesia disociativa dissociative amnesia.

amnesia emocional emotional amnesia.

amnesia episódica episodic amnesia.

amnesia generalizada generalized amnesia.

amnesia infantil infantile amnesia.

amnesia lacunar, amnesia lagunar lacunar amnesia.

amnesia orgánica organic amnesia.

amnesia poscontusional postcontussional amnesia.

amnesia posthipnótica posthypnotic amnesia.

amnesia postraumática post-traumatic amnesia.

amnesia retroanterógrada retroanterograde amnesia.

amnesia retrógada retrograde amnesia.

amnesia selectiva selective amnesia.

amnesia táctil tactile amnesia.

amnesia traumática traumatic amnesia.

amnesia verbal verbal amnesia.

amnesia visual visual amnesia.

amniocentesis *f.* amniocentesis.

amniocoriónico, -ca *adj.* amniochorial.

amnionitis *f.* amnionitis, amniotitis.

amniorrexis *f.* amniorrhexis.

amnios *m.* amnion.

amnioscopia *f.* amnioscopia.

amnioscopio *m.* amnioscope.

amniótico, -ca *adj.* amniotic.

amniotitis *f.* anmiotitis.

amoniaco, amoníaco *m.* ammonia.

amoniemia *f.* ammoniemia.

amoniuria *f.* ammoniuria.

amorfa *f.* amorpha.

amorfo *m.* amorphus.

amorfo, -fa *adj.* amorphous.

amortiguador *m.* buffer.

amortiguamiento¹ *m.* buffering.

amortiguamiento² *m.* damping.

amplificación *f.* amplification.

amplitud *f.* amplitude.

amplitud de convergencia amplitude of convergence.

ampolla¹ *f.* ampoule, ampule.

ampolla² *f.* ampulla.

ampolla³ *f.* bleb, blister.

ampollar *adj.* ampular, ampullary.

amputación *f.* amputation.

amputación abierta open amputation.

amputación amniótica amniotic amputation.

amputación aperióstica aperiosteal amputation.

amputación cerrada closed amputation.

amputación cervical cervical amputation.

amputación circular cirular amputation, circus amputation.

amputación con colgajos, amputación de colgajo flap amputation.

amputación sin colgajos flapless amputation.

amputación completa complete amputation.

amputación cuádruple quadruple amputation.

amputación por debajo de la rodilla below-knee (B-K) amputation.

amputación espontánea spontaneous amputation.

amputación excéntrica eccentric amputation.

amputación inmediata immediate amputation.

amputación intrauterina intrauterine amputation.

amputación menor minor amputation.

amputación musculocutánea musculocutaneous amputation.

amputación natural natural amputation, birth amputation.

amputación oblicua oblique amputation.

amputación operatoria operative amputation.

amputación oval oval amputation.

amputación parcial partial amputation.

amputación patológica pathologic amputation.

amputado, -da *m., f.* amputee.

anabolismo *m.* anabolism.

anabolito *m.* anabolite.

anaerobio, -a *adj.* anaerobe.

anaerobiótico, -ca *adj.* anaerobiotic.

anafase *f.* anaphase.

anafiláctico, -ca *adj.* anaphylactic.

anafilaxia *f.* anaphylaxis.

anafilaxia adquirida acquired anaphylaxis.

anafilaxia de antisuero antiserum anaphylaxis.

anafilaxia generalizada generalized anaphylaxis.

anafilaxia indirecta indirect anaphylaxis.

anafilaxia pasiva passive anaphylaxis.

anafilaxia sistémica systemic anaphylaxis.

anafilaxis *f.* anaphylaxis.

anágeno *m.* anagen.

anal *adj.* anal.

analgesia *f.* analgesia.

analgesia auditiva audio analgesia.

analgesia dolorosa analgesia dolorosa.

analgesia epidural epidural.

analgesia por infiltración infiltration analgesia.

analgesia por inhalación inhalation analgesia.

analgesia superficial surface analgesia.

analgésico, -ca *adj.* analgesic.

análisis *m.* analysis.

análisis de impedancia bioeléctrica (AIB) bioelectrical impedance analysis (BIA).

análisis de inmunoabsorción ligado a enzimas (ELISA) enzyme-linked immunosorbent assay.

análisis de orina urinalysis.

análisis de la varianza (ANOVA) analysis of variance.

análisis volumétrico volumetric analysis.

analizador *m.* analyzer.

analogía *f.* analogy.

análogo, -ga *adj.* analog.

anamnesis *f.* anamnesis.

anaplasia *f.* anaplasia.

anaplásico, -ca *adj.* anaplastic.

anasarca *f.* anasarca.

anastomosar *v.* anastomose.

anastomosis *f.* anastomosis.

anastomosis arteriovenosa arteriovenous anastomosis.

anastomosis iliorrectal iliorectal anastomosis.

anastomosis microneurovascular microneurovascular.

anastomosis microvascular microvascular anastomosis.

anastomosis terminoterminal termino-terminal anastomosis.

anastomosis transureteroureteral transureteroureteral anastomosis.

anastomosis ureteroureteral ureteroureteral anastomosis.

anastomótico, -ca *adj.* anastomotic.

anatomía *f.* anatomy.

anatomía aplicada applied anatomy.

anatomía clínica clinical anatomy.

anatomía comparada comparative anatomy.

anatomía dental dental anatomy.

anatomía descriptiva descriptive anatomy.

anatomía fisiológica physiological anatomy.

anatomía funcional functional anatomy.

anatomía general general anatomy.

anatomía histológica histological anatomy.

anatomía macroscópica gross anatomy, macroscopic anatomy.

anatomía microscópica microscopic anatomy, minute anatomy.

anatomía patológica pathological anatomy.

anatomía quirúrgica surgical anatomy.

anatómico, -ca *adj.* anatomic, anatomical.

anatomopatológico, -ca *adj.* anatomicopathological.

anclaje *m.* anchorage.

androgénesis *f.* androgenesis.

androgenización *f.* androgenization.

andrógeno *m.* androgen.

androsterona *f.* androsterone.

anéfrico, -ca *adj.* anephric.

anejos *m.* adnexa.

anemia *f.* anemia.

anemia aguda acute anemia.

anemia arregenerativa aregenerative anemia.

anemia carencial deficiency anemia.

anemia de células falciformes sickle cell anemia.

anemia por deficiencia de ácido fólico folic acid deficiency anemia.

anemia por deficiencia de hierro iron deficiency anemia.

anemia drepanocítica sickle cell anemia.

anemia eritroblástica de la infancia erythroblastic anemia of childhood.

anemia eritroblástica familiar familial erythroblastic anemia.

anemia eritrocítica pura pure red cell anemia.

anemia escorbútica scorbutic anemia.

anemia esferocítica spherocytic anemia.

anemia esplénica splenic anemia, anemia splenica.

anemia ferropénica iron deficiency anemia.

anemia fisiológica physiologic anemia.

anemia hemolítica hemolytic anemia.

anemia hemolítica aguda acute hemolytic anemia.

anemia hemolítica autoinmune autoimmune hemolytic anemia (AIHS).

anemia hemolítica congénita congenital hemolytic anemia.

anemia hemolítica infecciosa infectious hemolytic anemia.

anemia hemolítica inmune immune hemolytic anemia, immunohemolytic anemia.

anemia hemolítica inmune inducida por fármacos drug-induced immune hemolytic anemia.

anemia hemorrágica hemorrhagic anemia.

anemia hipoférrica hypoferric anemia.

anemia hipoplásica hypoplastic anemia.

anemia linfática anemia lymphatica.

anemia local local anemia.

anemia macrocítica macrocytic anemia.

anemia macrocítica del embarazo macrocytic anemia of pregnancy.

anemia macrocítica nutricional nutritional macrocytic anemia.

anemia maligna malignant anemia.

anemia megaloblástica megaloblastic anemia.

anemia megalocítica megalocytic anemia.

anemia metaplásica metaplastic anemia.

anemia de los mineros miners' anemia.

anemia de las montañas mountain anemia.

anemia neonatal anemia neonatorum.

anemia normocítica normocytic anemia.

anemia normocrómica normochromic anemia.

anemia nutricional nutritional anemia.

anemia perniciosa pernicious anemia.

anemia perniciosa juvenil juvenile pernicious anemia.

anemia poshemorrágica posthemorrhagic anemia.

anemia poshemorrágica neonatal posthemorrhagic anemia of the newborn.

anemia rebelde refractory anemia.

anemia refractaria refractory anemia.

anemia sideroacréstica sideroachrestic anemia.

anemia sideroblástica sideroblastic anemia.

anemia sideropénica sideropenic anemia.

anemia traumática traumatic anemia.

anémico, -ca *adj.* anemic.

anencefalia *f.* anencephalia.

anencefálico, -ca *adj.* anencephalic, anencephalous.

anencéfalo *m.* anencephalus.

anergia *f.* anergy.

  anergia específica specific anergy.

  anergia inespecífica non-specific anergy.

  anergia negativa negative anergy.

  anergia positiva positive anergy.

anérgico, -ca *adj.* anergic.

anestesia *f.* anesthesia.

  anestesia bloqueante, anestesia bloqueo block anesthesia.

  anestesia bulbar bulbar anesthesia.

  anestesia caudal caudal anesthesia.

  anestesia central central anesthesia.

  anestesia cerrada closed anesthesia.

  anestesia completa total anesthesia.

  anestesia por compresión compression anesthesia.

  anestesia por conducción conduction anesthesia.

  anestesia por congelación frost anesthesia.

  anestesia cruzada crossed anesthesia.

  anestesia disociada dissociated anesthesia.

  anestesia dolorosa anesthesia dolorosa.

  anestesia eléctrica electric anesthesia.

  anestesia epidural epidural anesthesia.

  anestesia epidural lumbar lumbar epidural anesthesia.

  anestesia espinal spinal anesthesia.

  anestesia facial facial anesthesia.

  anestesia faríngea pharyngeal anesthesia.

  anestesia general general anesthesia.

  anestesia hipotérmica hypothermic anesthesia.

  anestesia histérica hysterical anesthesia.

  anestesia por infiltración infiltration anesthesia.

  anestesia por inhalación inhalation anesthesia.

  anestesia intercostal intercostal anesthesia.

  anestesia intrabucal intraoral anesthesia.

  anestesia intranasal intranasal anesthesia.

  anestesia intraósea intraosseous anesthesia.

  anestesia intravenosa intravenous anesthesia.

  anestesia local local anesthesia.

  anestesia muscular muscular anesthesia.

  anestesia olfatoria olfactory anesthesia.

  anestesia paraneural paraneural anesthesia.

  anestesia paravertebral paravertebral anesthesia.

  anestesia peridural peridural anesthesia.

  anestesia periférica peripheral anesthesia.

  anestesia perineural perineural anesthesia.

  anestesia por presión pressure anesthesia.

anestesia quirúrgica surgical anesthesia.

anestesia raquídea spinal anesthesia.

anestesia rectal rectal anesthesia.

anestesia por refrigeración refrigeration anesthesia.

anestesia regional regional anesthesia.

anestesia sacra sacral anesthesia.

anestesia segmentaria segmental anesthesia.

anestesia en silla de montar saddle block anesthesia.

anestesia subaracnoidea subarachnoid anesthesia.

anestesia de superficie surface anesthesia.

anestesia táctil tactile anesthesia.

anestesia térmica thermal anesthesia, thermic anesthesia.

anestesia tópica topical anesthesia.

anestesia unilateral unilateral anesthesia.

anestesia visceral visceral anesthesia.

anestésico, -ca *m. y adj.* anesthetic.

anestésico endovenoso intravenous anesthetic.

anestésico general general anesthetic.

anestésico local local anesthetic.

anestésico raquídeo spinal anesthetic.

anestésico tópico topical anesthetic.

anestesiología *f.* anesthesiology.

anestesista *m., f.* anesthetist.

aneuploide *adj.* aneuploid.

aneuploidia *f.* aneuploidy.

aneurisma *m.* aneurysm.

aneurisma abdominal abdominal aneurysm.

aneurisma anastomático, aneurisma por anastomosis aneurysm by anastomosis.

aneurisma aórtico aortic aneurysm.

aneurisma arterioesclerótico atherosclerotic aneurysm.

aneurisma arteriovenoso arteriovenous aneurysm.

aneurisma bacteriano bacterial aneurysm.

aneurisma cardíaco cardiac aneurysm.

aneurisma cerebral cerebral aneurysm.

aneurisma cerebral congénito congenital cerebral aneurysm.

aneurisma compuesto compound aneurysm.

aneurisma disecante dissecting aneurysm.

aneurisma embólico embolic aneurysm.

aneurisma falso false aneurysm.

aneurisma infectado infected aneurysm.

aneurisma intracraneal intracranial aneurysm.

aneurisma lateral lateral aneurysm.

aneurisma micótico mycotic aneurysm.

aneurisma orbitario orbital aneurysm.

aneurisma **pélvico** pelvic aneurysm.

aneurisma **renal** renal aneurysm.

aneurisma **sifilítico** syphilitic aneurysm.

aneurisma **torácico** thoracic aneurysm.

aneurisma **traumático** traumatic aneurysm.

aneurisma **varicoso** varicose aneurysm.

aneurisma **ventricular** ventricular aneurysm.

aneurisma **verdadero** true aneurysm.

anexectomía *f.* adnexectomy.

anexitis *f.* adnexitis.

anexos *m.* adnexa.

angiectasia *f.* angiectasis, angiectasia.

angiitis *f.* angiitis, angitis.

angiitis **alérgica cutánea** allergic cutaneous angiitis.

angiitis **necrosante** necrotizing angiitis.

angina *f.* angina.

angina **aguda** angina acuta.

angina **catarral** angina catarrhalis.

angina **diftérica** angina diphtheritica.

angina **dispéptica** angina dyspeptica.

angina **exudativa** exudative angina.

angina **falsa** false angina.

angina **intestinal** intestinal angina.

angina **neutropénica** neutropenic angina.

angina **de pecho** angina pectoris.

angina **reumática** angina rheumatica.

angina **traqueal** angina trachealis.

angioblastoma *f.* angioblastoma.

angiocardiograma *f.* angiocardiogram.

angiocardiopatía *f.* angiocardiopathy.

angioedema *m.* angioedema.

angiogénesis *f.* angiogenesis.

angiogénico, -ca *adj.* angiogenic.

angiografía *f.* angiography.

angioma *m.* angioma.

angioma **arteriovenoso del cerebro** arteriovenous angioma of the brain.

angioma **capilar** capillary angioma.

angioma **cavernoso** cavernous angioma, angioma cavernosum.

angioma **en cereza** cherry angioma.

angioma **del cutis** angioma cutis.

angioma **en fresa** strawberry angioma.

angioma **linfático** angioma lymphaticum.

angioma **senil** angioma senile.

angioma **telangiectásico** telangiectatic angioma.

angiomatosis *f.* angiomatosis.

angiopatía *f.* angiopathy.

angiopático, -ca *adj.* angiopathic.

angioplastia *f.* angioplasty.

angioplastia **coronaria transluminal percutánea (ACTP)** percutaneous transluminal coronary angioplasty (PTCA).

angioscopia *f.* angioscopy.

angioscopio *m.* angioscope.

angor angor.

angular *adj.* angular.

ángulo *m.* angle, angulus.

  ángulo de aberración angle of aberration.

  ángulo de abertura angle of aperture.

  ángulo de apertura, ángulo de abertura angle of aperture.

angustia *f.* anxiety.

anhídrido *m.* anhydride.

anhidrosis *f.* anhidrosis.

anidación *f.* innidation.

anillo *m.* ring, annulus.

  anillo cervical cervical loop, neck ring.

  anillo umbilical umbilical ring, annulus umbilicalis.

  anillo vascular vascular ring.

ánima *f.* anima.

anión *m.* anion.

aniónico, -ca *adj.* anionic.

ano *m.* anus.

  ano artificial, ano contra natura artificial anus.

  ano ectópico ectopic anus.

  ano imperforado imperforate anus.

  ano vesical anus vesicalis.

  ano vestibular, ano vulvovaginal vestibular anus, vulvovaginal anus.

anococcígeo, -a *adj.* anococcygeal.

anocoxígeo, -a *adj.* anococcygeal.

anodinia *f.* anodynia.

anodino, -na *adj.* anodyne.

ánodo *m.* anode.

anoftalmía *f.* anophthalmia.

anomalía *f.* anomaly.

  anomalía cardíaca congénita congenital cardiac anomaly.

anomalía cromosómica chromosomal anomaly, chromosome anomaly.

  anomalía de desarrollo developmental anomaly.

  anomalía gestante gestant anomaly.

anorexia *f.* anorexia.

  anorexia nerviosa anorexia nervosa.

anoréxico, -ca *adj.* anoretic, anorexic.

anorexígeno *m.* anorexiant.

anorgasmia *f.* anorgasmy, anorgasmia.

anormal *adj.* abnormal.

anormalidad *f.* abnormality.

anorquia *f.* anorchia, anorchidism.

anorquidia *f.* anorchia, anorchidism.

anórquidico, -ca *adj.* anorchidic.

anórquido, -da *adj.* anorchid.

anorquismo *m.* anorchism.

anorrectal *adj.* anorectal.

anoscopia *f.* anoscopy.

anoscopio *m.* anoscope.

anosigmoidoscopia *f.* anosigmoidoscopy.

anosmia *f.* anosmia.

  anosmia gustatoria anosmia gustatoria.

  anosmia preferencial preferential anosmia.

  anosmia respiratoria anosmia respiratoria.

anósmico, -ca *adj.* anosmic.

anovulación *f.* anovulation.

anovulatorio, -a *adj.* anovulatory.

anoxia *f.* anoxia.

anoxia del neonato anoxia neonatorum.

anóxico, -ca *adj.* anoxic.

anquilopoyético, -ca *adj.* ankylopoietic.

anquilosado, -da *adj.* ankylosed.

anquilosis *f.* ankylosis.

anquilosis artificial artificial ankylosis.

anquilosis dental dental ankylosis.

anquilosis espuria spurious ankylosis.

anquilosis del estribo stapedial ankylosis.

anquilosis extracapsular extracapsular ankylosis.

anquilosis falsa false ankylosis.

anquilosis fibrosa fibrous ankylosis.

anquilosis intracapsular intracapsular ankylosis.

anquilosis ósea bony ankylosis.

anquilosis verdadera true ankylosis.

ansiedad *f.* anxiety.

ansiedad ante los extraños stranger anxiety.

ansiedad anticipatoria anticipatory anxiety.

ansiedad básica basic anxiety.

ansiedad presenil anxietas presenilis.

ansiedad de separación separation anxiety.

ansiedad de situación situation anxiety.

ansiedad traumática traumatic anxiety.

ansiolítico, -ca *adj.* anxiolytic.

antagonismo *m.* antagonism.

antagonista *adj.* antagonist.

antagonista del ácido fólico folic acid antagonist.

antagonista aldosterona aldosterone antagonist.

antagonista asociado associated antagonist.

antagonista del calcio calcium antagonist.

antagonista competitivo competitive antagonist.

antagonista directo direct antagonist.

antagonista enzimático enzyme antagonist.

antagonista de los narcóticos, antagonista narcótico narcotic antagonist.

antebraquial *adj.* antebrachial.

antebrazo *m.* forearm, antebrachium.

antecedentes *m.* background, history.

antecedentes médicos past health.

antecedentes personales y sociales personal and social history.

anteflexión *f.* anteflexion, anteflexio.

anteflexión del iris anteflexion of the iris.

anteflexión uterina, anteflexio uteri uterine anteflexion.

antenatal *adj.* antenatal.

anteojos *m.* spectacles.

anteojos bifocales bifocal spectacles.

anteojos trifocales trifocal spectacles.

anteparto *adj.* antepartum.

ante partum antepartum.

anterior *adj.* anterior.

anteroexterno, -na *adj.* anteroexternal.

anterógrado, -ra *adj.* anterograde.

anteroinferior *adj.* anteroinferior.

anterointerno, -na *adj.* anterointernal.

anterolateral *adj.* anterolateral.

anteromediano, -na *adj.* anteromedian.

anteromedio, -dia *adj.* anteromedial.

anteroposterior *adj.* anteroposterior.

anteroseptal *adj.* anteroseptal.

anterosuperior *adj.* anterosuperior.

anteroventral *adj.* anteroventral.

anteversión *f.* anteversion.

antiabortivo *m.* antiabortifacient.

antiácido, -da *m. y adj.* antacid, antiacid.

antiadrenérgico, -ca *m. y adj.* antiadrenergic.

antiálgico, -ca *adj.* antalgic, antalgesic.

antiandrógeno, -na *adj.* antiandrogenic.

anticuerpo *m.* antibody.

antiantídoto *m.* antiantidote.

antiarrítmico, -ca *adj.* antiarrhythmic.

antiartrítico, -ca *adj.* antiarthritic, antarthritic.

antiasmático, -ca *adj.* antiasthmatic, antasthmatic.

antibacteriano, -na *adj.* antibacterial.

antibiograma *m.* antibiogram.

antibiótico, -ca *adj.* antibiotic.

antibioticograma *m.* antibiogram.

antibioticorresistente *adj.* antibiotic-resistant.

anticalculoso, -sa *adj.* anticalculous.

anticanceroso, -sa *adj.* anticancer.

anticarcinogénico, -ca *adj.* anticarcinogenic.

anticarcinógeno, -na *adj.* anticarcinogen.

anticariogénico, -ca *adj.* anticariogenic.

anticatalizador, -ra *adj.* anticatalyzer.

anticatarral *adj.* anticatarrhal.

anticetogénico, -ca *adj.* antiketogenetic.

anticetógeno, -na *adj.* antiketogenic.

anticoagulación *f.* anticoagulation.

anticoagulante *adj.* anticoagulant.

anticolinérgico, -ca *adj.* anticholinergic.

anticolinesterasa *f.* anticholinesterase.

anticomplemento *m.* anticomplement.

anticoncepción *f.* contraception.

anticonceptivo, -va *adj.* contraceptive.

anticonceptivo de barrera barrier contraceptive.

anticonceptivo oral oral contraceptive.

anticonceptivo oral combinado combination oral contraceptive.

anticonceptivo oral secuencial sequential oral contraceptive.

anticonvulsivo, -va *adj.* anticonvulsive.

anticuerpo *m.* antibody.

anticuerpo aglutinante agglutinating antibody.

anticuerpo anafiláctico anaphylactic antibody.

anticuerpo anti-D anti-D antibody.

anticuerpo anti-ADN anti-DNA antibody.

anticuerpo antimembrana basal anti-basement membrane antibody.

anticuerpo antimembrana basal glomerular (anti-MBG) anti-glomerular basement membrane antibody.

anticuerpo antimicrosomal antimicrosomal antibody.

anticuerpo antimitocóndrico, anticuerpo antimitocondrial antimitochondrial antibody.

anticuerpo antinuclear (ANA) antinuclear antibody (ANA).

anticuerpo antirreceptor antireceptor antibody.

anticuerpo antitiroglobulina antithyroglobulin antibody.

anticuerpo antitiroideo antithyroid antibody.

anticuerpo antitreponema treponema-immobilizing antibody.

anticuerpo autólogo antologous antibody.

anticuerpo biespecífico bispecific antibody.

anticuerpo bivalente bivalent antibody.

anticuerpo bloqueante blocking antibody.

anticuerpo caliente, anticuerpo caliente-reactivo warm antibody, warm-reactive antibody.

anticuerpo circulante detectable circulating antibody.

anticuerpo citotóxico cytotoxic antibody.

anticuerpo completo complete antibody.

anticuerpo fijador del complemento complement-fixing antibody.

anticuerpo fijo a célula, anticuerpo ligado a la célula cell-fixed antibody, cell-bound antibody.

anticuerpo fluorescente fluorescent antibody.

anticuerpo frío, anticuerpo frío-reactivo cold antibody, cold-reactive antibody.

anticuerpo heterocitotrópico heterocytotropic antibody.

anticuerpo heteroclítico heteroclitic antibody.

anticuerpo heterófilo heterophil antibody, heterophile antibody.

anticuerpo heterogenético heterogenetic antibody.

anticuerpo híbrido hybrid antibody.

anticuerpo idiotipo idiotype antibody.

anticuerpo incompleto incomplete antibody.

anticuerpo inhibidor inhibiting antibody.

anticuerpo inmunitario immune antibody.

anticuerpo linfocitotóxico lymphocytotoxic antibody.

anticuerpo mitocondrial mitochondrial antibody.

anticuerpo monoclonal monoclonal antibody.

anticuerpo natural natural antibody.

anticuerpo neutralizante neutralizing antibody.

anticuerpo normal normal antibody.

anticuerpo policlonal polyclonal antibody.

anticuerpo protector protective antibody.

anticuerpo de reacción cruzada cross-reacting antibody.

anticuerpo reagínico reaginic antibody.

anticuerpo Rh Rh antibody.

anticuerpo salino saline antibody.

anticuerpo sensibilizante sensitizing antibody.

anticuerpo de tipo equino horse-type antibody.

anticuerpo treponémico treponemal antibody.

anticuerpo univalente univalent antibody.

antidepresivo, -va *adj.* antidepressant.

antidiabético, -ca *adj.* antidiabetic.

antidiarreico, -ca *adj.* antidiarrheal, antidiarrheic.

antidiurético, -ca *adj.* antidiuretic.

antídoto *m.* antidote.

antídoto fisiológico physiologic antidote.

antídoto mecánico mechanical antidote.

antídoto químico chemical antidote.

antídoto universal universal antidote.

antiemético, -ca *adj.* antiemetic.

antiepiléptico, -ca *adj.* antiepileptic.

antiescabioso, -sa *adj.* antiscabietic.

antiescabiético, -ca *adj.* antiscabietic.

antiescarlatinoso, -sa *adj.* antiscarlatinal.

antiescorbútico, -ca *adj.* antiscorbutic.

antiespasmódico *m.* antispasmodic.

antiespasmódico biliar billiary antispasmodic.

antiespasmódico bronquial bronchial antispasmodic.

antiespasmódico, -ca *adj.* antispasmodic.

antiespástico, -ca *adj.* antispastic.

antiestreptoquinasa *f.* antiestreptokinase.

antiestrógeno *m.* antiestrogen.

antifebril *adj.* antifebrile.

antiflatulento, -ta *adj.* antiflatulent.

antifúngico, -ca *adj.* antifungal.

antigénico, -ca *adj.* antigenic.

antígeno *m.* antigen.

antígeno alogénico allogenic antigen.

antígeno asociado a hepatitis hepatitis associated antigen (HAA).

antígeno asociado a las leucemias humanas human leukemia-associated antigen.

antígeno asociado a tumor tumor associated antigen.

antígeno Australia Australia antigen.

antígeno carcinoembrionario (CEA) carcinoembryonic antigen.

antígeno clase I class I antigen.

antígeno clase II class II antigen.

antígeno clase III class III antigen.

antígeno completo complete antigen.

antígeno común common antigen.

antígeno conjugado conjugated antigen.

antígeno de cubierta envelope antigen.

antígeno delta delta antigen.

antígeno específico de especie species-specific antigen.

antígeno específico de órgano organ-specific antigen.

antígeno específico de tejido tissue-specific antigen.

antígeno específico de tumor tumor-specific antigen (TSA).

antígeno específico specific antigen.

antígeno F F antigen.

antígeno febril febrile antigen.

antígeno de grupo group antigen.

antígeno de grupo sanguíneo blood group antigen.

antígeno heterógeno heterogenetic antigen.

antígeno heterólogo heterologous antigen.

antígeno hidrocarbonado carbohydrate antigen.

antígeno de histocompatibilidad histocompatibility antigen.

antígeno de histocompatibilidad mayor histocompatibility major antigen.

antígeno de histocompatibilidad menor histocompatibility minor antigen.

antígeno homólogo homologous antigen.

antígeno leucocitario común common leukocyte antigen.

antígeno leucocitario humano, antígeno de los linfocitos humanos (hla) human lymphocyte antigen (HLA).

antígeno nuclear nuclear antigen.

antígeno nuclear extraíble (ena) extractable nuclear antigen (ena).

antígeno o o antigen.

antígeno oncofetal oncofetal antigen.

antígeno parcial partial antigen.

antígeno del polen pollen antigen.

antígeno privado private antigen.

antígeno propio self-antigen.

antígeno prostático específico (psa) prostate specific antigen.

antígeno público public antigen.

antígeno de reacción cruzada cross-reacting antigen.

antígeno de recuerdo recall antigen.

antígeno secuestrado sequestered antigen.

antígeno sensibilizado sensitized antigen.

antígeno serodefinido (sd) serodefined antigen, serologically defined antigen.

antígeno de shock shock antigen.

antígeno Sm Sm antigens.

antígeno soluble soluble antigen.

antígeno somático somatic antigen.

antígeno SS-a SS-a antigen.

antígeno SS-b SS-b antigen.

antígeno de superficie del virus de la hepatitis b hepatitis b surface antigen (hbsag).

antígeno Tac Tac antigen.

antígeno Thy, antígeno theta Thy antigen, theta antigen.

antígeno de trasplante transplantation antigen.

antígeno de trasplante específico del tumor tumor-specific transplantation antigen (ttet).

antígeno tumoral tumor antigen.

antiglobulina *f.* antiglobulin.

antihemolítico, -ca *adj.* antihemolytic.

antihemorrágico, -ca *adj.* anthemorrhagic, antihemorrhagic.

antiherpético, -ca *adj.* antherpetic, antiherpetic.

antihigiénico, -ca *adj.* insanitary.

antihipercolesterolémico, -ca *adj.* antihypercholesteronemic.

antihiperglucémico, -ca *adj.* antihyperglycemic.

antihiperlipoproteico, -ca *adj.* antihyperlipoproteinemic.

antihipertensivo, -va *adj.* antihypertensive.

antihistamínico, -ca *adj.* antihistaminic.

antiinfeccioso, -sa *adj.* anti-infectious.

antiinflamatorio, -ria *adj.* anti-inflammatory.

antimicótico, -ca *adj.* antimycotic.

antimicrobiano, -na *adj.* antimicrobial, antimicrobic.

antineoplásico, -ca *adj.* antineoplastic.

antioncogen *m.* antioncogene.

antioxidante *m.* antioxidant.

antipalúdico, -ca *adj.* antipaludial.

antiparalítico, -ca *adj.* antiparalytic.

antiparasitario, -ria *adj.* antiparasitic.

antiparkinsoniano, -na *adj.* antiparkinsonian.

antipediculoso, -sa *adj.* antipedicular.

antiperistáltico, -ca *adj.* antiperistaltic.

antiperspirante *adj.* antiperspirant.

antipirético, -ca *adj.* antipyretic.

antiplaquetario, -ria *adj.* antiplatelet.

antipruriginoso, -sa *adj.* antipruritical.

antipsicótico, -ca *adj.* antipsychotic.

antiséptico, -ca *adj.* antiseptic.

antisocial *adj.* antisocial.

antispasmódico, -ca *adj.* antispasmodic.

antisuero *m.* antiserum.

antisuero específico specific antiserum.

antisuero de grupos sanguíneos blood group antiserum.

antisuero heterólogo heterologous antiserum.

antisuero homólogo homologous antiserum.

antisuero **monovalente** monovalent antiserum.

antisuero **polivalente** polyvalent antiserum.

antisuero **Rh** Rh antiserum.

antitérmico, -ca *adj.* antithermic.

antitetánico, -ca *adj.* antitetanic.

antitoxina *f.* antitoxin, antivenin.

antitoxina **botulínica** botulism antitoxin, botulinum antitoxin.

antitoxina **diftérica** diphtheria antitoxin.

antitripsina *f.* antitrypsin.

antitrombina *f.* antithrombin.

antitromboplastina *f.* antithromboplastin.

antitrombótico, -ca *adj.* antithrombotic.

antituberculoso, -sa *adj.* antitubercular, antituberculous.

antitusígeno, -na *adj.* antitussive.

antiulceroso, -sa *adj.* antiulcerative.

antivenenoso, -sa *adj.* antivenomous.

antivenéreo, -a *adj.* antivenereal.

antiviral *adj.* antiviral.

antocianidina *f.* anthocyanidin.

antojo¹ *m.* whim.

antojo² *m.* birthmark.

antracosis *f.* anthracosis.

ántrax *m.* carbuncle.

antro *m.* antrum.

antropología *f.* anthropology.

anuclear *adj.* anuclear.

anular¹ *m.* ring finger.

anular² *adj.* annular.

anuria *f.* anuria.

anuria **calculosa** calculus anuria.

anuria **obstructiva** obstructive anuria.

anuria **posrenal** postrenal anuria.

anuria **prerrenal** prerenal anuria.

anuria **renal** renal anuria.

anuria **por supresión** suppressive anuria.

aorta *f.* aorta.

aórtico, -ca *adj.* aortic.

aortitis *f.* aortitis.

aortografía *f.* aortography.

aparato¹ *m.* apparatus.

aparato **digestivo** digestive apparatus, apparatus digestorius.

aparato **locomotor** locomotor system.

aparato **reproductor** reproductive system.

aparato **respiratorio** respiratory apparatus, apparatus respiratorius.

aparato **urinario** urinary apparatus.

aparato² *m.* appliance.

aparato **ortodóncico** orthodontic appliance.

apareamiento *m.* mating, pairing.

apareamiento **al azar** random pairing.

apareamiento **de bases** base pairing.

apareamiento **concordante** assortative mating, assorted mating, assortive mating.

apareamiento **de los cromosomas** chromosome pairing.

apareamiento **selectivo** assortative mating, assorted mating, assortive mating.

apatía *f.* apathy.

apático, -ca *adj.* apathetic, apathic.

apéndice *m.* appendage, appendix.

apendicectomía *f.* appendicectomy.

apendicitis *f.* appendicitis.

  apendicitis aguda acute appendicitis.

  apendicitis crónica chronic appendicitis.

  apendicitis por cuerpo extraño foreign-body appendicitis.

  apendicitis destructiva perforating appendicitis.

  apendicitis focal focal appendicitis.

  apendicitis fulminante fulminating appendicitis.

  apendicitis gangrenosa gangrenous appendicitis.

  apendicitis izquierda left-sided appendicitis.

  apendicitis lumbar lumbar appendicitis.

  apendicitis obstructiva obstructive appendicitis.

  apendicitis perforante, apendicitis perforativa perforating appendicitis.

  apendicitis por contigüedad appendicitis by contiguity.

  apendicitis purulenta purulent appendicitis.

  apendicitis recurrente recurrent appendicitis.

  apendicitis segmentaria segmental appendicitis.

  apendicitis subperitoneal subperitoneal appendicitis.

  apendicitis supurada, apendicitis supurativa suppurative appendicitis.

  apendicitis traumática traumatic appendicitis.

  apendicitis verminosa verminous appendicitis.

apetencia *f.* appetition.

apetito *m.* appetite.

aplanamiento[1] *m.* saucerization.

aplanamiento[2] *m.* planing.

aplasia *f.* aplasia.

  aplasia ovárica ovarian aplasia, aplasia of the ovary.

  aplasia pilorum propia aplasia pilorum propia.

  aplasia tímica thymic aplasia.

aplásico, -ca *adj.* aplastic.

apnea *f.* apnea.

  apnea cardíaca cardiac apnea.

  apnea central central apnea.

  apnea central del sueño central sleep apnea.

  apnea de deglución deglutition apnea.

  apnea inducida induced apnea.

  apnea inducida por el sueño sleep-induced apnea.

  apnea neonatal apnea neonatorum.

  apnea obstructiva obstructive apnea.

  apnea obstructiva del sueño (SAOS) obstructive sleep apnea.

  apnea periférica peripheral apnea.

  apnea periódica del recién nacido periodic apnea of the newborn.

  apnea primaria primary apnea.

  apnea refleja reflex apnea.

  apnea secundaria secondary apnea.

  apnea del sueño sleep apnea.

  apnea del sueño mixta mixed sleep apnea.

apnea tardía late apnea.

apnea verdadera, apnea vera true apnea, apnea vera.

apneico, -ca *adj.* apneic.

apocrino, -na *adj.* apocrine.

apófisis *f.* apophysis.

apofisitis *f.* apophysitis.

apolipoproteína *f.* apolipoprotein.

aponeurosis *f.* aponeurosis.

apoplejía *f.* apoplexy, apoplexia.

apoplejía abdominal abdominal apoplexy.

apoplejía bulbar bulbar apoplexy.

apoplejía por calor heat apoplexy.

apoplejía cerebelar, apoplejía cerebelosa cerebellar apoplexy.

apoplejía cerebral cerebral hemorrhage.

apoplejía cutánea cutaneous apoplexy.

apoplejía embólica embolic apoplexy.

apoplejía espasmódica spasmodic apoplexy.

apoplejía funcional functional apoplexy.

apoplejía hipofisaria pituitary apoplexy.

apoplejía intestinal intestinal apoplexy.

apoplejía medular spinal apoplexy.

apoplejía neonatorum neonatal apoplexy.

apoplejía pancreática pancreatic apoplexy.

apoplejía placentaria placental apoplexy.

apoplejía pituitaria pituitary apoplexy.

apoplejía pontina pontile apoplexy, pontil apoplexy.

apoplejía renal renal apoplexy.

apoplejía trombótica thrombotic apoplexy.

apoplejía uterina apoplexia uterina.

apoplejía uteroplacentaria uteroplacental apoplexy.

apoptosis *f.* apoptosis.

apoyo[1] *m.* rest.

apoyo incisal incisal rest.

apoyo oclusal occlusal rest.

apoyo[2] *m.* support.

apoyo medio midstance support.

apraxia *f.* apraxia.

apraxia acinética akinetic apraxia.

apraxia amnésica amnestic apraxia.

apraxia cinética kinetic apraxia.

apraxia constructiva, apraxia de construcción constructional apraxia.

apraxia del desarrollo developmental apraxia.

apraxia ideatoria, apraxia de ideación, apraxia ideomotriz ideational apraxia.

apraxia ideomotora ideomotor apraxia.

apraxia de la marcha gait apraxia.

apraxia sensitiva sensory apraxia.

apráxico, -ca *adj.* apraxic.

aprendizaje *m.* learning.

aprendizaje psicomotor psychomotor learning.

aracnoidal *adj.* arachnoidal.

aracnoide *adj.* arachnoid.

aracnoides *f.* arachnoidea.

araña *f.* spider.

  *araña **arterial*** arterial spider.

  *araña **vascular*** vascular spider.

arcada *f.* arcade.

  *arcada **Alveolar**, arcada **dentaria*** dental arcade.

arco *m.* arch, arcus.

  *arco **faríngeo*** pharyngeal arch.

  *arco **reflejo*** reflex arch.

  *arco **senil*** arcus senilis.

ardor *m.* ardor.

  *ardor **epigástrico*** heartburn ardor.

areola, aréola *f.* areola.

  areola de la mama, areola del pezón areola mammae, areola of mammary gland, areola of the nipple.

  *areola **papilar*** areola papillaris.

  *areola **secundaria*** second areola.

  *areola **umbilical*** umbilical areola, areola umbilicus.

argiria *f.* argyria.

arritmia *f.* arrhythmia.

  *arritmia **cardíaca*** cardiac arrhythmia.

  *arritmia **continua*** continuous arrhythmia.

  *arritmia **fásica*** phasic arrhythmia.

  *arritmia **juvenil*** juvenile arrhythmia.

  *arritmia **perpetua*** perpetual arrhythmia.

  *arritmia **respiratoria*** respiratory arrhythmia.

  arritmia de seno, arritmia sinusal sinus arrhythmia.

arrítmico, -ca *adj.* arrhythmic.

arruga *f.* wrinkle, ruga.

artefacto *m.* artefact.

arteria *f.* artery, arteria.

arterial *adj.* arterial.

arterialización *f.* arterialization.

arteriocapilar *adj.* arteriocapillary, arterocapillary.

arteriodilatación *f.* arteriodilating.

arterioesclerosis *f.* arteriosclerosis.

  *arterioesclerosis **cerebral*** cerebral arteriosclerosis.

  *arterioesclerosis **coronaria*** coronary arteriosclerosis.

  *arterioesclerosis **hipertensiva*** hypertensive arteriosclerosis.

  *arterioesclerosis **periférica*** peripheral arteriosclerosis.

  *arterioesclerosis **presenil*** presenile arteriosclerosis.

  *arterioesclerosis **senil*** senile arteriosclerosis.

arterioesclerótico *adj.* arteriosclerotic.

arterioespasmo *m.* arteriospasm.

arterioestenosis *f.* arteriostenosis.

arteriogénesis *f.* arteriogenesis.

arteriografía *f.* arteriography.

  *arteriografía **cerebral*** cerebral arteriography.

  *arteriografía **espinal*** spinal arteriography.

  *arteriografía **selectiva coronaria*** selective coronary arteriography.

  *arteriografía **por sonda*** catheter arteriography.

arteriograma *m.* arteriogram.

arteriola *f.* arteriola, arteriole.

arteriolar *adj.* arteriolar.

arteriolitis *f.* arteriolitis.

  *arteriolitis **necrosante*** necrotizing arteriolitis.

arteriopatía *f.* arteriopathy.

arteriovenoso, -sa *adj.* arteriovenous, arteriovenosus.

arteritis *f.* arteritis.

  arteritis coronaria coronary arteritis.

  arteritis craneal cranial arteritis.

  arteritis reumática rheumatic arteritis.

articulación *f.* articulation, articulatio.

articulado, -da *adj.* articulated.

articulador *m.* articulator.

articular *v.* articulate.

artificial *adj.* artificial.

artralgia *f.* arthralgia.

artritis *f.* arthritis.

  artritis aguda acute arthritis.

  artritis climatérica climactic arthritis.

  artritis deformante arthritis deformans.

  artritis degenerativa degenerative arthritis.

  artritis exudativa exudative arthritis.

  artritis fúngica, artritis fungosa fungal arthritis, arthritis fungosa.

  artritis gonocócica, artritis gonorreica gonoccocal arthritis.

  artritis gotosa gouty arthritis.

  artritis gotosa aguda acute gouty arthritis.

  artritis infecciosa infectious arthritis.

  artritis inflamatoria crónica chronic inflammatory arthritis.

  artritis juvenil, artritis juvenil crónica juvenile arthritis, juvenile chronic arthritis.

  artritis de lyme lyme arthritis.

  artritis menopáusica menopausal arthritis.

  artritis micótica mycotic arthritis.

  artritis mutilante arthritis mutilans.

  artritis neuropática neuropathic arthritis.

  artritis nudosa arthritis nodosa.

  artritis reumática aguda acute rheumatic arthritis.

  artritis reumatoide rheumatoid arthritis.

  artritis reumatoide juvenil juvenile rheumatoid arthritis.

  artritis seca arthritis sicca.

  artritis séptica septic arthritis.

  artritis sifilítica syphilitic arthritis.

  artritis supurada suppurative arthritis.

  artritis tuberculosa tuberculous arthritis.

  artritis vírica viral arthritis.

artropatía *f.* arthropathy, arthropathia.

  artropatía de Charcot Charcot's arthropathy.

  artropatía diabética diabetic arthropathy.

  artropatía inflamatoria inflammatory arthropathy.

  artropatía neurógena neurogenic arthropathy.

  artropatía osteopulmonar osteopulmonary arthropathy.

  artropatía sifilítica syphilitic arthropathy.

  artropatía tabética tabetic arthropathy.

artrópodo *m.* arthropod.
artroscopia *f.* arthroscopy.
artroscopio *m.* arthroscope.
artrosis *f.* arthrosis.
  artrosis deformante, artrosis deformans arthrosis deformans.
  artrosis temporomandibular temporomandibular arthrosis.
asbestosis *f.* asbestosis.
ascítico, -ca *adj.* ascitic.
ascitis *f.* ascites.
  ascitis adiposa ascites adiposus.
  ascitis exudativa exudative ascites.
  ascitis grasa fatty ascites.
  ascitis hemorrágica hemorrhagic ascites.
  ascitis lechosa milky ascites.
  ascitis precoz ascites praecox.
  ascitis quiliforme chyliform ascites.
  ascitis quilosa chylous ascites, ascites chylosus.
  ascitis sanguinolenta bloody ascites.
asemia *f.* asemia.
asepsia *f.* asepsis.
aséptico, -ca *adj.* aseptic.
asfixia *f.* asphyxia.
  asfixia azul blue asphyxia.
  asfixia blanca white asphyxia.
  asfixia carbónica asphyxia carbonica.
  asfixia cianótica cyanotic asphyxia.
  asfixia fetal fetal asphyxia.
  asfixia lívida asphyxia livida.
  asfixia local local asphyxia.
  asfixia neonatal, asfixia neonatorum asphyxia neonatorum.
  asfixia pálida asphyxia pallida.
  asfixia reticular asphyxia reticularis.
  asfixia secundaria secondary asphyxia.
  asfixia traumática traumatic asphyxia.
asfixiante *adj.* asphyxiant.
asfixiar *v.* asphyxiate.
asimetría *f.* asymmetry.
asimétrico, -ca *adj.* asymmetric, asymmetrical.
asintomático, -ca *adj.* asymptomatic.
asistolia *f.* asystole, asystolia.
asistólico, -ca *adj.* asystolic.
asma *f.* asthma.
  asma abdominal abdominal asthma.
  asma alérgica allergic asthma.
  asma de los alfareros potter's asthma.
  asma alimentaria food asthma.
  asma alveolar alveolar asthma.
  asma atópica atopic asthma.
  asma bacteriana bacterial asthma.
  asma bronquial bronchial asthma.
  asma bronquítica bronchitic asthma.
  asma catarral catarrhal asthma.
  asma cardíaca cardiac asthma.
  asma convulsiva asthma convulsivum.
  asma enfisematosa Heberden's asthma.
  asma equina horse asthma.
  asma esencial essential asthma.
  asma espasmódica spasmodic asthma.
  asma extrínseca extrinsic asthma.

asma de los gatos cat asthma.

asma del heno hay asthma.

asma húmeda humid asthma.

asma infecciosa infective asthma.

asma intrínseca intrinsic asthma.

asma de los mineros miner's asthma.

asma nerviosa nervous asthma.

asma por polen pollen asthma.

asma por polvo dust asthma.

asma refleja reflex asthma.

asma renal renal asthma.

asma sexual sexual asthma.

asma tímica thymic asthma.

asma de verano summer asthma.

asma verdadera true asthma.

asmático, -ca *adj.* asthmatic.

asociación *f.* association.

asociación controlada controlled association.

asociación dirigida controlled association.

asociación genética genetic association.

asociación de ideas association of ideas.

asociación libre free association.

asociación onírica dream association.

asociación de sueño dream association.

asociado, -da *adj.* associated.

asonancia *f.* assonance.

aspecto *m.* aspect.

aspergiloma *m.* aspergilloma.

aspergilosis *f.* aspergillosis.

aspiración *f.* aspiration.

aspiración broncoscópica bronchoscopic aspiration.

aspiración meconial, aspiración de meconio meconium aspiration.

aspiración postusiva post-tussive aspiration.

aspiración al vacío vacuum aspiration.

aspirado, -da *adj.* aspirate.

aspirador *m.* aspirator.

aspirador de vacío vacuum aspirator.

astenia *f.* asthenia.

astenia miálgica myalgic asthenia.

astenia muscular myasthenia.

astenia nerviosa neurasthenia.

astenopía *f.* asthenopia.

astigmatismo *m.* astigmatism.

astigmatismo adquirido acquired astigmatism.

astigmatismo anormal astigmatism against the rule.

astigmatismo compuesto compound astigmatism.

astigmatismo congénito congenital astigmatism.

astigmatismo corneal corneal astigmatism.

astigmatismo directo direct astigmatism.

astigmatismo fisiológico physiological astigmatism.

astigmatismo hipermetrópico, astigmatismo hiperópico hypermetropic astigmatism, hyperopic astigmatism.

astigmatismo inverso inverse astigmatism.

astigmatismo irregular irregular astigmatism.

astigmatismo lenticular lenticular astigmatism.

astigmatismo mixto mixed astigmatism.

astilla *f.* splinter.

astrágalo *m.* astragalus.

astringente *m. y adj.* astringent.

astrocito *m.* astrocyte.

astrocitoma *m.* astrocytoma.

astroglia *f.* astroglia.

ataque *m.* attack, stroke.

ataque de calor heat stroke.

ataque cardíaco heart attack.

ataque isquémico transitorio transient ischemic attack.

ataque de pánico panic attack.

ataque de sol sunstroke.

ataque de sueño sleep attack.

ataque vagal vagal attack.

ataque vasovagal vasovagal attack.

ataxia *f.* ataxia.

ataxia aguda acute ataxia.

ataxia alcohólica alcoholic ataxia.

ataxia autónoma autonomic ataxia.

ataxia cardíaca, ataxia cordis ataxia cordis.

ataxia central central ataxia.

ataxia cerebelosa cerebellar ataxia.

ataxia cerebral cerebral ataxia.

ataxia cinética kinetic ataxia.

ataxia dinámica kinetic ataxia.

ataxia espinal spinal ataxia.

ataxia estática static ataxia.

ataxia frontal frontal ataxia.

ataxia hereditaria hereditary ataxia.

ataxia histérica hysterical ataxia.

ataxia laberíntica labyrinthic ataxia.

ataxia locomotora, ataxia locomotriz locomotor ataxia.

ataxia ocular ocular ataxia.

ataxia óptica optic ataxia.

ataxia sensitiva sensory ataxia.

atelectasia *f.* atelectasis.

atelectasia compresiva compression atelectasis.

atelectasia congénita congenital atelectasis.

atelectasia lobular lobular atelectasis.

atelectasia obstructiva obstructive atelectasis.

atelectasia segmentaria segmental atelectasis.

atención *f.* attention.

atenuación *f.* attenuation.

atenuar *v.* attenuate.

ateroembolia *m.* atheroembolism.

ateroembolismo *m.* atheroembolism.

ateroémbolo *m.* atheroembolus.

aterogénesis *f.* atherogenesis.

aterogenético, -ca *adj.* atherogenic.

aterogénico, -ca *adj.* atherogenic.

ateroma *m.* atheroma.

ateromatosis *f.* atheromatosis.

atetosis *f.* athetosis.

atipia *f.* atypia.

atípico, -ca *adj.* atypical.

atlas *m.* atlas.

átomo *m.* atom.

atonía *f.* atony.

atónico, -ca *adj.* atonic.

atopia *f.* atopia.

atópico, -ca *adj.* atopic.

atracción *f.* attraction.

atresia *f.* atresia.

atresia del ano anal atresia.

atresia aórtica aortic atresia.

atresia biliar biliary atresia.

atresia de las coanas choanal atresia.

atresia duodenal duodenal atresia.

atresia esofágica esophageal atresia.

atresia intestinal intestinal atresia.

atresia irídica, atresia del iris atresia iridis.

atresia mitral mitral atresia.

atresia pulmonar pulmonary atresia.

atresia tricúspide, atresia tricuspídea tricuspid atresia.

atresia vaginal vaginal atresia.

atrésico, -ca *adj.* atresic.

atrial *adj.* atrial.

atrio *m.* atrium.

atrofia *f.* atrophy, atrophia.

atrofia por agotamiento exhaustion atrophy.

atrofia cerebelosa cerebellar atrophy.

atrofia cutis atrophy cutis.

atrofia degenerativa degenerative atrophy.

atrofia espinal spinal atrophy.

atrofia gástrica gastric atrophy.

atrofia gingival gingival atrophy.

atrofia hemifacial hemifacial atrophy.

atrofia hemilingual hemilingual atrophy.

atrofia por inacción atrophy of disuse.

atrofia infantil infantile atrophy.

atrofia inflamatoria inflammatory atrophy.

atrofia miopática myopathic muscular atrophy.

atrofia muscular muscular atrophy.

atrofia ósea bone atrophy.

atrofia patológica pathologic atrophy.

atrofia periodontal periodontal atrophy.

atrofia ungueal atrophy unguium.

atrófico, -ca *adj.* atrophic.

atropismo *m.* atropinism.

aturdimiento *m.* dizziness.

audición *f.* audition.

audífono *m.* hearing aid.

audiograma *m.* audiogram.

audiometría *f.* audiometry.

auditivo, -va *adj.* auditive, auditory.

aura *f.* aura.

aura asmática aura asthmatica.

aura auditiva auditory aura.

aura cinestésica kinesthetic aura.

aura eléctrica electric aura.

aura epigástrica epigastric aura.

aura epiléptica epileptic aura.

aura histérica aura hysterica.

aura intelectual intellectual aura.

aura reminiscente reminiscent aura.

aura vertiginosa vertiginous aura.

aurícula *f.* atrium.

auricular *adj.* auricular.

auscultación *f.* auscultation.

auscultación directa direct auscultation.

auscultación inmediata immediate auscultation.

auscultación obstétrica obstetric auscultation.

auscultar *v.* auscultate, auscult.
ausencia *f.* absence.
  ausencia epiléptica epileptic absence.
autismo *m.* autism.
autista *adj.* autistic.
autoaglutinación *f.* autoagglutination.
autoaglutinina *f.* autoagglutinin.
autoanticuerpo *m.* autoantibody.
autoclave *m.* autoclave.
autoinmune *adj.* autoimmune.
autoinmunidad *f.* autoimmunity.
autoinmunitario, -ria *adj.* autoimmune.
autoinmunización *f.* autoimmunization.
autoinoculación *f.* autoinoculation.
automatismo *m.* automatism.
  automatismo ambulatorio ambulatory automatism.
  automatismo deambulante ambulatory automatism.
  automatismo de orden command automatism.
  automatismo postraumático inmediato immediate post-traumatic automatism.
automutilación *f.* autolesion.
autonomía *f.* autonomy.
autonómico, -ca *adj.* autonomic.
autopsia *f.* autopsy, autopsia.
autorregulación *f.* autoregulation.
autotransfusión *f.* autotransfusion.
autotrasplante *m.* autotransplant.
avascular *adj.* avascular.
axila *f.* axilla, armpit.
axilar *adj.* axillary.

axis *m.* axis.
axón *m.* axon.
axonal *adj.* axonal.
azoemia *f.* azotemia.
azoémico, -ca *adj.* azotemic.
azoospermia *f.* azoospermia, azoospermatism.
azúcar *f.* sugar.

B

baba *f.* slaver.
bacilar *adj.* bacillar, bacillary.
bacilemia *f.* bacillemia.
bacilífero, -ra *adj.* bacilleferous.
baciliforme *adj.* bacilliform.
bacilo *m.* bacillus.
bacteria *f.* bacterium.
bacteriano, -na *adj.* bacterial.
bactericida *m.* bactericide, bacteriocide.
bacteriemia *f.* bacteriemia.
bacteriófago *m.* bacteriophage.
bacteriología *f.* bacteriology.
  bacteriología clínica clinical diagnostic bacteriology.
  bacteriología higiénica public health bacteriology.
  bacteriología médica medical bacteriology.
  bacteriología sanitaria sanitary bacteriology.
  bacteriología sistemática systematic bacteriology.
bacteriológico, -ca *adj.* bacteriologic, bacteriological.
bacteriólogo, -ga *m., f.* bacteriologist.

bacteriosis *f.* bacteriosis.

bacteriuria *f.* bacteriuria, bacteruria.

 bacteriuria asintomática asymptomatic bacteriuria.

 bacteriuria gravídica pregnancy bacteriuria.

 bacteriuria significativa significant bacteriuria.

bacteriúrico, -ca *adj.* bacteriuric.

baile de San Vito *m.* Saint Vitus' dance.

baja estatura *f.* short stature.

baja visión *f.* low vision.

bajo peso *m.* underweight.

balance *m.* balance.

 balance acidobásico acid-base balance.

 balance cálcico calcium balance.

 balance calórico energy balance.

 balance electrolítico electrolyte balance.

 balance energético energy balance.

 balance enzimático enzyme balance.

 balance genético genic balance.

 balance glomérulo-tubular glomerulotubular balance.

 balance hídrico water balance.

 balance de inhibición y acción inhibition-action balance.

 balance líquido fluid balance.

 balance nitrogenado, balance de nitrógeno nitrogen balance.

 balance oclusal occlusal balance.

balanceo *m.* body rocking.

balanitis *f.* balanitis.

balneoterapia *f.* balneotherapeutics, balneotherapy.

balón *m.* balloon.

 angioplastia con balón balloon angioplasty.

balsámico, -ca *adj.* balsamic.

bálsamo *m.* balm.

banco *m.* bank.

 banco de embriones embryo bank.

 banco de esperma sperm bank.

 banco de genes gene bank.

 banco de ojos eye bank.

 banco de sangre blood bank.

 banco de semen semen bank.

 banco de suero serum bank.

banda *f.* band, bundle, stripe.

 banda abdominal belly band.

 banda abrazadera clamp band.

 banda amniótica amniotic band.

bandeja *f.* tray.

bandeo *m.* banding.

baño *m.* bath.

 baño de agua water bath.

 baño de agua de mar seawater bath.

 baño antipirético antipyretic bath.

 baño antiséptico antiseptic bath.

 baño de asiento sitz bath, hip bath.

 baño astringente astringent bath.

 baño de barro mud bath, moo bath.

 baño templado lukewarm bath.

barba *f.* beard, barba.

barbilla *f.* chin.

barbitúrico *m.* barbiturate.

bariatría *f.* bariatrics.

bariátrico, -ca *adj.* bariatric.

bario *m.* barium.

baroceptor *m.* baroceptor.

barorreceptor *m.* baroreceptor.

barotraumatismo *m.* barotrauma

barra *f.* bar.

barrera *f.* barrier.

   barrera cutánea skin barrier.

   barrera hematocerebral blood-brain barrier (BBB), blood-cerebral barrier.

   barrera hematocerebroespinal blood-cerebrospinal fluid barrier.

   barrera hematoencefálica (BHE) blood-brain barrier (BBB), blood-cerebral barrier.

   barrera mucosa, barrera de la mucosa gástrica gastric mucosal barrier.

   barrera placentaria placental barrier.

   barrera protectora protective barrier.

barrido *m.* scanning.

bartolinitis *f.* bartholinitis.

basal *adj.* basal.

base *f.* base.

   base de datos database.

   base nitrogenada nitrogenous base.

básico, -ca *adj.* basic.

basilar *adj.* basilar, basilaris.

basofilia *f.* basophilia.

basófilo, -la *m., f.* basophil.

bastón *m.* cane.

bastoncillo *m.* rod.

   bastoncillo retiniano retinal rod.

batería *f.* battery.

bazo *m.* spleen, splen, lien.

   bazo accesorio accessory spleen, lien accessorius, splen accesorius.

   bazo aumentado de tamaño enlarged spleen.

   bazo céreo waxy spleen.

   bazo cianótico cyanotic spleen.

   bazo errante wandering spleen.

   bazo flotante floating spleen.

   bazo moteado speckled spleen.

   bazo movible, bazo móvil movable spleen, lien mobilis.

bebé *m.* baby.

   bebé inmaduro immature baby.

   bebé probeta test-tube baby.

beneficio *m.* gain.

   beneficio primario de la enfermedad primary gain.

   beneficio secundario de la enfermedad secondary gain.

benigno, -na *adj.* benign.

beriberi *m.* beriberi.

berrinche *m.* tantrum.

beta *f.* beta.

   beta fetoproteína *f.* beta fetoprotein.

betabloqueante *m.* beta-blocker.

betacaroteno *m.* beta-carotene.

beta-lipoproteína *f.* beta-lipoprotein.

bezoar *m.* bezoar.

biarticulado, -da *adj.* biarticulate.

biarticular *adj.* biarticular.

biberón *m.* nursing bottle.

bicapa lipídica *f.* lipid bilayer.

bicarbonato *m.* bicarbonate.

   bicarbonato estándar standard bicarbonate.

   bicarbonato del plasma plasma bicarbonate.

   bicarbonato sanguíneo blood bicarbonate.

   bicarbonato sódico, bicarbonato de sodio sodium bicarbonate.

bíceps *m.* biceps.

bicipital *adj.* bicipital.

biclonal *adj.* biclonal.

bicóncavo, -va *adj.* biconcave.

biconvexo, -xa *adj.* biconvex.

bicorne *adj.* bicornate, bicornous, bicornuate.

bicúspide *m. y adj.* bicuspid.

bidé *m.* bidet.

bidimensional *adj.* bidimensional.

bienestar *m.* well-being, wellness.
  bienestar del enfermo well-being of the patient.
  bienestar de alto nivel high-level wellness.

bifásico, -ca *adj.* biphasic.

bifidobacteria *f.* bifidobacterium.

bifocal *adj.* bifocal.

bifurcación *f.* bifurcation, bifurcatio.
  bifurcación de la aorta, bifurcación aórtica bifurcation of the aorta, bifurcatio aortae, bifurcatio aortica.
  bifurcación de la carótida carotid bifurcation, bifurcatio carotidis.
  bifurcación de la tráquea bifurcation of trachea, bifurcatio tracheae.
  bifurcación del tronco pulmonar bifurcation of the pulmonary trunk, bifurcatio trunci pulmonalis.
  bifurcación radicular root furcation.

bifurcado, -da *adj.* bifurcate, bifurcated.

bigeminal *adj.* bigeminal.

bigeminismo *m.* bigeminy.

bilateral *adj.* bilateral.

bilateralismo *m.* bilateralism.

biliar *adj.* biliary.

biliosidad *f.* biliousness.

bilioso, -sa *adj.* bilious.

bilirrubina *f.* bilirubin.
  bilirrubina conjugada conjugated bilirubin.
  bilirrubina directa direct bilirubin.
  bilirrubina indirecta indirect bilirubin.
  bilirrubina libre free bilirubin.
  bilirrubina no conjugada unconjugated bilirubin.
  bilirrubina de reacción directa direct reacting bilirubin.
  bilirrubina de reacción indirecta indirect reacting bilirubin.
  bilirrubina total total bilirubin.

bilirrubinemia *f.* bilirubinemia.

bilis *f.* bile.

bilobulado, -da *adj.* bilobate, bilobed.

bilobular *adj.* bilobed.

binario, -ria *adj.* binary.

binuclear *adj.* binuclear.

bioactividad *f.* bioactivity.

bioanálisis *m.* bioassay.

biociencia *f.* bioscience.

biocompatibilidad *f.* biocompatibility.

biocompatible *adj.* biocompatible.

biodegradable *adj.* biodegradable.

biodisponibilidad *f.* bioavailability.

bioequivalente *adj.* bioequivalent.

bioestadística *f.* biostatistics.

bioética *f.* bioethics.

biofísica *f.* biophysics.

biogenia *f.* biogeny.

bioimplante *m.* bioimplant.

bioincompatibilidad *f.* bioincompatibility.

biología *f.* biology.

biomarcador *m.* biomarker.
biomecánica *f.* biomechanics.
biomedicina *f.* biomedicine.
bioprótesis *f.* bioprosthesis.
biopsia *f.* biopsy.
 biopsia por aguja needle biopsy.
 biopsia por aspiración aspiration biopsy.
 biopsia cerebral cerebral biopsy.
 biopsia citológica cytological biopsy.
 biopsia cónica, biopsia de cono cone biopsy.
 biopsia coriónica chorionic biopsy.
 biopsia del cuello uterino cervix uterinic biopsy.
 biopsia en cuña wedge biopsy.
 biopsia del endometrio endometrium biopsy.
 biopsia endoscópica endoscopic biopsy.
 biopsia por escisión, biopsia escisional excision biopsy.
 biopsia esternal sternal biopsy.
 biopsia de exploración exploratory biopsy.
 biopsia hepática liver biopsy.
 biopsia muscular muscular biopsy.
 biopsia negativa negative biopsy.
 biopsia ósea bone biopsy.
 biopsia percutánea percutaneous biopsy.
 biopsia positiva positive biopsy.
 biopsia por punción needle biopsy.
 biopsia por punción-aspiración con aguja fina fine-needle aspiration biopsy.
 biopsia quirúrgica surgical biopsy.
 biopsia renal renal biopsy.

 biopsia renal percutánea percutaneous renal biopsy.
 biopsia renal transvenosa transvenous renal biopsy.
 biopsia con sacabocados, biopsia de sacabocado punch biopsy.
 biopsia superficial, biopsia de superficie surface biopsy.
 biopsia por trepanación trephine biopsy.
 biopsia de vellosidad coriónica (BVC) chorionic villus biopsy (CVB).
bioquímica *f.* biochemistry.
bioquímico, -ca *adj.* biochemical.
biorretroalimentación *f.* biofeedback.
biorritmo *m.* biorhythm.
biosíntesis *f.* biosynthesis.
biotecnología *f.* biotechnology.
biotina *f.* biotin.
biotipo *m.* biotype.
biparietal *adj.* biparietal.
bipedestación *f.* orthostatism.
bipolar *adj.* bipolar.
birrefringencia *f.* birefringence.
biselar *v.* bevel.
bisexual *adj.* bisexual.
bisturí¹ *m.* bistoury.
bisturí² *m.* knife.
bivalente *adj.* bivalent.
biventricular *adj.* biventricular.
bizco, -ca *adj.* cross-eyed.
bizquear *v.* squint.
bizqueo *m.* squint.
 bizqueo de la acomodación accommodative squint.
 bizqueo concomitante comitant squint, concomitant squint.

bizqueo convergente convergent squint.

bizqueo divergente divergent squint.

bizqueo hacia arriba y hacia abajo upward and downward squint.

bizquera *f.* squint.

blanco[1] *m.* target.

blanco, -ca[2] *m. y adj.* white.

blanco del ojo white of the eye.

blanqueamiento *m.* bleaching.

blanqueo gingival *m.* gingival blanching.

blastémico, -ca *adj.* blastemic.

blastocele *m.* blastocele, blastocoele.

blastocisto *m.* blastocyst.

blastómero *m.* blastomere.

blastomicosis *f.* blastomycosis.

blástula *f.* blastula.

blefaritis *f.* blepharitis.

blefaritis rosácea blepharitis rosacea.

blefaritis seborreica seborrheic blepharitis.

blefaritis seborreica escamosa squamous seborrheic blepharitis.

blefaritis seca blepharitis sicca.

blefaritis ulcerosa ulcerative blepharitis, blepharitis ulcerosa.

blefaroespasmo *m.* blepharospasm, blepharospasmus.

blenorrea *f.* blennorrhea.

blister *m.* blister.

bloque *m.* block.

bloqueante *m.* blocker.

bloqueante alfa-adrenérgico alpha-adrenergic antagonist, alpha-blocker.

bloqueante beta-adrenérgico beta-adrenergic antagonist, beta-blocker.

bloqueante de los canales de calcio, bloqueante de la vía del calcio calcium channel blocker.

bloquear *v.* block.

bloqueo[1] *m.* block.

bloqueo de aire air block.

bloqueo auditivo ear block.

bloqueo auriculoventricular bloqueo A-V atrioventricular block, A-V block.

bloqueo cardíaco heart block.

bloqueo cardíaco congénito congenital heart block, congenital complete heart block.

bloqueo del corazón heart block.

bloqueo epidural epidural block.

bloqueo espinal spinal block.

bloqueo intercostal intercostal block.

bloqueo intraauricular intra-atrial block.

bloqueo intraespinal intraspinal block.

bloqueo nervioso nerve block.

bloqueo neuromuscular neuromuscular block.

bloqueo no despolarizante nondepolarizing block.

bloqueo paracervical paracervical block.

bloqueo perineural perineural block.

bloqueo presacro presacral block.

bloqueo protector protective block.

bloqueo de rama (BR) bundle-branch block (BBB), interventricular block.

bloqueo² *m.* blockade.

   bloqueo renal renal blockade.

   bloqueo vagal vagal blockade, vagus nerve blockade.

bloqueo³ *m.* blocking².

   bloqueo afectivo affective blocking.

   bloqueo emocional affective blocking.

   bloqueo mental mental blocking.

   bloqueo del pensamiento thought blocking.

boca *f.* mouth, os.

   boca saburral saburral mouth.

   boca seca dry mouth.

   boca ulcerada sore mouth.

   boca ulcerada por dentadura denture sore mouth.

bocio *m.* goiter.

   bocio agudo acute goiter.

   bocio de Basedow Basedow's goiter.

   bocio coloidal, bocio coloide colloid goiter.

   bocio congénito congenital goiter.

   bocio difuso diffuse goiter.

   bocio ectópico ectopic goiter.

   bocio endémico endemic goiter.

   bocio exoftálmico exophthalmic goiter.

   bocio familiar familial goiter.

   bocio folicular follicular goiter.

   bocio intratorácico intrathoracic goiter.

   bocio lingual lingual goiter.

   bocio multinodular multinodular goiter.

   bocio multinodular tóxico toxic multinodular goiter.

   bocio nodular nodular goiter.

   bocio nodular tóxico toxic nodular goiter.

   bocio no tóxico non-toxic goiter.

   bocio retrosternal substernal goiter.

   bocio simple simple goiter.

   bocio subesternal substernal goiter.

   bocio torácico thoracic goiter.

   bocio tóxico toxic goiter.

   bocio vascular vascular goiter.

   bocio por yoduro iodide goiter.

bola *f.* ball.

   bola adiposa de Bichat fatty ball of Bichat, buccal fat pad.

   bola alimentaria, bola de alimento food ball.

   bola micótica fungus ball.

bolo *m.* bolus.

   bolo alimenticio, bolo alimentario alimentary bolus.

   bolo intravenoso intravenous bolus.

bolsa¹ *f.* bag.

   bolsa de aguas bag of waters, forewaters bag.

   bolsa de colostomía colostomy bag.

   bolsa de ileostomía ileostomy bag.

   bolsa para micción micturition bag.

   bolsa testicular testicular bag.

bolsa² *f.* bursa.

bolsa³ *f.* pocket.

   bolsa gingival gingival pocket.

bolsa⁴ *f.* pouch.

   bolsa de Douglas Douglas's pouch, pouch of Douglas.

bolsa⁵ *f.* sac.

   bolsa amniótica amniotic sac.

bomba *f.* pump.

   bomba gástrica stomach pump.

   bomba de infusión infusion pump.

bomba para infusión constante constant infusion pump.

bomba de infusión y extracción infusion-withdrawal pump.

bomba de infusión de insulina insulin infusion pump.

bomba de insulina insulin pump.

bomba peristáltica peristaltic pump.

bomba de protones proton pump.

bomba sacaleches breast pump.

bomba de sodio sodium pump.

bomba de sodio-potasio, bomba de Na y K sodium-potassium pump.

borde¹ *m.* border.

borde estriado striated border.

borde² *m.* edge.

borde cortante cutting edge.

borde³ *m.* rim.

borde de oclusión occlusal rim, occlusion rim.

borderline *m.* borderline.

borrosidad *f.* blurring.

bostezo *m.* yawn.

bota *f.* boot.

botiquín *m.* first-aid kit.

botón¹ *m.* bouton.

botón sináptico synaptic bouton.

botón terminal terminal bouton, bouton terminale.

botón² *m.* button.

botón oriental, botón de Oriente Oriental button.

botulina *f.* botulin.

botulínico, -ca *adj.* botulinal.

botulismo *m.* botulism.

botulismo en heridas, botulismo por herida wound botulism.

bóveda *f.* vault.

bradicardia *f.* bradycardia.

bradicardia cardiomuscular cardiomuscular bradycardia.

bradicardia central central bradycardia.

bradicardia esencial essential bradycardia.

bradicardia fetal fetal bradycardia.

bradicardia idiopática idiopathic bradycardia.

bradicardia nodal nodal bradycardia.

bradicardia postinfecciosa, bradicardia posinfecciosa postinfectious bradycardia, postinfective bradycardia.

bradicardia sinoauricular sinoatrial bradycardia.

bradicardia sinusal sinus bradycardia.

bradicardia vagal vagal bradycardia.

bradicardia ventricular ventricular bradycardia.

bradicárdico, -ca *adj.* bradycardiac, bradycardic.

bradipnea *f.* bradypnea.

bradipsiquia *f.* bradypsychia.

bradiquinesia *f.* bradykinesia.

braguero¹ *m.* brace.

braguero² *m.* truss.

braille *m.* braille.

braquial *adj.* brachial.

braquialgia *f.* brachialgia.

braquialgia estática parestésica brachialgia statica paresthestica.

brazal *m.* cuff.

brazalete *m.* bracelet.

brazo *m.* arm.

brecha *f.* gap.

brecha de ADN DNA gap.

bromatología *f.* bromatology.

bromatólogo, -ga *m., f.* bromatologist.

broncoalveolitis *f.* bronchoalveolitis.

broncoaspiración *f.* bronchoaspiration.

broncoconstricción *f.* bronchoconstriction.

broncoconstrictor *m. y adj.* bronchoconstrictor.

broncodilatación *m.* bronchodilatation.

broncodilatador *m. y adj.* bronchodilator.

broncoespasmo *m.* bronchismus, bronchospasm.

broncofibroscopia *f.* bronchofiberscopy, bronchofibroscopy.

broncofibroscopio *m.* bronchofiberscope, bronchofibroscope.

bronconeumonía *f.* bronchopneumonia.

  bronconeumonía postoperatoria postoperative bronchopneumonia.

  bronconeumonía subaguda subacute bronchopneumonia.

  bronconeumonía tuberculosa tuberculous bronchopneumonia.

  bronconeumonía por virus virus bronchopneumonia.

bronconeumónico, -ca *adj.* bronchopneumonic.

bronconeumonitis *f.* bronchopneumonitis.

broncopatía *f.* bronchopathy.

broncorrea *f.* bronchorrhea.

broncoscopia *f.* bronchoscopy.

  broncoscopia de fibra óptica, broncoscopia fibroóptica fiberoptic bronchoscopy.

  broncoscopia láser laser bronchoscopy.

broncospasmo *m.* bronchospasm.

bronquial *adj.* bronchial.

bronquiectasis *f.* bronchiectasia, bronchiectasis.

bronquiectásico, -ca *adj.* bronchiectasic.

bronquiectático, -ca *adj.* bronchiectatic.

bronquio *m.* bronchus.

  bronquio fuente, bronquio de sostén stem bronchus.

  bronquio traqueal tracheal bronchus.

bronquiolitis *f.* bronchiolitis.

  bronquiolitis aguda obliterante acute obliterating bronchiolitis.

  bronquiolitis obliterante bronchiolitis obliterans.

bronquiolo, bronquíolo *m.* bronchiole, bronchiolus.

  bronquiolo lobulillar lobular bronchiole.

  bronquiolo terminal terminal bronchiole, bronchiolus terminalis.

bronquitis *f.* bronchitis.

  bronquitis aguda acute bronchitis.

  bronquitis asmática infecciosa infectious asthmatic bronchitis.

  bronquitis catarral catarrhal bronchitis.

  bronquitis crónica chronic bronchitis.

  bronquitis crupal croupous bronchitis.

  bronquitis epidémica epidemic bronchitis.

bronquitis estafilocócica staphylococcus bronchitis.

bronquitis estreptocócica streptococcal bronchitis.

bronquitis exudativa exudative bronchitis.

bronquitis fétida putrid bronchitis.

bronquitis membranosa membranous bronchitis.

bronquitis obliterante obliterative bronchitis, bronchitis obliterans.

bronquitis productiva productive bronchitis.

bronquitis seca dry bronchitis.

brote[1] *m.* bout.

brote[2] *m.* bud.

brote bronquial bronchial bud.

brote caudal tail bud.

brote pulmonar lung bud.

brote vascular vascular bud.

brucelosis *f.* brucellosis.

bruxismo *m.* bruxism.

buba *f.* buba, bubas.

bubón *m.* bubo.

bucal *adj.* buccal.

bucle *m.* loop.

buffer *m.* buffer.

bujía *f.* bougie.

bujía auditiva ear bougie.

bulbar *adj.* bulbar.

bulbitis *f.* bulbitis.

bulbo *m.* bulb, bulbus.

bulimia *f.* bulimia.

bulimia nerviosa bulimia nervosa.

bulímico, -ca *adj.* bulimic.

bulla *f.* bulla.

bulla enfisematosa emphysematous bulla.

bulla etmoidal ethmoid bulla, ethmoidal bulla, bulla ethmoidalis.

bulla ossea bulla ossea.

bulla pulmonar pulmonary bulla.

bullosis *f.* bullosis.

bulloso, -sa *adj.* bullous.

burbuja de aire *f.* venous air trap.

bursitis *f.* bursitis.

bursitis aquilea, bursitis aquiliana Achilles bursitis.

bursitis oleocraniana, bursitis del olécranon olecranal bursitis.

bursitis poplítea popliteal bursitis.

bursitis prerrotuliana prepatellar bursitis.

bursitis radiohumeral radiohumeral bursitis.

bursitis retrocalcánea retrocalcaneal bursitis.

bursitis subacromial subacromial bursitis.

bursitis subdeltoidea subdeltoid bursitis.

C

cabalgamiento *m.* overriding.

cabalgamiento del dedo gordo overtoe.

cabello *m.* hair, capillus, pilus.

cabestrillo *m.* sling.

cabeza *f.* head, caput.

cabeza de medusa medusa head, caput medusae.

cadáver *m.* cadaver.

cadavérico, -ca *adj.* cadaveric, cadaverous.

cadena *f.* chain.

cadera *f.* hip, coxa.

caduca *f.* caduca.

caída de espaldas *f.* swayback.

calambre *m.* cramp.

  calambre por calor heat cramp.

  calambre por decúbito recumbency cramp.

  calambre de los escritores writers' cramp.

  calambre intermitente intermittent cramp.

  calambre de minero miner's cramp.

  calambre de músico musician's cramp.

  calambre de pianista pianist's cramp.

  calambre de relojero watchmaker's cramp.

  calambre de los sastres tailor's cramp.

  calambre de violinista violinist's cramp.

calasia *f.* chalasia, chalasis.

calcáneo *m.* calcaneus.

calcemia *f.* calcemia.

calcificación *f.* calcification.

  calcificación patológica pathologic calcification.

  calcificación de la pulpa pulp calcification.

calcinosis *f.* calcinosis.

calcio *m.* calcium.

calciuria *f.* calciuria.

cálculo *m.* gallstone, calculus.

  cálculo de ácido úrico uric acid calculus.

  cálculo articular articular calculus.

  cálculo artrítico arthritic calculus.

  cálculo biliar biliary calculus.

  cálculo bronquial bronchial calculus.

  cálculo cardíaco cardiac calculus.

  cálculo cerebral cerebral calculus.

  cálculo de cistina cystine calculus.

  cálculo de colesterol cholesterol calculus.

  cálculo dental, cálculo dentario dental calculus.

  cálculo enquistado encysted calculus.

  cálculo faríngeo pharyngeal calculus.

  cálculo de fibrina fibrin calculus.

  cálculo gástrico gastric calculus, stomachic calculus.

  cálculo hepático hepatic calculus.

  cálculo intestinal intestinal calculus.

  cálculo pancreático pancreatic calculus.

  cálculo renal renal calculus.

  cálculo salival salivary calculus.

  cálculo de urato urate calculus.

  cálculo urinario urinary calculus.

  cálculo de la vejiga bladder calculus.

  cálculo vesical vesical calculus.

  cálculo xantínico xanthic calculus.

caldo *m.* bouillon, broth.

calentura *f.* calentura, calenture.

calibrador *m.* gauge.

caliemia *f.* kaliemia.

cáliz *m.* calyx.

callo *m.* callus.

  callo duro hard callus.

callosidad *f.* callosity, callositas.

calloso, -sa[1] *adj.* callous.

calloso, -sa[2] *adj.* callosal.

calmante *m.* calmative.

calor *m.* heat, calor.

caloría *f.* calorie.

calórico, -ca *adj.* caloric.

calostro *m.* colostrum.

calostro gravídico colostrum gravidum.

calostro puerperal colostrum puerperarum.

calvario m. calvaria.

calvicie f. baldness, calvities.

calvicie congénita congenital baldness.

calvicie de distribución masculina male pattern baldness.

calvicie masculina común common male baldness.

calvicie del pubis pubic baldness.

calvo, -va adj. bald.

cámara f. chamber, camera.

cámara pulpar pulp camera, pulp chamber.

cambio m. change.

cambio trófico trophic change.

campo m. field.

campo auditivo auditory field.

campo de visión, campo visual visual field.

canal m. canal, canalis.

canal iónico ion channel.

canalículo m. canaliculus.

canalización f. canalization.

canceloso, -sa adj. cancellated, cancellous.

cáncer m. cancer.

cáncer familiar familial cancer.

cáncer de los fumadores de pipa pipe-smoker's cancer.

cáncer de hígado liver cancer.

cáncer in situ cancer in situ.

cáncer latente latent cancer.

cáncer de mama breast cancer.

cáncer medular medullary cancer.

cáncer del muñón stump cancer.

cáncer oculto occult cancer.

cáncer óseo bone cancer.

cáncer de pulmón lung cancer.

cancerígeno, -na adj. cancerigenic, cancerogenic.

canceroso, -sa adj. cancerous.

Candida f. Candida.

candidemia f. candidemia.

candidiasis f. candidiasis.

candidiasis cutánea cutaneous candidiasis.

candidiasis endocárdica endocardial candidiasis.

candidosis f. candidosis.

canino m. canine.

cannabis m. cannabis.

cánula f. cannula.

cánula de traqueostomía tracheostomy cannula.

canulización f. cannulization.

capa¹ f. coat.

capa² f. layer.

capacidad f. capacity.

capacidad buffer buffer capacity.

capacidad de fijación de hierro (CFH) iron-binding capacity (IBC).

capacidad hipnótica hypnotic capacity.

capacidad inspiratoria inspiratory capacity.

capacidad de oxígeno oxygen capacity.

capacidad pulmonar total (CPT) total lung capacity (TLC).

capacidad residual residual capacity.

capacidad respiratoria respiratory capacity.

capacidad térmica heat capacity, thermal capacity.

capacidad vital (CV), capacidad vital forzada (CVF) vital capacity (VC), forced vital capacity (FVC).

capacitación *f.* capacitation.

capilar *m.* capillary.

capilaridad *f.* capillarity.

cápsida *f.* capsid.

cápside *m.* capsid.

cápsula, capsula *f.* capsule, capsula.

cápsula nasal nasal capsule.

cápsula óptica optic capsule.

cápsula ótica otic capsule.

capsulitis *f.* capsulitis.

capsulitis adhesiva adhesive capsulitis.

capsulitis hepática hepatic capsulitis.

captura *f.* capture.

capuchón *m.* cap.

caquéctico, -ca *adj.* cachectic.

caquexia *f.* cachexia.

caquexia nerviosa anorexia nervosa.

caquexia palúdica malarial cachexia.

caquexia suprarrenal cachexia suprarrenalis.

caquexia tiroidea cachexia thyroidea.

cara *f.* face.

cara articular facies articularis.

cara hipocrática hippocratic face.

cara de luna llena moon face.

cara de máscara masklike face.

cara de pájaro bird face.

cara de plato dish face.

cara de sapo frog face.

cara de vaca cow face.

carácter *m.* character.

carácter dominante dominant character.

carácter hereditario inherited character.

carácter ligado al sexo sex-linked character.

carácter mendeliano Mendelian character.

carácter recesivo recessive character.

carácter sexual primario primary sex character.

carácter sexual secundario secondary sex character.

característica *f.* characteristic.

caracterización *f.* characterization.

carbono *m.* carbon.

carbunco *m.* anthrax.

carbunco cerebral cerebral anthrax.

carbunco cutáneo cutaneous anthrax.

carbunco gastrointestinal gastrointestinal anthrax.

carbunco por inhalación inhalational anthrax.

carbunco intestinal intestinal anthrax.

carbunco meníngeo meningeal anthrax.

carbunco pulmonar pulmonary anthrax.

carcinoembrionario, -ria *adj.* carcinoembryonic.

carcinogénesis *f.* carcinogenesis.

carcinogénico, -ca *adj.* carcinogenic.

carcinógeno *m.* carcinogen.

carcinoide *m.* carcinoid.

carcinoma *m.* carcinoma.

  carcinoma in situ carcinoma in situ.

  carcinoma oculto occult carcinoma.

  carcinoma preinvasivo preinvasive carcinoma.

  carcinoma primario primary carcinoma.

cardíaco, -ca *adj.* cardiac.

cardias *m.* cardia.

cardinal *adj.* cardinal.

cardioesofágico, -ca *adj.* cardioesophageal.

cardioespasmo *m.* cardiospasm.

cardiógrafo *m.* cardiograph.

cardiograma *m.* cardiogram.

cardiología *f.* cardiology.

cardiólogo, -ga *m., f.* cardiologist.

cardiomegalia *f.* cardiomegaly.

cardiomiopatía *f.* cardiomyopathy.

  cardiomiopatía alcohólica alcoholic cardiomyopathy.

  cardiomiopatía congestiva congestive cardiomyopathy.

  cardiomiopatía de dilatación dilated cardiomyopathy.

  cardiomiopatía hipertrófica hypertrophic cardiomyopathy.

  cardiomiopatía idiopática idiopathic cardiomyopathy.

  cardiomiopatía posparto, cardiomiopatia postpartum postpartum cardiomyopathy.

  cardiomiopatía restrictiva restrictive cardiomyopathy.

cardiópata *m., f.* cardiopath.

cardiopatía *f.* cardiopath, cardiopathia.

cardiopulmonar *adj.* cardiopulmonary.

cardiotónico, -ca *adj.* cardiotonic.

cardiotóxico, -ca *adj.* cardiotoxic.

cardiovascular *adj.* cardiovascular.

cardiovasculorrenal *adj.* cardiovasculorenal.

cardioversión *f.* cardioversion.

cardioversor *m.* cardioverter.

carditis *f.* carditis.

carencia *f.* deficiency.

carga *f.* burden.

  carga corporal body burden.

  carga salina salt loading.

  carga tumoral tumor burden.

caries *f.* caries.

  caries bucal buccal caries.

  caries incipiente incipient caries.

  caries oclusal occlusal caries.

  caries recurrente recurrent caries.

carilla *f.* facing.

carina *f.* carina.

cariotipo *m.* karyotype.

caroteno *m.* carotene.

carótida *f.* carotid.

carotídeo, -a *adj.* carotid.

carpiano, -na *adj.* carpal.

carpo *m.* carpus.

carpocarpiano, -na *adj.* carpocarpal.

carpofalángico, -ca *adj.* carpophalangeal.

carpometacarpiano, -na *adj.* carpometacarpal.

cartilaginoso *m.* cartilaginous.

cartílago *m.* cartilage, cartilago.

  cartílago calcificado calcified cartilage.

  cartílago de crecimiento metaphyseal cartilage.

caseoso, -sa *adj.* caseous.
caso *m.* case.
caspa *f.* dandruff.
castración *f.* castration.
castrar[1] *v.* castrate.
castrar[2] *v.* spay.
catabólico, -ca *adj.* catabolic.
catabolismo *m.* catabolism.
catabolito *m.* catabolite.
catalepsia *f.* catalepsy.
cataléptico, -ca *adj.* cataleptic.
catálisis *f.* catalysis.
catalizador *m.* catalyst, catalyzer.
cataplasma *m.* cataplasm.
catarata *f.* cataract, cataracta.
  catarata blanda soft cataract.
  catarata capsular capsular cataract.
  catarata completa complete cataract.
  catarata complicada complicated cataract.
  catarata cristalina crystalline cataract.
  catarata diabética diabetic cataract.
  catarata dura hard cataract.
  catarata glaucomatosa glaucomatous cataract.
  catarata incipiente incipient cataract.
  catarata infantil infantile cataract.
  catarata inmadura immature cataract.
  catarata juvenil juvenile cataract.
  catarata madura mature cataract, ripe cataract.
  catarata membranosa membranous cataract.
  catarata periférica peripheral cataract.

  catarata perinuclear perinuclear cataract.
  catarata progresiva progresssive cataract.
  catarata por rubéola rubella cataract.
  catarata secundaria secondary cataract.
  catarata senil senile cataract.
  catarata supermadura overripe cataract.
  catarata traumática traumatic cataract.
  catarata vascular vascular cataract.
catarro *m.* catarrh.
  catarro bronquial bronchitis.
  catarro intestinal endoenteritis.
  catarro laríngeo laryngitis.
catarsis *f.* catharsis.
catártico, -ca *adj.* cathartic.
catatonía *f.* catatonia.
catatónico, -ca *adj.* catatonic.
catecolaminas *f.* catecholamine.
catequina *f.* catechin.
catéter *m.* catheter.
  catéter venoso central central venous catheter.
cateterismo *m.* catheterization.
catgut *m.* catgut.
catión *m.* cation.
cátodo *m.* cathode.
caudado, -da *adj.* caudate.
caudal *adj.* caudal.
causa *f.* cause.
  causa específica specific cause.
  causa local local cause.
  causa necesaria necessary cause.
  causa predisponente predisposing cause.

causa primaria primary cause.

causa secundaria secondary cause.

causa suficiente sufficient cause.

causa última ultimate cause.

cáustico, -ca *adj.* caustic.

cauterización *f.* cauterization.

caverna *f.* cavern.

cavernoso, -sa *adj.* cavernous.

cavidad *f.* cavity, cavitas.

cavidad amniótica amniotic cavity.

cavidad cariosa, cavidad de caries tooth-decay cavity.

cavitación *f.* cavitation.

cefalalgia *f.* cephalalgia.

cefalea *f.* headache.

cefalea acuminada cluster headache.

cefalea de Horton Horton's headache.

cefalea migrañosa migraine headache.

cefalea en racimo cluster headache.

cefalea tensional tension headache, tension-type headache.

cefálico, -ca *adj.* cephalic.

ceguera *f.* blindness.

ceguera para los colores color blindness.

ceguera mental mind blindness.

ceguera musical music blindness.

ceguera nocturna night blindness.

ceguera para el olfato smell blindness.

ceguera psíquica psychic blindness.

ceja *f.* eyebrow.

celiaquía *f.* celiac disease.

célula *f.* cell.

célula adiposa adipose cell.

célula asesina killer cell.

célula B B-cell.

célula bronquial bronchic cell.

célula cigoto egg cell.

célula diana target cell.

célula endotelial endothelial cell.

célula epitelial epithelial cell.

célula madre brood cell, mother cell.

célula miocárdica cardiac muscle cell of the myocardium.

célula muscular estriada striated muscle cell.

célula muscular estriada cardíaca cardiac muscle cell.

célula muscular estriada esquelética skeletal muscle cell.

célula muscular lisa smooth muscle cell.

célula necrótica necrotic cell.

célula nerviosa nerve cell.

célula ósea osseous cell, bone cell.

célula pigmentaria pigment cell.

célula T T cell.

célula T citotóxica, célula TC T cytotoxic cell, TC cell.

célula T colaboradora, célula TH T-helper cell, TH cell.

célula T supresora, célula TS T-suppressor cell, TS cell.

celularidad *f.* cellularity.

celulitis *f.* cellulitis.

celulitis gangrenosa gangrenous cellulitis.

celulitis necrotizante necrotizing cellulitis.

celulitis orbitaria orbital cellulitis.

celulitis pélvica pelvic cellulitis.

central *adj.* central.

céntrico, -ca *adj.* centric.

centro *m.* center, centrum.

centro activo active center.

centro de la alimentación feeding center.

centro espiratorio expiratory center.

centro inspiratorio inspiratory center.

centro de osificación ossific center, center of ossification.

centro de la saciedad satiety center.

centro secundario de osificación secondary center of ossification.

centro vasomotor vasomotor center.

centro vitales vital center.

cenuriasis *f.* cenuriasis, coenurasis.

cepa *f.* strain.

cepa tipo salvaje wild type strain.

cepillo *m.* brush.

cepillo dental denture brush.

ceramida *f.* ceramide.

cerclaje *m.* cerclage.

cerebelitis *f.* cerebellitis.

cerebelo *m.* cerebellum.

cerebral *adj.* cerebral.

cerebritis *f.* cerebritis.

cerebro *m.* brain, cerebrum.

cerebro anterior forebrain.

cerebro medio midbrain.

cerebro posterior hindbrain.

cerebrovascular *adj.* cerebrovascular.

cero absoluto *m.* absolute zero.

cerumen *m.* cerumen.

cervical *adj.* cervical.

cervicitis *f.* cervicitis.

cérvix *m.* cervix.

cesárea *f.* cesarean.

cestoideo, -a *adj.* cestoid.

cetoacidosis *f.* ketoacidosis.

cetoaciduria *f.* ketoaciduria.

cetona *f.* ketone.

cetonemia *f.* ketonemia.

cetónico, -ca *adj.* ketonic.

cetonuria *f.* ketonuria.

cetosis *f.* ketosis.

chalazión *m.* chalazion.

chancro *m.* chancre.

chancro sifilítico hard chancre.

choque *m.* shock.

choque anafiláctico anaphylactic shock.

choque anafilactoide anaphylactoid shock.

choque por anestesia, choque anestésico anesthetic shock.

choque bacteriémico bacteriemic shock.

choque cardiogénico cardiogenic shock.

choque crónico chronic shock.

choque cultural cultural shock.

choque delirante delirious shock.

choque por descompresión declamping shock.

choque eléctrico electric shock.

choque por endotoxinas endotoxin shock.

choque endotóxico endotoxic shock.

choque hemorrágico hemorrhagic shock.

choque hipovolémico hypovolemic shock.

choque histamínico histamine shock.

choque insulínico insulin shock.

choque irreversible irreversible shock.

choque medular spinal shock.

choque quirúrgico surgical shock.

choque reversible reversible shock.

choque séptico septic shock.

choque sérico serum shock.

choque traumático traumatic shock.

cianosis *f.* cyanosis.

cianosis por compresión compression cyanosis.

cianótico, -ca *adj.* cyanotic.

ciática *f.* sciatica.

cicatriz *f.* scar, cicatrix.

cicatrización *f.* cicatrization.

cicatrizante *adj.* cicatrizant.

cíclico, -ca *adj.* cyclic.

ciclo *m.* cycle.

ciclo anovulatorio anovulatory cycle.

ciclo cardíaco cardiac cycle.

ciclo celular cell cycle.

ciclo menstrual menstrual cycle.

ciclo del pelo hair cycle.

ciclo visual visual cycle.

ciclo vital life cycle.

ciclope, ciclope *adj.* cyclops.

ciclotímico, -ca *adj.* cyclothymiac, cyclotymic.

ciego *m.* caecum.

ciego, -ga *adj.* blind.

cierre *m.* closure.

cifoescoliosis *f.* kyphoscoliosis.

cifosis *f.* kyphosis.

cigomático, -ca *adj.* zygomatic.

cigoto *m.* zygote.

ciliado *m.* ciliate.

ciliar *adj.* ciliary.

cilíndrico, -ca *adj.* cylindrical.

cilindro *m.* cast, cylinder.

cilindro renal renal cast.

cilio *m.* cilium.

cinesia *f.* kinesia, kinesis.

cinesis *f.* kinesia, kinesis.

cinestesia *f.* kinesthesia.

cinestésico, -ca *adj.* kinesthetic.

cinética *f.* kinetics.

cinta *f.* ribbon, tape.

cinta adhesiva adhesive tape.

cinta dental dental tape.

cintura *f.* girdle, waist.

cintura escapular shoulder girdle.

cintura torácica thoracic girdle.

circuito *m.* circuit.

circulación *f.* circulation.

circulación capilar capillary circulation.

circulación colateral collateral circulation.

circulación coronaria coronary circulation.

circulación embrionaria embryonic circulation.

circulación extracorpórea extracorporeal circulation.

circulación fetal fetal circulation.

circulación general systemic circulation.

circulación linfática lymph circulation.

circulación mayor greater circulation.

circulación menor lesser circulation.

circulación placentaria placental circulation.

*circulación **portal*** portal circulation.

*circulación **pulmonar*** pulmonary circulation.

*circulación **sanguínea*** bloodstream.

*circulación **sistémica*** systemic circulation.

*circulación **de la vena porta*** portal circulation.

circulatorio, -ria *adj.* circulatory.

circular *adj.* circular.

círculo *m.* circle, circulus.

*círculo **vicioso*** vicious circle.

circuncisión *f.* circumcision.

cirrosis *f.* cirrhosis.

*cirrosis **alcohólica*** alcoholic cirrhosis.

*cirrosis **biliar*** biliary cirrhosis.

*cirrosis **biliar primaria*** primary biliary cirrhosis.

*cirrosis **grasa*** fatty cirrhosis.

*cirrosis **periportal*** periportal cirrhosis.

*cirrosis **posnecrótica*** postnecrotic cirrhosis.

cirugía *f.* surgery.

*cirugía **abdominal*** abdominal surgery.

*cirugía **ambulatoria*** ambulatory surgery.

*cirugía **antiséptica*** antiseptic surgery.

*cirugía **aséptica*** aseptic surgery.

*cirugía **bucal*** oral surgery.

*cirugía **cardíaca*** cardiac surgery.

*cirugía **cerrada*** closed surgery.

*cirugía **conservadora*** conservative surgery.

*cirugía **cosmética*** cosmetic surgery.

*cirugía **dental*** dental surgery.

*cirugía **estética*** esthetic surgery.

*cirugía **general*** general surgery.

*cirugía **mayor*** major surgery.

*cirugía **menor*** minor surgery.

*cirugía **operatoria*** operative surgery.

*cirugía **oral*** oral surgery.

*cirugía **ortopédica*** orthopedic surgery.

*cirugía **ótica**, cirugía **otológica*** aural surgery.

*cirugía **plástica*** plastic surgery.

*cirugía **radical*** radical surgery.

*cirugía **reconstructora**, cirugía **reconstructiva*** reconstructive surgery.

*cirugía **transexual*** transsexual surgery.

cirujano, -na *m., f.* surgeon.

cistadenoma *m.* cystadenoma, cystoadenoma.

cistectomía *f.* cystectomy.

cisticercosis *f.* cysticercosis.

cístico, -ca *adj.* cystic, cystous.

cistinuria *f.* cystinuria.

cistitis *f.* cystitis.

*cistitis **aguda*** acute catarrhal cystitis.

*cistitis **alérgica*** allergic cystitis.

*cistitis **bacteriana*** bacterial cystitis.

*cistitis **diftérica*** diphtheritic cystitis.

*cistitis **hemorrágica*** hemorrhagic cystitis.

*cistitis **quística*** cystitis cystica.

*cistitis **senil*** cystitis senilis.

cistitis vírica viral cystitis.

cistograma *m.* cystogram.

cistoma *m.* cystoma.

cistoscopia *f.* cystocopy.

cistoscopio *m.* cystoscope.

cistostomía *f.* cystostomy.

citocida[1] *m.* cytocide.

citocida[2] *adj.* cytocidal.

citocina *f.* cytokine.

citogenética *f.* cytogenetics.

citólisis *f.* cytolysis.

citología *f.* cytology.

citología cervicovaginal cervicovaginal cytology.

citomegalovirus *m.* cytomegalovirus.

citopatología *f.* cytopathology.

citoplasma *m.* cytoplasm.

citoplasmático, -ca *adj.* cytoplasmic.

citosis *f.* cytosis.

citotoxicidad *f.* cytotoxicity.

citotóxico, -ca *adj.* cytotoxic.

citotoxina *f.* cytotoxin.

clamidia *f.* Chlamydia.

clamp *m.* clamp.

clamp de Gaskell Gaskell's clamp.

clasificación *f.* classification.

claudicación *f.* claudication.

claudicación intermitente intermittent claudication.

claudicación venosa venous claudication.

claustrofobia *f.* claustrophobia.

claustrofóbico, -ca *adj.* claustrophobic.

clavícula *f.* clavicle, clavicula.

cleptómano *m.* kleptomaniac.

clima *m.* climate, weather.

climaterio *m.* climacterium.

clímax *m.* climax.

clínica *f.* clinic.

clínico, -ca[1] *adj.* clinical.

clínico, -ca[2] *m., f.* clinician.

clinicopatológico, -ca *adj.* clinicopathologic.

clítoris *m.* clitoris.

cloasma *m.* chloasma.

clon *m.* clone.

clonación *f.* cloning.

clonal *adj.* clonal.

clonar *v.* clone.

clónico, -ca *adj.* clonic.

clonus *m.* clonus.

cloroformo *m.* chloroform.

clorosis *f.* chlorosis.

clostridio *m.* clostridium.

coadyuvante *adj.* adjuvant.

coagulación *f.* coagulation.

coagulación intravascular difusa diffuse intravascular coagulation.

coagulación intravascular diseminada (CID) disseminated intravascular coagulation (DIC).

coagulación masiva massive coagulation.

coagulación plasmática plasmatic coagulation.

coagulación sanguínea blood clotting.

coagulante *adj.* coagulant.

coágulo *m.* clot, coagulum.

coágulo ante mortem antemortem clot.

coágulo cardíaco heart clot.

coágulo distal distal clot.

coágulo externo external clot.

coágulo en grasa de pollo chicken fat clot.

coágulo interno internal clot.

coágulo post mortem post mortem clot.

coágulo proximal proximal clot.

coágulo sanguíneo blood clot.

coagulopatía *f.* coagulopathy.

coana *f.* choana.

coaptación *f.* coaptation.

coartación *f.* coarctation.

coartación de la aorta, coartación aórtica coarctation of the aorta.

coartación aórtica de tipo adulto adult type coarctation of the aorta.

coartación aórtica de tipo infantil infantile type coarctation of the aorta.

coartación invertida reversed coarctation.

coartado, -da *adj.* coarctate.

coarticulación *f.* coarticulation.

cobaltosis *f.* cobaltosis.

cobertura funcional *f.* functional overlay.

cocaína *f.* cocaine, cocain.

cocainómano, -na *m., f.* cocainist.

cóccix *m.* coccyx.

cóxis *m.* coccyx.

cóclea *f.* cochlea.

coclear *adj.* cochlear.

cocobacilo *m.* coccobacillus.

cóctel *m.* cocktail.

código *m.* code.

código analógico analogical code.

código digital digital code.

código genético genetic code.

codo *m.* elbow.

codo dislocado pulled elbow.

codo del estudiante student elbow.

codo de golfista golfer's elbow.

codo de lanzador baseball pitcher's elbow.

codo de los mineros miner's elbow.

codo de las niñeras nursemaid's elbow.

codo péndulo dropped elbow.

codo de tenista tennis elbow.

codón *m.* codon.

coeficiente *m.* coefficient.

coenzima *f.* coenzyme.

cofactor *m.* cofactor.

cognición *f.* cognition.

cognitivo, -va *adj.* cognitive.

cohorte *f.* cohort.

coital *adj.* coital.

coitalgia *f.* coitalgia.

coito *m.* coitus.

cojera *f.* lameness, limp.

cojo -ja *adj.* lame.

cola *f.* tail.

colágeno *m.* collagen.

colágeno tipo I type I collagen.

colágeno tipo II type II collagen.

colágeno tipo III type III collagen.

colágeno tipo IV type IV collagen.

colágeno, -na *adj.* collagenous.

colagenosis *f.* collagenosis.

colangiocolecistografía *f.* cholangiocholecystography.

colangiografía *f.* cholangiography.

colangiograma *m.* cholangiogram.

colangiohepatitis *f.* cholangiohepatitis.

colangiopancreatografía *f.* cholangiopancreatography.

colangiopancreatografía endoscópica retrógrada, colangiopancreatografía retrógrada endoscópica (CPRE) ERCP, endoscopic retrograde cholangiopancreatography (ERCP).

colangioscopia *f.* cholangioscopy.

colangitis *f.* cholangitis, cholangeitis.

  colangitis esclerosante sclerosing cholangitis.

colapso *m.* collapse.

  colapso circulatorio circulatory collapse.

  colapso masivo massive collapse.

  colapso nervioso nervous breakdown.

  colapso pulmonar pulmonary collapse, collapse of the lung.

colateral *adj.* collateral.

colecistectomía *f.* cholecystectomy.

colecistitis *f.* cholecystitis.

colédoco *m.* choledoch.

cólera *m.* cholera.

  cólera infantil cholera infantum.

  cólera tífico, cólera tifoídico typhoid cholera.

colestasis *f.* cholestasis.

colestático -ca *adj.* cholestatic.

colesteatoma *m.* cholesteatoma.

colesterol *m.* cholesterol.

colesterolemia *f.* cholesterolemia.

colgajo *m.* flap.

cólico *m.* colic.

  cólico biliar, cólico bilioso biliary colic.

  cólico por cálculo biliar gallstone colic.

  cólico gástrico gastric colic.

  cólico hepático hepatic colic.

  cólico intestinal intestinal colic.

  cólico del lactante infantile colic.

  cólico menstrual menstrual colic.

  cólico nefrítico nephritic colic.

  cólico pancreático pancreatic colic.

  cólico renal renal colic.

cólico -ca *adj.* colic.

colinefritis *f.* cholinephritis.

colinérgico, -ca *adj.* cholinergic.

colítico, -ca *adj.* kolytic.

colitis *f.* colitis.

  colitis ulcerosa ulcerative colitis, colitis ulcerativa.

collar *m.* collar.

  collar ortopédico cervical collar.

collarín cervical *m.* cervical collar.

colocación *f.* placement.

colon *m.* colon.

  colon gigante giant colon.

  colon inactivo inactive colon.

  colon irritable irritable colon.

  colon perezoso lazy colon.

colonia *f.* colony.

colonitis *f.* colonitis.

colonización *f.* colonization.

colonorragia *f.* colonorrhagia.

colonorrea *f.* colonorrhea.

colonoscopia *f.* colonoscopy.

colonoscopio *m.* colonoscope.

color *m.* color.

colorante *adj.* staining, dyeing.

colorimetría *f.* colorimetry.

colorrectal *adj.* colorectal.

colosigmoidoscopia *f.* colosigmoidoscopy.

colostomía *f.* colostomy.

colostomizado, -da *adj.* colostomate.

colposcopia *f.* colposcopy.

colposcopio *m.* colposcope.

columna *f.* column, columna.

  columna vertebral vertebral column.

coluria *f.* choluria.

colúrico, -ca *adj.* choluric.

colutorio *m.* collutory, mouthwash, collutorium.

coma *m.* coma.

  coma alcohólico alcoholic coma.

  coma por barbitúricos barbiturate coma.

  coma diabético diabetic coma.

  coma hepático hepatic coma, coma hepaticum.

  coma hiperosmolar hyperosmolar coma.

  coma hipoclorémico coma hypochloraemicum.

  coma hipoglucémico hypoglycemic coma.

  coma irreversible irreversible coma.

  coma de Kussmaul Kussmaul's coma.

  coma metabólico metabolic coma.

  coma tirotóxico thyrotoxic coma.

  coma de trance trance coma.

  coma urémico uremic coma.

  coma vigil coma vigil.

comadrona *f.* midwife.

comatoso, -sa *adj.* comatose.

combinación *f.* combination.

  combinación nueva new combination.

comedogénico, -ca *adj.* comedogenic.

comedón *m.* comedo.

  comedón abierto open comedo.

  comedón blanco whitehead comedo.

  comedón cerrado closed comedo.

comensal *m.* commensal.

comezón *m.* itch.

comida *f.* food, meal.

comisura *f.* commissura, commisure.

comorbilidad *f.* comorbidity.

compacta *f.* compacta.

compacto, -ta *adj.* compact.

comparador *m.* comparator.

compartimento *m.* compartment.

compatibilidad *f.* compatibility.

compatible *adj.* compatible.

compensación *f.* compensation.

  compensación de dosis dosage compensation.

compensador, -ra *adj.* compensatory.

competencia *f.* competence.

  competencia cardíaca cardiac competence.

  competencia embrionaria embryonic competence.

  competencia inmunológica immunological competence.

competición *f.* competition.

complejo, -ja *m. y adj.* complex.

  complejo aberrante aberrant complex.

  complejo anómalo anomalous complex.

  complejo antigénico antigenic complex.

  complejo antígeno-anticuerpo antigen-antibody complex.

  complejo apical apical complex.

  complejo auricular atrial complex, auricular complex.

  complejo bifásico diphasic complex.

  complejo demencia SIDA (CDS) AIDS dementia complex (ADC).

  complejo de Edipo Oedipus complex.

  complejo de Gohn Gohn's complex.

  complejo de Golgi Golgi complex.

  complejo hemoglobina-haptoglobina hemoglobin-haptoglobin complex.

  complejo HLA HLA complex.

complejo materno mother complex.

complejo mayor de histocompatibilidad (CMH) major histocompatibility complex (MHC).

complejo paterno father complex.

complejo principal de histocompatibilidad major histocompatibility complex.

complejo QRS QRS complex.

complejo QRST QRST complex.

complejo relacionado con el SIDA (CRS) AIDS related complex (ARC).

complejo de superioridad superiority complex.

complementación *f.* complementation.

complementariedad *f.* complementarity.

complementario, - ria *adj.* complementary.

complemento *m.* complement.

complexión *f.* complexion.

compliancia *f.* compliance.

compliancia cerebral brain compliance.

compliancia del corazón compliance of the heart.

compliancia específica specific compliance.

compliancia estática static compliance.

compliancia pulmonar lung compliance.

compliancia torácica thoracic compliance.

compliancia ventilatoria ventilatory compliance.

complicación *f.* complication.

complicación médica medical complication.

complicación quirúrgica surgical complication.

complicación vascular vascular complication.

complicado, -da *adj.* complicated.

componente *m.* constituent.

componente del complemento constituent of complement.

componente metabólico metabolic constituent.

componente de la oclusión constituent of occlusion.

componente respiratorio respiratory constituent.

componente secretor secretory constituent.

componente somático motor somatic motor constituent.

componente somático sensitivo somatic sensory constituent.

componente visceral motor splanchnic motor constituent.

componente visceral sensitivo splanchnic sensory constituent.

comportamiento *m.* behavior.

comportamiento impulsivo acting out.

comportamiento sexual sexual behavior.

composición *f.* composition.

comprensión *f.* comprehension.

compresa *f.* compress.

compresa caliente hot compress.

compresa fría cold compress.

compresa ginegológica gynecologic compress.

compresa graduada graduated compress.

compresa húmeda wet compress.

compresa perineal perinal compress.

compresión *f.* compression.

compresión cardíaca cardiac compression.

compresión cerebral, compresión del cerebro cerebral compression, compression of the brain.

compresión digital digital compression.

compresión espinal spinal compression.

compresión instrumental instrumental compression.

compresión de la médula espinal spinal cord compression.

compresión medular medullar compression.

compresión nerviosa nerve compression.

compresión raquídea spinal compression.

compresor *m.* compressor.

compresor de aire air compressor.

comprimido *m.* tablet.

comprobación *f.* ascertainment.

comprobación completa complete ascertainment.

comprobación incompleta incomplete ascertainment.

comprobación múltiple multiple ascertainment.

comprobación única single ascertainment.

comprobación truncada truncate ascertainment.

compuesto, -ta *adj.* compound.

compulsión *f.* compulsion.

compulsivo *adj.* compulsive.

comunicación *f.* communication.

comunicación congruente congruent communication.

comunicación disfuncional dysfunctional communication.

comunicación incongruente incongruent communication.

comunicación verbal alterada impaired verbal communication.

comunicante *adj.* communicans.

comunidad *f.* community.

comunidad terapéutica therapeutic community.

concavidad *f.* concavity.

cóncavo, -va *adj.* concave.

concebir *v.* conceive.

concentración *f.* concentration.

concentración bactericida mínima minimal bactericidal concentration.

concentración celular máxima (CM) maximum cell concentration (MC).

concentración de hemodiálisis hemodialysate concentration.

concentración letal mínima (MCL) minimal lethal concentration (MLC).

concentración molar molar concentration.

concentración normal normal concentration.

concentración sérica de oxigeno oxygen concentration in blood.

concentración de la solución ratio solution.

concentración urinaria máxima (CUM) maximum urinary concentration (MUC).

concentrado, -da *adj.* concentrated.

concentrado *m.* concentrate.

concentrado celular packed cell concentrate.

concentrado de hematíes red blood cell concentrate.

concentrado de hígado liver concentrate.

concentrado de plaquetas platelet concentrate.

concentrado vitamínico vitamin concentrate.

concentrar *v.* concentrate.

concéntrico, -ca *adj.* concentric.

concepción *f.* conception.

concepción imperativa imperative conception.

conceptivo, -va *adj.* conceptive.

concepto *m.* concept.

concepto de no umbral no-threshold concept.

conceptual *adj.* conceptual.

conciencia *f.* consciousness.

conciencia doble double consciousness, dual consciousness.

conciencia moral moral consciousness.

conciencia nublada clouding consciousness.

conciencia de la realidad reality awareness.

concordancia *f.* concordance.

concordante *adj.* concordant.

concreción *f.* concretion, concretio.

concreción calculosa calculous concretion.

concreción cardiaca concretio cordis.

concreción prostática prostatic concretion.

concreción tofácea, concreción tófica tophic concretion.

concusión *f.* concussion.

concusión abdominal abdominal concussion.

concusión del cerebro, concusión cerebral concussion of the brain.

concusión del laberinto concussion of the labyrinth.

concusión de la médula espinal concussion of the spinal cord.

concusión pulmonar pulmonary concussion.

concusión de la retina concussion of the retina.

condensación *f.* condensation.

condensador *m.* condenser.

condición *f.* condition.

condición basal basal condition.

condicionamiento *m.* conditioning.

condicionamiento operante, condicionamiento operativo operant conditioning.

condicionamiento de Pavlov, condicionamiento pavloviano Pavlovian conditioning.

condilar *adj.* condylar.

condíleo, -a *adj.* condylar.

condilectomía *f.* condylectomy.

cóndilo *m.* condyle.

condiloma *m.* condyloma.

condón *m.* condom.

condritis *f.* chondritis.

condrocito *m.* chondrocyte.

condrodisplasia *f.* chondrodysplasia.

condrodisplasia punteada, condrodisplasia puntiforme, condrodisplasia punctata chondrodysplasia punctata.

condroesqueleto *m.* chondroskeleton.

condrogénesis *f.* chondrogenesis.

condroma *m.* chondroma.

condromatosis *f.* chondromatose.

condropatía *f.* chondropathia.

conducción *f.* conduction.

  conducción **acelerada** accelerated conduction.

  conducción **anterior** forward conduction.

  conducción **anterógrada** anterograde conduction.

  conducción **anómala** anomalous conduction.

  conducción **auriculoventricular (A-V)** atrioventricular conduction (A-V).

  conducción **decreciente** decremental conduction.

  conducción **demorada** delayed conduction.

  conducción **del impulso nervioso** conduction of the nervous impulse.

  conducción **intraventricular** intraventricular conduction.

  conducción **nerviosa** nerve conduction.

  conducción **ósea** bone conduction.

  conducción **retardada** delayed conduction.

  conducción **retrógrada** retrograde conduction.

  conducción **saltatoria** saltatory conduction.

  conducción **sináptica** synaptic conduction.

  conducción **supranormal** supranormal conduction.

  conducción **ventricular** ventricular conduction.

  conducción **ventricular aberrante** aberrant ventricular conduction.

  conducción **ventriculoauricular (V-A)** ventriculoatrial conduction (V-A).

conducta *f.* behavior.

conductismo *m.* behaviorism.

conductista *adj.* behaviorist.

conducto *m.* duct, ductus.

  conducto **aberrante** aberrant duct, ductus aberrans.

  conducto **hipofisario** hypophyseal duct.

  conducto **neural** neural canal.

  conducto **tirogloso** thyroglossal duct.

  conducto **tirolingual** thyrolingual duct.

  conducto **tubotimpánico** tubotympanic canal.

  conducto **urogenital** urogenital canal.

conductor, -ra *adj.* conductive.

conductor *m.* conductor.

conectivo, -va *adj.* connective.

conector *m.* connector.

conexión *f.* connection, connexus.

confianza *f.* confidence.

conflicto *m.* conflict.

  conflicto **de acercamiento-acercamiento** approach-approach conflict.

  conflicto **de acercamiento-evitación** approach-avoidance conflict.

  conflicto **doble** double conflict.

  conflicto **enfoque-evitación** approach-avoidance conflict.

conflicto de evitación-evitación avoidance-avoidance conflict.

conflicto intrapersonal intrapsychic conflict.

conflicto intrapsíquico intrapsychic conflict.

conflicto motivación motivational conflict.

conformación *f.* conformation.

congelación[1] *f.* freezing.

congelación[2] *f.* frostbite.

congelación profunda deep frostbite.

congelación superficial superficial frostbite.

congelación-desecación *f.* freeze-drying.

congelación-sustitución *f.* freeze-substitution.

congénito, -ta *adj.* congenital.

congestión *f.* congestion.

congestión bronquial bronchial congestion.

congestión cerebral brain congestion.

congestión esplácnica splanchnic engorgement.

congestión fisiológica physiologic congestion.

congestión funcional functional congestion.

congestión hipostática hypostatic congestion.

congestión mamaria caked breast.

congestión neurotónica neurotonic congestion.

congestión ocular bloodshot.

congestión pasiva passive congestion.

congestión pulmonar pulmonary congestion.

congestión de rebote rebound congestion.

congestionado, -da *adj.* congested.

congestivo, -va *adj.* congestive.

cónico, -ca *adj.* conic, conical.

conización *f.* conization.

conización cervical cervical conization.

conización por cauterio cautery conization.

conización en frío cold conization.

conjugación *f.* conjugation.

conjugado *m.* conjugate.

conjugado, -da *adj.* conjugate.

conjuntiva *f.* conjunctiva.

conjuntiva bulbar bulbar conjunctiva.

conjuntiva palpebral palpebral conjunctiva.

conjuntival *adj.* conjunctival.

conjuntivitis *f.* conjunctivitis.

conjuntivitis aguda acute conjunctivitis.

conjuntivitis aguda contagiosa epidemic conjunctivitis.

conjuntivitis alérgica allergic conjunctivitis.

conjuntivitis anafiláctica allergic conjunctivitis.

conjuntivitis angular angular conjunctivitis.

conjuntivitis atópica atopic conjunctivitis.

conjuntivitis atropínica atropine conjunctivitis.

conjuntivitis bacteriana bacterial conjunctivitis.

conjuntivitis blenorrágica blenorrheal conjunctivitis.

conjuntivitis calcárea calcareous conjunctivitis.

conjuntivitis catarral, conjuntivitis catarral aguda catarrhal conjunctivitis, acute catarrhal conjunctivitis.

conjuntivitis cicatricial, conjuntivitis cicatrizal cicatricial conjunctivitis.

conjuntivitis contagiosa aguda acute contagious conjunctivitis.

conjuntivitis diftérica diphtheritic conjunctivitis.

conjuntivitis epidémica epidemic conjunctivitis.

conjuntivitis flictenular phlyctenular conjunctivitis.

conjuntivitis gonocócica gonococcal conjunctivitis.

conjuntivitis gonorreica gonorrheal conjunctivitis.

conjuntivitis hemorrágica aguda acute hemorrhagic conjunctivitis.

conjuntivitis de inclusión inclusion conjunctivitis.

conjuntivitis infantil purulenta infantile purulent conjunctivitis.

conjuntivitis lagrimal lacrimal conjunctivitis.

conjuntivitis leñosa ligneous conjunctivitis.

conjuntivitis litiásica lithiasis conjunctivitis.

conjuntivitis medicamentosa conjunctivitis medicamentosa.

conjuntivitis de Meibomio Meibomian conjunctivitis.

conjuntivitis membranosa membranous conjunctivitis.

conjuntivitis meningocócica meningococcus conjunctivitis.

conjuntivitis neonatal neonatal conjunctivitis.

conjuntivitis de las piscinas swimming pool conjunctivitis.

conjuntivitis de las praderas prairie conjunctivitis.

conjuntivitis primaveral spring conjunctivitis.

conjuntivitis purulenta purulent conjunctivitis.

conjuntivitis purulenta infantil infantile purulent conjunctivitis.

conjuntivitis química chemical conjunctivitis.

conjuntivitis del recién nacido, conjuntivitis de los recién nacidos conjunctivitis of the newborn.

conjuntivitis seudomembranosa pseudomembranous conjunctivitis.

conjuntivitis simple simple conjunctivitis.

conjuntivitis de soldador welder's conjunctivitis.

conjuntivitis toxicogénica toxicogenic conjunctivitis.

conjuntivitis tracomatosa trachomatous conjunctivitis.

conjuntivitis tularémica, conjuntivitis tularensis tularemic conjunctivitis, conjunctivitis tularensis.

conjuntivitis urática uratic conjunctivitis.

conjuntivitis vacunal vaccinial conjunctivitis.

conjuntivitis vírica viral conjunctivitis.

conjuntivo, -va *adj.* conjunctive.

conminuto, -ta *adj.* comminuted.

conmoción *f.* commotio.

  conmoción cerebral commotio cerebri.

cono *m.* cone, conus.

  cono congénito congenital cone.

conos *m.* cones.

  conos y bastones rods and cones.

consanguíneo, -a *adj.* consanguineous.

consanguinidad *f.* consanguinity, sibship.

consciencia *f.* conscience.

consciente *adj.* conscious.

consecutivo, -va *adj.* consecutive.

consensual *adj.* consensual.

consentimiento informado *m.* informed consent.

conservación *f.* conservation, preservation.

  conservación de la energía conservation of energy.

  conservación en frío cold preservation.

  conservación en máquina perfusion system.

  conservación de la materia conservation of matter.

conservador, -ra *adj.* conservative.

conservante *m.* preservative.

consistencia *f.* consistence.

  consistencia gingival gingival consistence.

consolidación *f.* consolidation.

consolidado, -da *adj.* consolidate.

consolidante *adj.* consolidant.

constancia *f.* constancy.

constante *f. y adj.* constant.

  constante de asociación association constant.

  constante de conjugación binding constant.

  constante de desactivación desintegration constant.

  constante de desintegración desintegration constant.

  constante de difusión diffusion constant.

  constante de disociación dissociation constant.

  constante de equilibrio equilibrium constant.

  constante de velocidad velocity constant.

constitución *f.* constitution.

  constitución cromosómica chromosome set.

  constitución linfática lymphatic constitution.

constitucional *adj.* constitutional.

constricción *f.* constriction.

  constricción duodenopilórica duodenopyloric constriction.

  constricción primaria primary constriction.

  constricción secundaria secondary constriction.

constrictivo, -va constrictive.

constrictor *m.* constrictor.

constructivo, -va *adj.* constructive.

consumo *m.* consumption.

  consumo de oxígeno oxygen consumption.

  consumo pasivo de tabaco passive smoking consumption.

consumo perjudicial damaging consumption.

consumo sistémico de oxígeno systemic oxygen consumption.

contacto *m.* contact.

contacto completo complete contact.

contacto débil weak contact.

contacto directo direct contact.

contacto indirecto mediate contact.

contacto inicial initial contact.

contacto inmediato immediate contact.

contacto oclusal occlusal contact.

contacto prematuro premature contact.

contacto proximal, contacto próximo proximal contact, proximate contact.

contacto con la realidad contact with reality.

contacto de trabajo working contact.

contador *m.* counter.

contagio *m.* contagion.

contagio directo, contagio inmediato immediate contagion.

contagio indirecto mediate contagion.

contagio mental psychic contagion.

contagio psíquico psychic contagion.

contagioso, -sa *adj.* contagious.

contaminación *f.* contamination.

contaminante *adj.* contaminant.

contenido *m.* content.

continencia *f.* continence.

continencia fecal fecal continence.

continencia urinaria urinary continence.

contracción *f.* contraction, twitch.

contracción Braxton Hicks Braxton-Hicks contraction.

contracción espasmódica twiching contraction.

contracción isométrica isometric contraction.

contracción isotónica isotonic contraction.

contracción isovolumétrica isovolumetric contraction.

contracción paradójica paradoxical contraction.

contracción postural postural contraction.

contracción prematura premature contraction.

contracción de sacudida twich contraction.

contracción tetánica tetanic contraction.

contracción tónica tonic contraction.

contracción uterina uterine contraction.

contracción ventricular automática automatic ventricular contraction.

contracción ventricular de escape escaped ventricular contraction.

contracción ventricular prematura (CVP) premature ventricular contraction (PVC).

contracepción *f.* contraception.

contracepción hormonal hormonal contraception.

contracepción intrauterina intrauterine contraception.

contraceptivo *m.* contraceptive.

contracorriente *f.* countercurrent.

contráctil *adj.* contractile.

contractilidad *f.* contractility.

contractilidad cardíaca cardiac contractility.

contractilidad idiomuscular idiomuscular contractility.

contractura *f.* contracture.

contractura de defensa defense contracture.

contractura dolorosa painful contracture.

contractura de Dupuytren Dupuytren's contracture.

contractura fisiológica physiologic contracture.

contractura funcional functional contracture.

contractura hipertónica hypertonic contracture.

contractura histérica hysterical contracture.

contractura isquémica ischemic contracture.

contractura isquémica del ventrículo izquierdo ischemic contracture of the left ventricle.

contractura de Volkmann Volkmann's contracture.

contraestímulo *m.* contrastimulus.

contrafuerte *m.* abutment.

contraindicación *f.* contraindication.

contraindicado, -da *adj.* contraindicated.

contraste *m.* contrast.

contraste baritado baric contrast.

contraste doble double contrast.

contraste liposoluble liposoluble contrast.

contraste negativo negative contrast.

contraste de la película film contrast.

contraste radiográfico radiographic contrast.

contraste yodado, contraste iodado iodate contrast.

control *m.* control.

control automático automatic control.

control biológico biological control.

control de calidad quality control.

control del estrés stress management.

control de la hemorragia control of hemorrhage.

control local local control.

control natal, control de la natalidad birth control.

control con placebo en investigación control with placebo in investigation.

control por presión nudge control.

control reflejo reflex control.

control respiratorio respiratory control.

control por retroalimentación feedback control.

control sinérgico synergic control.

control social social control.

control tónico tonic control.

control vestibuloequilibratorio vestibulo-equilibratory control.

control volitivo, control voluntario volitional control, voluntary control.

contusión *f.* contusion.

contusión cerebral brain contusion.

contusión del cuero cabelludo scalp contusion.

contusión por contragolpe countercoup contusion.

contusión del lóbulo temporal temporal lobe contusion.

contusión de la médula espinal contusion of the spinal cord.

contusión medular medullar contusion.

contusión por piedra stone contusion.

contusión renal renal contusion.

convalecencia *f.* convalescence.

convaleciente *adj.* convalescent.

convergencia *f.* convergence.

convergencia de acomodación, convergencia acomodativa accommodative convergence.

convulsión *f.* convulsion, seizure.

convulsión clónica clonic convulsion, clonic seizure.

convulsión estática static convulsion.

convulsión febril febrile convulsion, febrile seizure.

convulsión focal focal seizure.

convulsión histérica, convulsión histeroide hysterical convulsion, hysteroid convulsion, hysterical seizure.

convulsión infantil infantile convulsion.

convulsión mímica mimetic convulsion, mimic convulsion.

convulsión neonatal neonatal seizure.

convulsión parcial partial convulsion, partial seizure.

convulsión parcial compleja complex partial convulsion.

convulsión postraumática inmediata immediate post-traumatic convulsion.

convulsión puerperal puerperal convulsion.

"convulsión en salaam" salaam convulsion.

convulsión tetánica tetanic convulsion.

convulsión tónica tonic convulsion, tonic seizure.

convulsión tónico-clónica generalizada generalized tonic-clonic convulsion, generalized tonic-clonic seizure.

convulsionante *adj.* convulsant.

convulsivo, -va *adj.* convulsive.

convulsoterapia *f.* convulsotherapy.

coordinación *f.* coordination.

coordinación motora motor coordination.

coordinación visualmotora visualmotor coordination.

coprocultivo *m.* coproculture.

corazón *m.* heart, cor.

corazón adiposo fat heart, fatty heart, cor adiposum.

corazón artificial artificial heart.

corazón de atleta, corazón atlético athlete's heart, athletic heart.

corazón colgante hanging heart.

corazón congelado frosted heart.

corazón derecho right heart.

corazón errante wandering heart.

corazón graso fat heart, fatty heart.

corazón hipoplásico hypoplastic heart.

corazón horizontal horizontal heart.

corazón izquierdo left heart.

corazón móvil movable heart, cor mobile.

corazón pulmonar pulmonary heart, cor pulmonale.

corazón sistémico systemic heart.

corazón suspendido suspended heart.

corazón de tres cavidades three-chambered heart, cor triloculare.

corazón venoso venous heart.

corazón vertical vertical heart.

corazón en zueco sabot heart.

corditis *f.* chorditis, corditis.

corditis de los cantantes chorditis cantorum.

corditis nudosa chorditis nodosa.

corditis tuberosa chorditis tuberosa.

corditis vocal chorditis vocalis.

corditis vocal inferior chorditis vocalis inferior.

cordura *f.* sanity.

corea *f.* chorea.

corea aguda acute chorea.

corea crónica chronic chorea.

corea danzante dancing chorea.

corea degenerativa degenerative chorea.

corea epidémica epidemic chorea.

corea festinante chorea festinans.

corea histérica hysteric chorea, hysterical chorea.

corea de Huntington Huntington's chorea.

corea juvenil juvenile chorea.

corea mayor, corea major chorea major.

corea menor, corea minor chorea minor.

corea reumática rheumatic chorea.

corea unilateral onesided chorea.

corion *m.* chorion, corium.

corion velloso shaggy chorion.

coriónico, -ca *adj.* chorionic.

coriza *f.* coryza.

coriza alérgica allergic coryza.

coriza espasmódica coryza spasmodica.

coriza del polen pollen coryza.

córnea *f.* cornea.

córnea cónica conical cornea.

corneal *adj.* corneal.

corneítis *f.* corneitis.

coroides *f.* choroidea.

coroiditis *f.* choroiditis.

coroiditis anterior anterior choroiditis.

coroiditis multifocal multifocal choroiditis.

coroiditis posterior posterior choroiditis.

coroiditis proliferante proliferative choroiditis.

coroiditis serosa serous choroiditis.

corona *f.* crown, corona.

corona artificial artificial crown.

corona funda jacket crown.

corona parcial partial crown.

corona radiada, corona radiante radiate crown, corona radiata.

coronal *adj.* coronal, coronale.

coronario, -ria *adj.* coronary.

corpóreo, -a *adj.* corporeal.

corpus corpus.

corpus albicans corpus albicans.

corpus luteum corpus luteum.

corpuscular *adj.* corpuscular.

corpúsculo *m.* corpuscle, corpusculum.

corrección *f.* correction.

corrector, -ra *adj.* corrective.

corrector *m.* corrector.

corrector de función function corrector.

corredera *f.* groove.

correlación *f.* correlation.

correspondencia *f.* correspondence.

correspondencia anómala anomalous correspondence.

correspondencia armoniosa harmonious correspondence.

correspondencia inarmónica dysharmonious correspondence.

correspondencia retiniana retinal correspondence.

corrosión *f.* corrosion.

corrosivo, -va *adj.* corrosive.

corsé *m.* brace, jacket, corset.

corte *m.* cut, section.

corteza *f.* cortex.

cortical *adj.* cortical.

corticomedular *adj.* corticospinal.

corticosteroide *m.* corticosteroid.

cortisol *m.* cortisol.

cortisolemia *f.* cortisolemia.

costilla, costa *f.* rib, costa.

costra *f.* crust, crusta.

costra inflamatoria crusta inflammatoria.

costra láctea, costra de leche milk crust, crusta lactea.

costroso, -sa *adj.* costrous, crustal.

cotiledón *m.* cotyledon.

coxa *f.* coxa.

coxalgia *f.* coxalgia.

craneal *adj.* cranial.

craneano, -na *adj.* cranial.

cráneo *m.* skull, cranium.

craneotomía *f.* craniotomy.

cráter *m.* crater.

cráter gingival gingival crater.

cráter interdental interdental crater.

craurosis *f.* kraurosis.

creatina *f.* creatine.

creatinemia *f.* creatinemia.

creatinina *f.* creatinin, creatinine.

creatinina de 24 horas creatinine height index.

creatinuria *f.* creatinuria.

crecimiento *m.* growth.

crecimiento absoluto absolute growth.

crecimiento compensador catch-up growth.

crecimiento condíleo condylar growth.

crecimiento diferencial differential growth.

crecimiento interno ingrowth.

crecimiento intrauterino retardado intrauterine retarded growth.

crecimiento nuevo new growth.

crecimiento relativo relative growth.

crema *f.* cream.

crepitación *m.* crepitation, crepitus.

  crepitación articular, crépito articular articular crepitus, joint crepitus.

  crepitación dolorosa de los tendones painful tendon crepitus.

  crepitación ósea, crépito óseo bony crepitus.

crepitante *adj.* crepitant.

cretinismo *m.* cretinism.

  cretinismo bocioso goitrous cretinism.

  cretinismo espontáneo, cretinismo esporádico spontaneous cretinism, sporadic cretinism.

  cretinismo esporádico bocioso sporadic goitrous cretinism.

  cretinismo familiar familial cretinism.

cretino, -na[1] *m., f.* cretin.

cretino, -na[2] *adj.* cretinous.

cretinoide *adj.* cretinoid.

criba *f.* crib.

cribado *m.* cribration.

crioconservación *f.* cryopreservation.

crioglobulina *f.* cryoglobulin.

criptorquidia *f.* cryptorchidy.

crisis[1] *f.* seizure.

  crisis de ansiedad anxiety attack.

  crisis atónica atonic seizure.

  crisis de ausencia absence seizure.

  crisis convulsiva convulsive seizure.

  crisis epiléptica epileptic seizure.

  crisis jacksoniana Jacksonian seizure.

  crisis generalizada generalized seizure.

  crisis generalizada secundaria secondarily generalized seizure.

  crisis generalizada tónico-clónica tonic-clonic seizure.

  crisis de gran mal grand mal seizure.

  crisis mioclónica myoclonic seizure.

  crisis motora motor seizure.

  crisis parcial partial seizure.

  crisis parcial compleja partial complex seizure.

  crisis parcial simple partial simple seizure.

  crisis de pequeño mal petit mal seizure.

crisis[2] *f.* crisis.

  crisis de Adam Stokes Adam-Stokes syndrome.

  crisis de Addison, crisis addisoniana Addison crisis, Addisonian crisis.

  crisis de adolescencia adolescent crisis.

  crisis adrenal adrenal crisis.

  crisis bronquial bronchial crisis.

  crisis cardiaca cardiac crisis.

  crisis de catatimia catathymic crisis.

  crisis colinérgica colinergic crisis.

  crisis del desarrollo developmental crisis.

  crisis drepanocítica sickle cell crisis.

  crisis falsa false crisis.

  crisis faríngea pharyngeal crisis.

  crisis febril febrile crisis.

  crisis gástrica gastric crisis.

  crisis genital del neonato genital crisis of the newborn.

crisis hepática hepatic crisis.

crisis hipertensiva hypertensive crisis.

crisis de identidad identity crisis.

crisis intestinal intestinal crisis.

crisis laríngea laryngeal crisis.

crisis de maduración maturational crisis.

crisis ocular ocular crisis.

crisis con pérdida salina salt-losing crisis.

crisis puberal puberal crisis.

crisis de rechazo rejection crisis.

crisis renal renal crisis.

crisis sanguínea blood crisis.

crisis de situación situational crisis.

crisis suprarrenal adrenal crisis.

crisis tabética tabetic crisis.

crisis terapéutica therapeutic crisis.

crisis tiroidea, crisis tirotóxica thyroid crisis, thyrotoxic crisis.

crisis torácica thoracic crisis.

crisis visceral visceral crisis.

cristal[1] *m.* glass.

cristal[2] *m.* crystal.

cristalina *f.* crystallin.

cristalino *m.* lens.

cristalización *f.* crystallization.

criterio *m.* criterion.

criterio de normalidad normality criterion.

criterio de normalidad de frecuencia frequency normality criterion.

criterio de normalidad funcional functional normality criterion.

criterio de normalidad ideal ideal normality criterion.

criterio de normalidad social social normality criterion.

criterio de normalidad subjetivo subjective normality criterion.

crítico, -ca *adj.* critical.

cromático, -ca *adj.* chromatic.

cromátida *f.* chromatid.

cromátide *f.* chromatid.

cromatina *f.* chromatin.

cromatina asociada al núcleo nucleolar-associated chromatin, nucleus-associated chromatin.

cromatina nuclear nucleolar chromatin, nucleous chromatin.

cromatina sexual sex chromatin.

cromatografía *f.* chromatography.

cromosoma *m.* chromosome.

cromosómico, -ca *adj.* chromosomal.

cronicidad *f.* chronicity.

crónico, -ca *adj.* chronic.

crup *m.* croup.

cruzado, -da *adj.* crossed.

cruádriceps *adj.* quadriceps.

cuadro *m.* chart.

cuarentena *f.* quarantine.

cubital *adj.* cubital.

cúbito *m.* cubitus, ulna.

cuclillas *f.* squatting.

cuchicheo *m.* whisper.

cuchilla *f.* knife.

cuello *m.* neck, cervix, collum.

cuenca *f.* watershed.

cuenca del ojo eyesocket.

cuentagotas *m.* dropper.

cuerda *f.* cord, chorda.

cuerda vocal vocal cord.

cuerdo, -da *m., f.* sane.

cuerno *m.* horn, cornu.

cuero cabelludo scalp.

cuerpo *m.* body, corpus.

   cuidado *m.* care.

   cuidado intensivo intensive care.

   cuidado paliativo palliative care.

   cuidado posparto postpartal care.

   cuidado posoperatorio postoperative care.

cultivo *m.* culture.

cuña *f.* wedge, cuneus.

cura *f.* cure.

curación *f.* healing.

   curación por primera intención healing by first intention.

   curación por segunda intención healing by second intention.

   curación por tercera intención healing by third intention.

curativo, -va *adj.* curative.

curvado, -da *adj.* curvated.

curvatura *f.* curvature.

cúspide *f.* cusp, cuspis.

cutáneo, -a *adj.* cutaneous.

cutaneomucoso, -sa *adj.* cutaneomucosal.

cutícula *f.* cuticle, cuticula.

cutis *m.* cutis.

D

dactilar *adj.* dactilar.

dactilitis *f.* dactylitis.

daltónico, -ca *adj.* daltonian.

daltonismo *m.* daltonism.

danza *f.* dance.

   danza de san Vito Saint Vitus dance.

dato aberrante *m.* outlier.

debilidad *f.* debility, weakness.

   debilidad mental mental debility, feeblemindedness, mild mental retardation.

debilitación *f.* debilitation, weakening.

decalaje *m.* rotational deformity, displacement.

decalcificación *f.* decalcification.

decalcificante *m.* decalcifying.

deceso *m.* decease, death.

decidua *f.* decidua, membranae deciduae.

decoloración *f.* decoloration.

decorticación *f.* decortication, decortization.

decrecimiento *m.* degrowth.

decúbito *m.* decubitus.

   decúbito supino supine decubitus position.

dedo¹ *m.* finger.

   dedo en martillo hammer finger.

   dedo en resorte spring finger.

dedo² *m.* toe.

   dedo del pie de tenista tennis toe.

defecación *f.* defecation.

defecto *m.* defect.

   defecto adquirido acquired defect.

   defecto del campo visual visual field defect.

   defecto congénito birth defect.

   defecto genético genetic defect.

   defecto de llenado filling defect.

   defecto de nacimiento birth defect.

   defecto del tubo neural neural-tube defect.

defectuoso, -sa *adj.* defective.

defeminización *f.* defeminization.

defensa *f.* defense.

   defensa abdominal abdominal guarding.

   defensa muscular muscular defense.

deferente *adj.* deferent.

deficiencia *f.* deficiency.

   deficiencia de inmunidad, deficiencia inmunitaria, deficiencia inmunológica inmune deficiency.

déficit *m.* deficit.

   déficit sensitivo sensory deficit.

   déficit vitamínico vitamin deficit.

definición *f.* definition.

definitivo, -va *adj.* definitive.

deflexión *f.* deflection.

deformación *f.* deformation.

deformante *adj.* deforming.

deformidad *f.* deformity.

degeneración *f.* degeneration, degeneratio.

   degeneración combinada subaguda de la médula espinal subacute combined degeneration of the spinal cord.

   degeneración macular macular degeneration.

deglución *f.* deglutition.

deglutir *v.* swallow.

degradación *f.* degradation.

degustación *f.* degustation.

dehiscencia *f.* dehiscence.

   dehiscencia de una herida wound dehiscence.

déjà entendu déjà entendu.

déjà pensé déjà pensé.

déjà vécu déjà vécu.

déjà vu déjà vu.

delactación *f.* delactation.

deleción *f.* deletion.

   deleción cromosómica chromosomal deletion.

delgadez *f.* leanness, thinness.

delimitación *f.* delimitation.

delirante *adj.* deliriant.

delirio *m.* delusion.

   delirio traumático traumatic delusion.

deltoideo, -a, deltoide *adj.* deltoide.

demanda *f.* request.

demencia *f.* dementia.

   demencia de Alzheimer Alzheimer's dementia.

   demencia senil senile dementia.

   demencia vascular vascular dementia.

demente *adj.* demented.

demografía *f.* demography.

dendrita *f.* dendrite.

densidad *f.* density.

densitometría *f.* densitometry.

   densitometría ósea bone densitometry.

densitómetro *m.* densitometer.

dentado, -da *adj.* dentatum.

dentadura *f.* denture.

dentición *f.* dentition, teething.

   dentición primaria, primera dentición primary dentition, first dentition.

   dentición secundaria, segunda dentición secondary dentition.

dentina *f.* dentin.

dentista *m., f.* dentist.

dependencia *f.* dependence.

depigmentación *f.* depigmentation.

depilación *f.* depilation.

depleción *f.* depletion.

deposición *f.* stool.

depósito *m.* deposit.

depresión *f.* depression.

depresión mental mental depression.

depresión posparto postnatal depression.

depresor, -ra *m. y adj.* depressant.

deprimido, -da *adj.* depressed.

derivación[1] *f.* by pass.

derivación[2] *f.* derivation, revulsion.

derivación[3] *f.* lead.

derivación aVF aVF lead.

derivación[4] *f.* referral.

derivación[5] *f.* shunt.

derivación arteriovenosa (AV) arteriovenous (A-V) shunt.

dermabrasión *f.* dermabrasion.

dermatitis *f.* dermatitis.

dermatitis alérgica allergic dermatitis.

dermatitis del área del pañal napkin dermatitis.

dermatitis atópica atopic dermatitis.

dermatología *f.* dermatology.

dermatológico, -ca *adj.* dermatologic.

dermatólogo, -ga *m., f.* dermatologist.

dermatosis *f.* dermatosis.

dermatosis acarina acarine dermatosis.

dermatosis seborreica seborrheic dermatosis.

dermatosis ulcerosa ulcerative dermatosis.

dérmico, -ca *adj.* dermic.

dermis *f.* dermis.

dermoabrasión *f.* dermabrasion.

dermografismo *m.* dermographism.

dermoide *m. y adj.* dermoid.

derramamiento *m.* spill.

derrame *m.* effusion.

derrame articular articular effusion, joint effusion.

derrame cerebral cerebral effusion.

desaceleración *f.* deceleration.

desarreglo *m.* derangement.

desarrollo *m.* development.

desarrollo físico y psicomotor de los lactantes psychomotor and physical development of infants.

desarrollo infantil child development.

desarrollo embrionario embryologic development.

desarrollo prenatal prenatal development.

desarrollo psicosocial psychosocial development.

desarticulación *f.* disarticulation.

desaturación *f.* desaturation.

desbridamiento *m.* débridement, wound excision.

desbridamiento quirúrgico surgical débridement.

descamación *f.* desquamation.

descamativo, -va *adj.* desquamative.

descanso *m.* rest.

descarga *f.* discharge.

descarga epiléptica epileptic discharge.

descendente *adj.* descending.

descenso *m.* descent, descensus.

descentrar *v.* decenter.

descompensación *f.* decompensation.

descomposición¹ *f.* abbau.

descomposición² *f.* decay.

descomposición³ *f.* decomposition.

descompresión *f.* decompression.

descongestionante *m. y adj.* decongestant.

descongestivo *m.* decongestant.
  descongestivo nasal nasal decongestant.

descontrol *m.* dyscontrol.

desdoblamiento *m.* splitting.

desecación *f.* desiccation, exsiccation.

desecho¹ *m.* débris.

desecho² *m.* detritus.

desencadenante *m.* trigger.

desensibilización *f.* desensitization.

desensibilizar *v.* desensitize.

desequilibrado, -da *adj.* imbalanced.

desequilibrio *m.* imbalance, disequilibrium.

desfallecimiento *m.* faint.

desfibrilación *f.* defibrillation.

desfibrilador *m.* defibrillator.

desgarro *m.* tear.
  desgarro ligamentoso ligamental tear.
  desgarro vaginal vaginal tear.

desgaste *m.* detrition, fretting, grinding, wear.

deshidratación *f.* dehydration.

deshidratar *v.* dehydrate.

desinfección *f.* disinfection.

desinfectante *m.* disinfectant.

desinfectar *v.* disinfect.

desinfestación *f.* disinfestation.

desinhibición *f.* disinhibition.

desintoxicación *f.* detoxication, detoxification.

desintoxicar *v.* detoxicate, detoxify.

desmayo *m.* blackout, faint.

desmielinación *f.* demyelination.
  desmielinación segmentaria segmentary demyelination.

desmielinización *f.* demyelinization.

desmineralización *f.* demineralization.

desnaturalización *f.* denaturation.
  desnaturalización de proteínas protein denaturation.

desnaturalizado, -da *adj.* denatured.

desnutrición *f.* denutrition, malnutrition.

desodorante *m.* deodorant.

desodorizante *m.* deodorizer.

desodorizar *v.* deodorize.

desorganización *f.* disorganization.

desorientación *f.* disorientation.

despersonalización *f.* depersonalization.

despertar¹ *m.* arousal.

despertar² *m.* emergence.

despigmentación *f.* depigmentation.

desplazamiento¹ *m.* displacement.
  desplazamiento condíleo condylar displacement.
  desplazamiento fetal fetal displacement.
  desplazamiento pélvico lateral lateral pelvic displacement.

desplazamiento tisular tissue displacement.

desplazamiento[2] *m.* drift.

desplazamiento antigénico antigenic drift.

desplazamiento genético genetic drift.

desplazamiento[3] *m.* drifting.

desplazamiento[4] *m.* shift.

desplazamiento axial axis shift.

desplazamiento hacia la derecha shift to the right.

desplazamiento de Doppler Doppler shift.

desplazamiento hacia la izquierda shift to the left.

desplazamiento del umbral threshold shift.

despoblación *f.* depopulation.

despolarización *f.* depolarization.

despolarización diastólica lenta slow diastolic depolarization.

despolarizador *m.* depolarizer.

despolarizar *v.* depolarize.

desprendimiento *m.* detachment.

desprendimiento de coroides choroidal detachment.

desprendimiento epifisario epiphytical detachment.

desprendimiento exudativo de la retina exudative retinal detachment.

desprendimiento de los miembros detachment of members.

desprendimiento de la placenta, desprendimiento placentario detachment of the placenta, placental detachment.

desprendimiento posterior del vítreo posterior vitreous detachment.

desprendimiento regmatógeno de la retina rhegmatogenous retinal detachment.

desprendimiento de la retina, desprendimiento de retina, desprendimiento retiniano detachment of the retina, retinal detachment.

desprendimiento de retina exudativo exudative retinal detachment.

desprendimiento vítreo vitreous detachment.

desproporción *f.* disproportion.

desproporción cefalopélvica (DCP) cephalopelvic disproportion (CPD).

destello *m.* flicker.

destetado, -da *m., f.* weanling.

destetar *v.* wean.

destete *m.* weaning.

destilación *f.* distillation.

destino *m.* fate.

destoxicación *f.* detoxication.

destoxicar *v.* detoxicate.

destreza *f.* skill.

destructivo, -va *adj.* destructive.

destubación *f.* detubation.

desviación[1] *f.* bias.

desviación[2] *f.* deviance, deviation.

desviación[3] *f.* deviation.

desviación de la columna vertebral spinal column deviation.

desviación del complemento complement deviation.

desviación a la derecha, desviación hacia la derecha deviation to the right.

desviación derecha del eje right axis deviation (RAD).

desviación de los dientes deviation of the teeth.

desviación estándar (DE) standard deviation (SD).

desviación estándar de una muestra sample standard deviation.

desviación estrábica strabismal deviation, strabismic deviation, squint deviation.

desviación inmunitaria, desviación inmunológica immune deviation.

desviación a la izquierda, desviación hacia la izquierda deviation to the left.

desviación izquierda del eje left axis deviation (LAD).

desviación latente latent deviation.

desviación de la lengua deviation of the tongue.

desviación manifiesta manifest deviation.

desviación mínima minimal deviation, minimum deviation.

desviación de la norma deviation from normal.

desviación oblicua skew deviation.

desviación del ojo eye deviation.

desviación orgánica organic deviation.

desviación primaria primary deviation.

desviación secundaria secondary deviation.

desviación sesgada skew deviation.

desviación sexual sexual deviation.

desviación social social deviation.

desviación uterina uterine deviation.

desviación vertical disociada dissociated vertical deviation.

desviación⁴ *f.* drift.

desviación antigénica antigenic drift.

desviación cubital ulnar drift.

desviación genética genetic drift.

desviación⁵ *f.* shift.

desviación axial axis shift.

desviación hacia la derecha shift to the right.

desviación hacia la izquierda shift to the left.

desviación luteoplacentaria luteoplacental shift.

desviación química chemical shift.

desviación sanguínea regenerativa regenerative blood shift.

desviado, -da *adj.* deviant.

desviado sexual sexual deviant.

desvisceración *f.* devisceration.

desvitalización *f.* devitalization.

desvitalización pulpar pulp devitalization.

desvitalizado, -da *adj.* devitalized.

desvitalizar *v.* devitalize.

detección *f.* counting, detection, screening.

detectar *v.* detect.

detector *m.* detector.

detergente *adj.* detergent.

deterioro *m.* deterioration, impairment, loss.

deterioro alcohólico alcoholic deterioration.

deterioro auditivo hearing loss.

deterioro mental mental impairment.

deterioro senil senile deterioration.

determinación[1] *f.* ascertainment.

determinación aislada single ascertainment.

determinación completa complete ascertainment.

determinación incompleta incomplete ascertainment.

determinación[2] *f.* determination, measurement.

determinación directa de la tensión arterial direct measurement of blood pressure.

determinación de gases en sangre blood gas determination.

determinación del sexo, determinación sexual sex determination.

determinante *m. y adj.* determinant.

determinante antigénico antigenic determinant.

determinante de enfermedad disease determinant.

determinante genético genetic determinant.

determinante inmunogénico immunogenic determinant.

determinante isoalotípico isoallotypic determinant.

determinante de la marcha gait determinant.

determinante de oclusión determinant of occlusion.

determinante oculto hidden determinant.

determinante psíquico psychic determinant.

determinante secuencial sequential determinant.

determinismo *m.* determinism.

determinismo psíquico psychic determinism.

detrusor *adj.* detrusor.

deuda *f.* debt.

deuda de oxígeno oxygen debt.

deuda de oxígeno aláctico alactic oxygen debt.

deuda de oxígeno lactácido lactacid oxygen debt.

dextrocardia *f.* dextrocardia.

dextrocardia aislada isolated dextrocardia.

dextrocardia corregida corrected dextrocardia.

dextrocardia falsa false dextrocardia.

dextrocardia en imagen en espejo mirror-image dextrocardia.

dextrocardia secundaria secondary dextrocardia.

dextrocardia con situs inversus dextrocardia with situs inversus.

dextrocardia tipo 1 type 1 dextrocardia.

dextrocardia tipo 2 type 2 dextrocardia.

dextrocardia tipo 3 type 3 dextrocardia.

dextrocardia tipo 4 type 4 dextrocardia.

dextrocardiograma *m.* dextrocardiogram.

dextrocerebral *adj.* dextrocerebral.

dextroversión *f.* dextroversion.

dextroversión del corazón dextroversion of the heart.

diabetes *f.* diabetes.

diabetes del adulto type II diabetes.

diabetes albuminúrica diabetes albuminurinicus.

diabetes alimentaria alimentary diabetes.

diabetes artificial artificial diabetes.

diabetes azucarada diabetes mellitus.

diabetes bronceada bronze diabetes.

diabetes calcinúrica calcinuric diabetes.

diabetes cerebroespinal cerebrospinal diabetes.

diabetes clínica clinical diabetes.

diabetes de comienzo en el crecimiento growth-onset diabetes.

diabetes de comienzo en la edad adulta adult-onset diabetes.

diabetes de comienzo en la juventud juvenile onset diabetes.

diabetes de comienzo en la madurez maturity-onset diabetes.

diabetes de comienzo en la madurez de la juventud maturity-onset diabetes of youth (MODY).

diabetes cutánea skin diabetes.

diabetes con deficiencia de insulina insulin-deficient diabetes.

diabetes por derramamiento overflow diabetes.

diabetes disimulada masked diabetes.

diabetes del embarazo pregnancy diabetes.

diabetes insípida diabetes insipidus.

diabetes insípida nefrogénica nephrogenic diabetes insipidus.

diabetes insulinodependiente insulin-dependent diabetes.

diabetes no insulinodependiente non-insulin dependent diabetes.

diabetes juvenil juvenile diabetes.

diabetes mellitus (DM) diabetes mellitus (DM).

diabetes mellitus endocrina endocrine diabetes mellitus.

diabetes mellitus gestacional (DMG) gestational diabetes mellitus (GDM).

diabetes mellitus insulinodependiente (DMID) insulin-dependent diabetes mellitus (IDDM).

diabetes mellitus no insulinodependiente (DMNID) non-insulin-dependent diabetes mellitus (NIDDM).

diabetes no insulinodependiente (DNID) non-insulin dependent diabetes (NIDD).

diabetes tipo I type I diabetes.

diabetes tipo II type II diabetes.

diabético, -ca *adj.* diabetic.

diabetología *f.* diabetology.

díada *f.* dyad.

diafragma¹ *m.* diaphragm.

diafragma² *m.* diaphragm.

diafragma anticonceptivo contraceptive diaphragm.

diafragma anticonceptivo de espiral arcing spring contraceptive diaphragm.

diafragma anticonceptivo de

muelle espiral coil-spring contraceptive diaphragm.

diafragma anticonceptivo de resorte plano flat spring contraceptive diaphragm.

diafragma vaginal vaginal diaphragm.

diafragmático, -ca *adj.* diaphragmatic.

diagnosticar *v.* diagnose.

diagnóstico *m.* diagnosis.

diagnóstico antenatal antenatal diagnosis.

diagnóstico citológico, diagnóstico citohistológico cytohistologic diagnosis.

diagnóstico clínico clinical diagnosis.

diagnóstico diferencial differencial diagnosis.

diagnóstico directo direct diagnosis.

diagnóstico por exclusión diagnosis by exclusion.

diagnóstico físico physical diagnosis.

diagnóstico de laboratorio laboratory diagnosis.

diagnóstico neonatal neonatal diagnosis.

diagnóstico patológico pathologic diagnosis.

diagnóstico prenatal prenatal diagnosis.

diagnóstico serológico serum diagnosis.

diagnóstico topográfico topographic diagnosis.

diagrama *m.* diagram.

diagrama de Punnet Punnett square.

diálisis *f.* dialysis.

diálisis peritoneal ambulatoria continua (DPAC) continuous ambulatory peritoneal dialysis (CAPD).

diálisis renal renal dialysis.

dializador, -ra *m., f.* dialysate.

dializador *m.* dialyzer.

dializar *v.* dialyze.

diámetro *m.* diameter.

diapasón *m.* diapason.

diarrea *f.* diarrhea.

diarrea acuosa watery diarrhea.

diarrea aguda acute diarrhea.

diarrea del destete diarrhea ablactatorum.

diarrea disentérica dysentric diarrhea.

diarrea entérica enteral diarrhea.

diarrea epidémica del neonato, diarrea epidémica del recién nacido epidemic diarrhea of the newborn.

diarrea estival summer diarrhea.

diarrea gastrógena gastrogenous diarrhea.

diarrea grasa fatty diarrhea.

diarrea infantil infantile diarrhea.

diarrea intestinal enteral diarrhea.

diarrea irritativa irritative diarrhea.

diarrea lientérica lienteric diarrhea.

diarrea matinal morning diarrhea.

diarrea mecánica mecanical diarrhea.

diarrea membranosa membranous diarrhea.

*diarrea **mucosa*** mucous diarrhea.

*diarrea **neonatal*** neonatal diarrhea.

*diarrea **nocturna*** nocturnal diarrhea.

*diarrea **osmótica*** osmotic diarrhea.

*diarrea **pancreatógena*** pancreatogenous diarrhea.

*diarrea **paradójica*** paradoxical diarrhea.

*diarrea **parenteral*** parenteral diarrhea.

*diarrea **purulenta*** purulent diarrhea.

*diarrea **putrefactiva*** putrefactive diarrhea.

*diarrea **quilosa*** diarrhea chylosa.

*diarrea **simple*** simple diarrhea.

*diarrea **tropical*** tropical diarrhea.

*diarrea **del viajero*** traveler's diarrhea.

diarreico, -ca *adj.* diarrheal, diarrheic.

diartrosis *f.* diarthrosis.

diastema *m.* diastema.

diástole *f.* diastole.

*diástole **cardíaca*** cardiac diastole.

diastólico, -ca *adj.* diastolic.

diatermia *f.* diathermy.

*diatermia **quirúrgica*** surgical diathermy.

diatérmico, -ca *adj.* diathermal.

diatermocoagulación *f.* diathermocoagualtion.

diátesis *f.* diathesis.

diente *m.* tooth, dens.

*diente **anatómico*** anatomic tooth.

*diente **no anatómico*** non-anatomic tooth.

*diente **artificial*** artificial tooth.

*diente **decidual*** deciduous tooth.

*diente **desvitalizado*** devitalized tooth.

*diente **errante*** wandering of a tooth.

*diente **fusionado*** fused tooth.

*diente **impactado*** impacted tooth.

*diente **del juicio*** wisdom tooth.

*diente **de leche*** milk tooth, dens lacteus.

*diente **en malposición*** malposed tooth.

*diente **manchado*** mottled tooth.

*diente **migratorio*** migrating tooth.

*diente **muerto*** dead tooth.

*diente **en mordida cruzada*** crossbite tooth.

*diente **natal*** natal tooth.

*diente **neonatal*** neonatal tooth.

*diente **no anatómico*** non-anatomic tooth.

*diente **no vital*** non-vital tooth.

*diente **permanente*** permanent tooth.

*diente **en posición normal*** normally posed tooth.

*diente **prematuro*** premature tooth.

*diente **primario*** primary tooth.

*diente **prominente*** buck tooth.

*diente **protruido*** protruding tooth.

*diente **de resina acrílica*** acrylic resin tooth.

*diente **salido*** buck tooth.

*diente **secundario*** second tooth.

*diente **vital*** vital tooth.

diestro, -tra *adj.* dextromanual.
dieta *f.* diet.
  dieta absoluta absolute diet.
  dieta adecuada adequate diet.
  dieta de adelgazamiento reduction diet.
  dieta alcalina alkali-ash diet.
  dieta de arroz rice diet.
  dieta baja en calorías low calorie diet.
  dieta basal basal diet.
  dieta básica basic diet.
  dieta blanda soft diet.
  dieta cetógenica ketogenic diet.
  dieta completa full diet.
  dieta de conservación de proteínas protein sparing diet.
  dieta diabética, dieta para diabéticos diabetic diet.
  dieta de eliminación elimination diet.
  dieta equilibrada balanced diet.
  dieta para gotosos gouty diet.
  dieta hídrica clear liquid diet.
  dieta hipocalórica low-caloric diet.
  dieta láctea milk diet.
  dieta libre de gluten gluten-free diet.
  dieta ligera light diet.
  dieta líquida liquid diet.
  dieta líquida clara clear liquid diet.
  dieta líquida completa full liquid diet.
  dieta mixta mixed diet.
  dieta óptima optimal diet.
  dieta pobre en calcio low-calcium diet.
  dieta pobre en calorías low calorie diet.

  dieta pobre en colesterol low-cholesterol diet.
  dieta pobre en grasas low fat diet.
  dieta pobre en grasas saturadas low-saturated-fat diet.
  dieta pobre en oxalato low oxalate diet.
  dieta pobre en purina low purine diet.
  dieta pobre en residuos low residue diet.
  dieta de provocación challenge diet.
  dieta raquítica rachitic diet.
  dieta reductora reducing diet.
  dieta regular regular diet.
  dieta con restricción de purina purine restricted diet.
  dieta rica en calorías high calorie diet.
  dieta rica en fibra high fiber diet.
  dieta rica en grasas high fat diet.
  dieta rica en potasio high-potassium diet.
  dieta rica en proteínas high protein diet.
  dieta rica en vitaminas high-vitamin diet.
  dieta sin gluten gluten-free diet.
  dieta sin sal salt-free diet.
  dieta de subsistencia subsistence diet.
dietética *f.* dietetics.
dietético, -ca *adj.* dietetic.
dietista *m.* dietitian.
diferencia *f.* difference.
  diferencia individual individual difference.
  diferencia luminosa light difference.

diferenciación *f.* differentiation.
diferenciado, -da *adj.* differentiated.
difteria *f.* diphtheria.
  difteria cutánea cutaneous diphtheria.
  difteria dérmica cutaneous diphtheria.
  difteria faríngea pharyngeal diphtheria.
  difteria gangrenosa gangrenous diphtheria.
  difteria grave diphtheria gravis.
  difteria laríngea laryngeal diphtheria.
  difteria maligna malignant diphtheria.
  difteria nasal nasal diphtheria.
  difteria nasofaríngea nasopharyngeal diphtheria.
  difteria quirúrgica surgical diphtheria.
  difteria séptica septic diphtheria.
  difteria umbilical umbilical diphtheria.
difusión *f.* diffusion.
digestión *f.* digestion.
digestivo, -va *adj.* digestant.
digital *adj.* digital.
dilatación *f.* dilatation, dilation.
dioptría *f.* diopter.
diplopía *f.* diplopia.
disartria *f.* dysarthria.
discapacidad *f.* disability.
disco *m.* disc, disk, discus.
  disco protruido protruded disc.
discordancia *f.* discordance.
disección *f.* dissection.
  disección aórtica aortic dissection.

disentería *f.* dysentery.
disfagia *f.* dysphagy, dysphagia.
disfonía *f.* dysphonia.
disfunción *f.* dysfunction.
  disfunción eréctil erectile dysfunction.
  disfunción sexual sexual dysfunction.
dislexia *f.* dyslexia.
disléxico, -ca *adj.* dyslexic.
dislipidemia *f.* dyslipidemia.
dismenorrea *f.* dysmenorrhea.
disminución *f.* decrease.
disnea *f.* dyspnea.
disociación *f.* dissociation.
disolvente *m. y adj.* dissolvent.
dispareunia *f.* dispareunia.
disparidad *f.* disparity.
dispepsia *f.* dyspepsia.
displasia *f.* dysplasia.
dispositivo¹ *m.* appliance.
  dispositivo ortodóncico orthodontic appliance.
dispositivo² *m.* device.
  dispositivo anticonceptivo contraceptive device.
disrupción *f.* disruption.
distal *adj.* distal, distalis.
distancia *f.* distance.
distensibilidad *f.* distensibility.
distensión *f.* distension, distention.
distimia *f.* dysthymia.
distocia *f.* dystocia.
distonía *f.* dystonia.
  distonía deformante muscular, distonía deformante progresiva dystonia deformans progressiva, dystonia musculorum deformans.
distorsión *f.* distortion.

distrés *m.* distress.
 distrés respiratorio del adulto adult respiratory distress.
distribución *f.* distribution.
 distribución del fármaco drug distribution.
 distribución normal normal distribution.
distrofia *f.* dystrophy, dystrophia.
 distrofia endotelial de la córnea endothelial dystrophy of the cornea, dystrophia endothelialis corneae.
 distrofia muscular muscular dystrophy.
 distrofia muscular de Duchenne Duchenne's muscular dystrophy.
disuria *f.* dysuria, dysury.
diuresis *f.* diuresis.
diverticulitis *f.* diverticulitis.
divertículo *m.* diverticulum.
división *f.* division, divisio.
 división celular cell division.
doble *adj.* double.
doctor, -ra *m., f.* doctor.
dolencia *f.* ache, infirmity.
dolor *m.* pain, dolor.
 dolor abdominal abdominal pain.
 dolor agudo acute pain.
 dolor de cabeza, dolor capitis headache, dolor capitis.
 dolor en cinturón girdle pain.
 dolor crónico chronic pain.
 dolor epigástrico epigastric pain.
 dolor de espalda backache.
 dolor intermenstrual intermenstrual pain.
 dolor de parto labor pain.
 dolor referido referred pain.
 dolor sordo dull pain.

 dolor urente burning pain.
doloroso, -sa *adj.* dolorific.
 doloroso a la presión tender.
dominancia *f.* dominance.
 dominancia genética genetic dominance.
dominante *adj.* dominant.
donante *m.* donor.
 donante de cadáver cadaveric donor.
 donante de sangre blood donor.
 donante vivo living donor.
 donante xenogénico xenogenic donor.
Doppler Doppler.
dorsalgia *f.* dorsalgia, backache.
dorso *m.* back, dorsum.
dosificación *f.* dosage.
dosis *f.* dose, dosis.
 dosis de ataque loading dose.
 dosis equivalente equivalent dose.
 dosis inicial initial dose.
 dosis máxima maximal dose, maximal dose.
 dosis mínima minimal dose, minimum dose.
drenaje¹ *m.* drain.
drenaje² *m.* drainage.
drepanocitemia¹ *f.* drepanocytemia.
drepanocitemia² *f.* sicklemia.
drepranocítico, -ca *adj.* drepanocytic.
drepanocito *m.* drepanocyte, sickle cell.
droga *f.* drug.
drogadicto, -ta *adj.* drug addict.
drogodependencia *f.* drug dependence.

dualismo *m.* dualism.

duelo *m.* bereavement, grief, mourning.

duodeno *m.* duodenum.

duplicación *f.* duplication.

   duplicación cromosómica duplication of chromosomes.

duramadre *f.* dura mater.

dureza *f.* hardness.

E

ebrio, -a *adj.* ebrious.

eccema *m.* eczema.

   eccema atópico atopic eczema.

   eccema de contacto contact eczema.

   eccema seborreico seborrheic eczema.

eclampsia *f.* eclampsia.

ecografía *f.* echography.

ecografista *m., f.* echographist.

ecógrafo *m.* echographer.

ecolalia *f.* echolalia, echo speech.

ectasia, *f.* ectasia, ectasis.

ectopia *f.* ectopy, ectopia.

ectópico, -ca *adj.* ectopic.

ectropión *m.* ectropion.

edad *f.* age.

   edad adulta adulthood.

   edad fértil childbearing age.

   edad fetal fetal age.

   edad gestacional gestational age.

   edad de la menarquia menarcheal age, menarchial age.

   edad mental mental age.

   edad ósea bone age.

edema *m.* edema.

efecto *m.* effect.

   efecto colateral side effect.

   efecto secundario secundary effect.

eferente *adj.* efferent.

eficacia *f.* effectiveness.

   eficacia anticonceptiva contraceptive effectiveness.

eje *m.* axis.

elasticidad *f.* elasticity, resilience.

electrocardiografía *f.* electrocardiography.

electrocardiograma (ECG) *m.* electrocardiogram (ECG).

elefantiasis *f.* elephantiasis.

elevador *m.* elevator, levator.

embarazada *adj.* pregnant.

embarazo *m.* pregnancy.

   embarazo ectópico ectopic pregnancy.

   embarazo extrauterino extrauterine pregnancy.

   embarazo gemelar twin pregnancy.

   embarazo molar molar pregnancy.

   embarazo múltiple multiple pregnancy.

   embarazo ovárico ovarian pregnancy.

   embarazo tubárico tubal pregnancy.

   embarazo uterino uterine pregnancy.

embolia[1] *f.* embole, emboly.

embolia[2] *f.* embolism.

   embolia cerebral cerebral embolism.

   embolia pulmonar pulmonary embolism.

   embolia venosa venous embolism.

embólico, -ca *adj.* embolic.

emboliectomía *f.* embolectomy.

embolización *f.* embolization.

émbolo *m.* embolus.

embriaguez *f.* drunkenness, inebriation.

embriología *f.* embryology.

embrión *m.* embryo.

embriopatía *f.* embryopathia, embriopathy.

emergencia *f.* emergency.

emesis *f.* emesia, emesis.

emético, -ca *m. y adj.* emetic.

emocional *adj.* emotional.

emoliente *adj.* emollient.

emotividad *f.* emotivity.

emparejamiento *m.* coupling.

empiema *m.* empyema.

empírico, -ca *adj.* empirical, empiric.

enajenación *f.* abalienation.

  enajenación mental mental abalienation.

enanismo *m.* dwarfism.

  enanismo acondroplásico achondroplastic dwarfism.

  enanismo hipofisario hypophyseal dwarfism.

enano, -na *m., f.* dwarf, midget.

  enano acondroplásico achondroplasic dwarf.

encajamiento *m.* engagement.

encapsulado, -da *adj.* encapsulated, encapsuled.

encefálico, -ca *adj.* encephalic.

encefalina *f.* enkephalin.

encefalitis *f.* encephalitis.

encéfalo *m.* brain, encephalon.

encefalomielitis *f.* encephalomyelitis.

encefalopatía *f.* encephalopathy, encephalopathia.

encía *f.* gum, gingiva.

enclavamiento *m.* nailing.

endémico, -ca *adj.* endemic.

enderezamiento *m.* redressement.

endocarditis *f.* endocarditis.

endocrinología *f.* endocrinology.

endocrinólogo, -a *m., f.* endocrinologist.

endodoncia *f.* endodontics, endodontia.

endodoncista *m., f.* endodontist.

endometrio *m.* endometrium.

endometriosis *f.* endometriosis.

endometritis *f.* endometritis.

endoscopia *f.* endoscopy.

endoscopio *m.* endoscope.

endoscopista *m., f.* endoscopist.

endotelial *adj.* endothelial.

endotelio *m.* endothelium.

endurecimiento *m.* hardening.

enema *m.* enema.

  enema baritado barium enema.

energía *f.* energy.

enfermedad *f.* disease, illness, sickness.

  enfermedad de Addison Addison's disease.

  enfermedad por almacenamiento storage disease.

  enfermedad de Alzheimer Alzheimer's disease.

  enfermedad autoinmune autoimmune disease.

  enfermedad celíaca celiac disease.

  enfermedad de Chagas, enfermedad de Chagas-Cruz Chagas' disease, Chagas-Cruz disease.

enfermedad contagiosa contagious disease.

enfermedad de Crohn Crohn's disease.

enfermedad de Cushing Cushing's disease.

enfermedad por deficiencia deficiency disease.

enfermedad drepanocítica sickle cell disease.

enfermedad específica specific disease.

enfermedad exantemática exanthematous disease.

enfermedad hipertensiva crónica chronic hypertensive disease.

enfermedad infecciosa infectious disease, infective disease.

enfermedad inflamatoria de la pelvis pelvic inflammatory disease.

enfermedad de injerto versus huésped graft versus host disease.

enfermedad mental mental disease, mental illness.

enfermedad molecular molecular disease.

enfermedad notificable notifiable disease.

enfermedad ocupacional occupational disease.

enfermedad orgánica organic disease.

enfermedad parasitaria parasitic disease.

enfermedad periódica periodic disease.

enfermedad primaria primary disease.

enfermedad por radiaciones radiation disease.

enfermedad del sueño sleeping sickness.

enfermedad de transmisión sexual (ETS) sexually transmitted disease (STD).

enfermedad venérea venereal disease.

enfermedad de von Willebrand von Willebrand's disease.

enfermería *f.* nursing.

enfermero, -ra *m., f.* male nurse, nurse.

enfermizo, -za *adj.* infirm.

enfermo, -ma *adj.* ill, sick.

enfermo, -ma *m., f.* ill person, sick person.

enfisema *m.* emphysema.

enfisema pulmonar pulmonary emphysema.

enfisematoso, -sa *adj.* emphysematous.

enfriamiento *m.* cold.

enmascarado, -da *adj.* masked.

enoftalmos *m.* enophthalmos.

enquistado, -da *adj.* encysted, saccate.

enriquecimiento *m.* enrichment.

enrojecimiento *m.* flare.

ensayo *m.* assay, trial.

entablillado *m.* splinting.

enteral *adj.* enteral.

entérico, -ca *adj.* enteric.

enteritis *f.* enteritis.

enterocito *m.* enterocyte.

enterocolitis *f.* enterocolitis.

enterotoxina *f.* enterotoxin.

enterovirus *m.* enterovirus.

entidad *f.* entity.

entrada *f.* inlet.

entrecruzamiento *m.* crossing-over, intercross.

entrenamiento *m.* training.

entrevista *f.* interview.

entuertos *m.* afterpains.

entumecimiento *m.* numbness.

enuresis *f.* enuresis.

  enuresis diurna diurnal enuresis.

  enuresis nocturna nocturnal enuresis.

envejecimiento *m.* aging.

envenenamiento *m.* poisoning.

envoltura *f.* envelope.

enyesado *m.* cast.

enzima *f.* enzyme.

eosinofilia *f.* eosinophilia.

eosinófilo *m.* eosinophil, eosinophile.

ependimitis *f.* ependymitis.

ependimo *m.* ependyma.

epicardias *m.* epicardia.

epicardio *m.* epicardium.

epicarditis *f.* epicarditis.

epicondíleo, -a *adj.* epicondylian, epicondylic.

epicondilitis *f.* epicondylitis.

epidemia *f.* epidemic.

epidémico, -ca *adj.* epidemic.

epidemiología *f.* epidemiology.

epidérmico, -ca *adj.* epidermic.

epidermis *f.* epiderm, epidermis.

epidermólisis *f.* epidermolysis.

epididimitis *f.* epididymitis.

epidídimo *m.* epididymis.

epidural *adj.* epidural.

epífisis *f.* epiphysis.

epigáster *m.* epigaster.

epigástrico, -ca *adj.* epigastric.

epiglotis *f.* epiglottis.

epilepsia *f.* epilepsy, epilepsia.

  epilepsia focal focal epilepsy.

  epilepsia generalizada generalized epilepsy.

  epilepsia de grand mal, epilepsia de gran mal grand mal epilepsy.

  epilepsia histérica hysterical epilepsy.

  epilepsia parcial partial epilepsy.

  epilepsia de petit mal, epilepsia de pequeño mal petit mal epilepsy.

epiléptico, -ca *adj.* epileptic.

episiotomía *f.* episiotomy.

episodio *m.* episode.

epistaxis *f.* epistaxis, nosebleed.

epitelio *m.* epithelium.

equilibrio *m.* balance, equilibrium.

  equilibrio ácido-base, equilibrio acidobásico acid-base equilibrium, acid-base balance.

equimosis *f.* ecchymosis.

erección *f.* erection.

erisipela *f.* erysipelas.

eritema *m.* erythema.

eritroblasto *m.* erythroblast.

eritrocito *m.* erythrocyte.

eritrocitopoyesis *f.* erythrocytopoiesis.

eritrocitosis *f.* erythrocytosis.

eritrodermia *f.* erythroderma.

eritropoyesis *f.* erythropoiesis.

eritropoyético, -ca *adj.* erythropoietic.

erosión *f.* erosion.

error *m.* error.

  error médico medical error.

eructo *m.* belch, ructus.

erupción *f.* eruption.

escabiasis *f.* scabies.

escafoide *adj.* scaphoid.

escala *f.* scale.

escalofrío *m.* chill.

escalpro *m.* scalprum.

escama¹ *f.* squame, squama.

escama² *f.* scale.

escamado, -da *adj.* squamate.

escamoso, -sa *adj.* scaly, squamate, squamous.

escáner *m.* scanner.

escápula *f.* scapula.

escarificación¹ *f.* scarification.

escarificación² *f.* scaling.

escarlatina *f.* scarlatina, scarlet fever.

escatología *f.* scatologia, scatology.

escatoma *m.* scatoma.

escayola *f.* cast.

   escayola de yeso plaster cast.

escayolar *v.* casting.

esclera *f.* sclera.

escleritis *f.* scleritis.

esclerodermia *f.* scleroderma.

esclerosado, -da *adj.* sclerosed.

esclerosante *adj.* sclerosant, sclerosing.

esclerosis *f.* sclerosis.

   esclerosis lateral amiotrófica (ELA) amyotrophic lateral sclerosis (ALS).

esclerótica *f.* sclerotica.

escoliosis *f.* scoliosis.

escorbuto *m.* scurvy.

escotoma *m.* scotoma.

escozor *m.* ardor.

escroto *m.* scrotum.

esencial *adj.* essential.

esfenoides *m.* sphenoid.

esfigmomanómetro *m.* sphygmomanometer.

esfínter *m.* sphincter.

esguince *m.* sprain.

   esguince de tobillo o de pie sprain of the ankle or foot.

esmalte *m.* enamel.

esmegma *m.* smegma.

esofagitis *f.* esophagitis.

esófago *m.* esophagus.

espaciador *m.* spreader.

espacio *m.* space, spatium.

espalda *f.* back.

espasmo *m.* spasm, spasmus.

espasmolítico, -ca *adj.* spasmolytic.

espasticidad *f.* spasticity.

espástico, -ca *adj.* spastic.

espátula *f.* spatula.

especialista *m., f.* specialist.

especificidad *f.* specificity.

específico, -ca *m. y adj.* specific.

espéculo *m.* speculum.

espejo *m.* mirror.

espermatogénesis *f.* spermatogenesis.

espermatozoide *m.* spermatozoid.

espermicida *m.* spermicide.

espina *f.* spine, spina.

espinilla *f.* shin.

espiración *f.* expiration.

espirometría *f.* spirometry.

espirómetro *m.* spirometer.

esplenectomía *f.* splenectomy.

esplenomegalia *f.* splenomegaly.

espondilartrosis *f.* spondylarthrosis.

espondilitis *f.* spondylitis.

espondilopatía *f.* spondylopathy.

esprue *f.* sprue.

esputo *m.* sputum.

esquelético, -ca *adj.* skeletal.

esqueleto *m.* framework, skeleton.

esquema *m.* schema, scheme.

esquistocito *m.* schistocyte.

esquistosoma *m.* schistosome.

esquistosomiasis *f.* schistosomiasis.

esquizofrenia *f.* schizophrenia.

esquizofrénico, -ca *adj.* schizophrenic.

estabilización *f.* stabilization.

estable *adj.* stabile, stable.

estadio *m.* stage.

  estadio tumoral tumor stage.

estadística *f.* statistics.

estado *m.* state, status.

  estado mental mental status.

  estado de reposo resting stage.

  estado vegetativo vegetative state.

estancamiento *m.* stagnation.

estándar *m.* standard.

estasia *f.* stasis.

estatura *f.* height, stature.

esteatorrea *f.* steatorrhea.

esteatosis *f.* steatosis.

estenosis *f.* stenosis.

  estenosis aórtica aortic stenosis.

  estenosis valvular valvular stenosis.

estéril *adj.* sterile.

esterilidad *f.* sterility, sterilitas.

esterilización *f.* sterilization.

esterilizador *m.* sterilizer.

esternoclavicular *adj.* sternoclavicular.

esternocleido, -da *adj.* sternocleidal.

esternón *m.* sternum.

estertor *m.* rattle, stertor.

  estertor crepitante crepitant rattle.

estetoscopio *m.* stethoscope.

estigma *m.* stigma.

estimación *f.* estimate.

estimulación *f.* stimulation.

estimulante *m. y adj.* stimulant.

estímulo *m.* stimulus.

estiramiento *m.* stretching.

estoma *m.* stoma.

estómago *m.* stomach.

estomatitis *f.* stomatitis.

estornudo *m.* sneeze, sternutatio, sternutation.

estrábico, -ca *adj.* strabismal.

estrabismo *m.* cross-eye, strabismus.

estrangulación *f.* strangle, strangulation.

estrangulado, -da *adj.* strangulated.

estrechez *f.* stricture.

estrecho *m.* strait.

estreñimiento *m.* constipation, costiveness.

estreptococo *m.* streptococcus.

estrés *m.* stress.

estría *f.* streak, stria.

estribo *m.* stapes.

estridor *m.* stridor.

estriol *m.* estriol.

estrogénico, -ca *adj.* estrogenic.

estrógeno *m.* estrogen.

estructura *f.* structure.

estruma *m.* struma.

estudio *m.* study.

  estudio prospectivo prospective study.

  estudio retrospectivo retrospective study.

estudio simple ciego single-blind study.

estudio transversal cross sectional study, cross-selectional study.

estupefaciente *adj.* stupefacient, stupefactive.

etapa *f.* stage.

ética *f.* ethics.

etilismo *m.* ethylism.

etiología *f.* etiology.

etiológico, -ca *adj.* etiologic, etiological.

etiopático, -ca *adj.* etiopathic.

etiopatogenia *f.* etiopathogenesis, etiology and pathogenesis.

etmoidal *adj.* ethmoidal, ethmoidale.

etmoide *adj.* ethmoid.

etmoides *m.* ethmoid bone.

etología *f.* ethology.

etológico, -ca *adj.* ethological.

eucariota *m.* eucaryote, eukaryote.

euforia *f.* euphoria.

eunuco *m.* eunuch.

eutanasia *f.* euthanasia.

eutónico, -ca *adj.* eutonic.

evacuación *f.* evacuation.

evaluación *f.* evaluation.

evaporación *f.* evaporation.

eventración *f.* eventration.

eversión *f.* eversion.

evisceración *f.* evisceration, exenteration.

evolución *f.* evolution.

evolutivo, -va *adj.* evolutive.

exacerbación *f.* exacerbation.

examen *m.* examination.

examen citológico cytologic examination.

examen de Papanicolaou Papanicolaou examination.

examen post mortem postmortem examination.

exanguinación *f.* exsanguination.

exantema *m.* rash, exanthema.

exceso *m.* excess.

excrecencia *f.* excrescence.

excreción *f.* excretion.

exfoliación *f.* exfoliation.

exocérvix *f.* exocervix.

exodoncia *f.* exodontics.

exoftalmía *f.* exophthalmia.

exoftalmos *m.* exophthalmos, exophtalmus.

exostosis *f.* exostosis.

expansor *m.* expander.

expansor del plasma plasma expander.

expectoración *f.* expectoration.

expectorante *m. y adj.* expectorant.

experiencia *f.* experience.

exploración *f.* exploration.

exploración física physical exploration.

exploración ginecológica gynecological exploration.

exposición *f.* exposure.

expulsión *f.* expulsion.

expulsivo, -va *adj.* expulsive.

éxtasis *m.* ecstasy.

extensión *f.* extension.

exterior *m. y adj.* exterior.

externalización *f.* externalization.

extracción *f.* extraction, delivery.

extracorpóreo, -a *adj.* extracorporeal, extracorpored.

extraño, -ña *adj.* extraneous, foreign.

extrasístole *f.* extrasystole.

extravasación *f.* extravasation.
extremo *m.* end, extreme.
extrusión *f.* extrusion.
extubar *v.* extubate.
exudación *f.* exudation.
exudado *m.* exudate.
eyaculación *f.* ejaculation, ejaculatio.
eyección *f.* ejection.

F

fabulación *f.* fabulation.
facies face, facies.
facoemulsión *f.* phacoemulsification.
facticio, -cia *adj.* factitious, factitial.
factor *m.* factor.
facultad *f.* faculty.
fagocito *m.* phagocyte.
faja *f.* binder.
   faja abdominal abdominal binder.
falange *f.* phalanx.
fallo *f.* failure.
falso, -sa *adj.* false.
falsonegativo *m.* false negative.
falsopositivo *m.* false positive.
familia *f.* family.
faringe *f.* pharynx.
faringitis *f.* pharyngitis.
farmacéutico, -ca[1] *m., f.* pharmaceutist, pharmacist.
farmacéutico, -ca[2] *adj.* pharmaceutic, pharmaceutical.
farmacia *f.* pharmaceutics, pharmacy.
fármaco *m.* drug.
farmacocinética *f.* pharmacokinetics.

farmacocinético, -ca *adj.* pharmacokinetic.
farmacología *f.* pharmacology.
farmacológico, -ca *adj.* pharmacologic, pharmacological.
farmacoterapia *f.* pharmacotherapy.
fascia *f.* fascia.
fascitis *f.* fasciitis.
fase *f.* phase, stage.
fatiga *f.* fatigue.
fecal *adj.* fecal.
fecaloma *m.* fecaloma.
feculento, -ta *adj.* feculent.
fecundación *f.* fecundation, fecundatio.
fecundar *v.* fecundate.
fecundidad *f.* fecundity.
feedback *m.* feedback.
femenino, -na *adj.* femenine.
feminización *f.* feminization.
femoral *adj.* femoral.
fémur *m.* femur.
fenestración *f.* fenestration.
fenilcetonuria (FCU) *f.* phenylketonuria (FKU).
fenómeno *m.* phenomenon.
fenotípico, -ca *adj.* phenotypic.
fenotipo *m.* phenotype.
fermentación *f.* fermentation.
feromonas *f.* pheromone.
ferritina *f.* ferritin.
fértil *adj.* fertile.
fertilidad *f.* fertility.
férula *f.* splint.
   férula quirúrgica surgical splint.
   férula de sostén abutment splint.
   férula de yeso plaster splint.
ferulización *f.* splinting.

fetal *adj.* fetal.

fetichismo *m.* fetishism.

fetidez *f.* mephitis.

fétido, -da *adj.* fetid.

feto *m.* fetus.

fetopatía *f.* fetopathy.

fetoproteína *f.* fetoprotein.

fetoscopia *f.* fetoscopy.

fiabilidad *f.* reliability.

fibrilación *f.* fibrillation.

fibrina *f.* fibrin.

fibrinogénesis *f.* fibrinogenesis.

fibrinógeno *m.* fibrinogen.

fibrinólisis *f.* fibrinolysis.

fibroblasto *m.* fibroblast.

fibrogénesis *f.* fibrogenesis.

fibroma *m.* fibroma.

   fibroma mixomatodes, fibroma mixomatoide, fibroma mixomatoso fibroma myxomatodes.

fibromatosis *f.* fibromatosis.

fibromatoso, -sa *adj.* fibromatous.

fibromioma *f.* fibromyoma.

fibrosis *f.* fibrosis.

fiebre *f.* fever.

   fiebre periódica periodic fever.

   fiebre recidivante relapsing fever.

   fiebre recurrente recurrent fever.

figura *f.* figure.

fijación *f.* fixation.

filariasis *m.* filariasis.

filiación *f.* filiation.

fimosis *f.* phimosis.

fisiología *f.* physiology.

fisiológico, -ca *adj.* physiologic, physiological.

fisiopatología *f.* physiopathology.

fisiopatológico, -ca *adj.* physiopathologic.

fisioterapeuta *m., f.* physiotherapeutist, physiotherapist.

fisioterapia *f.* physiotherapy.

fístula *f.* fistula.

   fístula ciega blind fistula.

   fístula completa complete fistula.

   fístula externa external fistula.

   fístula interna internal fistula.

   fístula intestinal intestinal fistula.

fistulización *f.* fistulization.

fisura *f.* fissure, fissura.

fitoterapia *f.* phytotherapy.

fláccido, -da *adj.* flaccid.

flato *m.* flatus.

flatulencia *f.* flatulence.

flatulento, -ta *adj.* flatulent.

flebectomía *f.* phlebectomy, strip.

flebítico, -ca *adj.* phlebitic.

flebitis *f.* phlebitis.

flebografía *f.* phlebography.

flebotomía *f.* phlebotomy.

flema *f.* phlegm.

flemón *m.* phlegmon.

flexibilidad *f.* flexibility.

flexible *adj.* flexible.

flexión[1] *f.* flexion.

flexión[2] *f.* flexure, flexura.

flexionar *v.* flex.

flora *f.* flora.

   flora intestinal intestinal flora.

fluctuación *f.* fluctuation.

fluctuante *adj.* fluctuant.

fluido *m.* fluid.

flujo[1] *m.* flow.

flujo[2] *m.* flux.

   flujo menstrual menstrual flux.

   flujo vaginal vaginal discharge.

flúter *m.* flutter.

fobia *f.* phobia.

foco *m.* focus.

focomelia *f.* phocomelia.

folicular *adj.* follicular.

foliculitis *f.* folliculitis.

foliculo *m.* follicle.

fomite *f.* fomite.

fonación *f.* phonation.

fondo *m.* fundus.

  fondo de ojo fundus oculi.

  fondo de saco cul de sac.

  fondo uterino, fondo del útero fundus of the uterus, fundus uteri.

  fondo de la vagina fundus of the vagina, fundus vaginae.

fonendoscopio *m.* phonendoscope.

fontanela *f.* fontanel.

foramen *m.* foramen.

fórceps *m.* forceps.

  fórceps obstétrico obstetrical forceps.

forense *m., f.* forensic scientist.

forense *adj.* forensic.

forma *f.* form.

formación *f.* formation.

fosa *f.* fosso.

fosfatemia *f.* phosphatemia.

fosfolípido *m.* phospholipid.

fotofobia *f.* photophobia.

fotosensibilización *f.* photosensitization.

fóvea *f.* fovea.

fracción *f.* fraction.

  fracción de eyección (FE), fracción de eyección sistólica ejection fraction (EF), systolic ejection fraction.

  fracción de filtración (FF) filtration fraction (FF).

fractura *f.* fracture.

  fractura abierta open fracture.

  fractura astillada splintered fracture.

  fractura por avulsión avulsion fracture.

  fractura en caña verde greenstick fracture, hickory-stick fracture.

  fractura cerrada closed fracture.

  fractura completa complete fracture.

  fractura complicada complicated fracture.

  fractura conminuta comminuted fracture.

  fractura en cuña wedge fracture.

  fractura epifisaria epiphyseal fracture.

  fractura espiral, fractura espiroidea spiral fracture.

  fractura espontánea spontaneous fracture.

  fractura estable stable fracture.

  fractura fisurada fissured fracture.

  fractura incompleta incomplete fracture.

  fractura inestable unstable fracture.

  fractura por luxación dislocation fracture.

  fractura parcial incomplete fracture.

  fractura simple simple fracture.

  fractura en tallo verde greenstick fracture, hickory stick fracture.

fragilidad *f.* fragility, fragilitas.

  fragilidad de los huesos fragility of bone, fragilitas ossium.

fragmentación *f.* fragmentation.

fragmento *m.* fragment.

franco, -ca *adj.* frank.

frecuencia *f.* frequency.
  frecuencia cardiaca heart rate.
  frecuencia cardiaca fetal fetal heart rate.
frémito *m.* fremitus.
frénico, -ca *adj.* phrenic.
frente *f.* forehead.
fricción *f.* friction.
frigidez *f.* frigidity.
frígido, -da *adj.* frigid.
frío *m.* cold.
frotis *m.* smear.
  frotis cervical cervical smear.
  frotis de Pap, frotis de Papanicolaou Pap smear.
  frotis sanguíneo blood smear.
fuerza[1] *f.* force.
  fuerza vital vital force.
fuerza[2] *f.* strength.
fulminante *adj.* fulminant.
función *f.* function.
funcional *adj.* functional.
funda *f.* jacket.
fundamental *adj.* fundamental.
fungicida *m.* funcigide.
furúnculo *m.* furuncle, boil.
furunculosis *f.* furunculosis.
fusiforme *adj.* fusiform.
fusión *f.* fusion.

G

gabaminérgico, -ca *adj.* gabaergic, GABAergic.
gabinete *m.* cabinet.
gafas *f.* glasses, spectacles.
  gafas bifocales Fran-klin glasses.

galactorrea *f.* galactorrhea.
galope *m.* gallop.
  galope auricular atrial gallop.
gameto *m.* gamete, germ cell.
gametogénesis *f.* gametogenesis.
gamma-angiografía *f.* radioisotope angiography.
gammagrafía *f.* gammagraphy.
gammapatía *f.* gammopathy.
ganancia *f.* gain.
gangliectomía *f.* gangliectomy.
gangliitis *f.* gangliitis.
ganglio *m.* ganglion.
ganglión *m.* ganglion.
ganglionar *adj.* ganglionic.
gangosa *f.* gangosa.
gangrena *f.* gangrene.
  gangrena gaseosa gas gangrene, gaseous gangrene.
  gangrena progresiva progressive gangrene.
garganta *f.* throat.
gárgaras *f.* gargle.
gargarismo *m.* gargarism, mouthwash.
gargoilismo *m.* gargoylysm.
garra *f.* claw.
gas *m.* gas.
  gas intestinal intestinal gas.
gasa *f.* gauze.
gasometría *f.* gasometry.
gasto *m.* output.
  gasto cardíaco cardiac output.
gástrico, -ca *adj.* gastric.
gastritis *f.* gastritis.
gastroduodenal *adj.* gastroduodenal.
gastroenteritis *f.* gastroenteritis.
gastroplastia *f.* gastroplasty.

gatillo¹ *m.* ferrule.

gatillo² *m.* trigger.

gel *m.* gel.

gelatina *f.* gelatin, jelly.

gemelar *adj.* gemellary.

gemelo, -la *m., f.* twin, geminus.
  gemelo idéntico identical twin.

gen *m.* gene.
  gen autosómico autosomal gene.
  gen dominante dominant gene.
  gen ligado a X X-linked gene.
  gen ligado a Y Y-linked gene.

generación *f.* generation.

general *adj.* general.

generalista *m., f.* general practitioner.

género¹ *m.* genus.

género² *m.* gender.

génesis *f.* genesis.

genética *f.* genetics.
  genética molecular molecular genetics.

genético, -ca *adj.* genetic.

genetista *m., f.* geneticist.

genital *adj.* genital.

genitales *m.* genitals, genitalia.
  genitales externos external genitalia.
  genitales internos internal genitalia.

genoma *m.* genome.

genómico, -ca *adj.* genomic.

genotipo *m.* genotype.

geoda *f.* geode.

geriatra *m., f.* geriatrician.

geriatría *f.* geriatrics.

geriátrico, -ca *adj.* gerontal, geriatric.

germen *m.* germ.

germicida¹ *m.* germicide.

germicida² *adj.* germicidal.

gerontología *f.* gerontology.

gerontólogo, -ga *m., f.* gerontologist.

gestación *f.* gestation.

gestacional *adj.* gestational.

gestágeno *m.* gestagen.

gestágeno, -na *adj.* gestagenic.

gigante *m., f.* giant.

gigantismo *m.* gigantism.

gimnasia *f.* gymnastics.

ginecología *f.* gynecology.

ginecológico, -ca *adj.* gynecologic, gynecological.

ginecólogo, -ga *m., f.* gynecologist.

ginecomanía *f.* gynecomania.

gingival *adj.* gingival.

gingivitis *f.* gingivitis.

glabela *f.* glabella, glabellum.

glande *m.* glans.

glándula *f.* gland, glandula.
  glándula apocrina apocrine gland.
  glándula ecrina eccrine gland.
  glándula exocrina exocrine gland.
  glándula heterocrina heterocrine gland.
  glándula holocrina holocrine gland.
  glándula lagrimal lacrimal gland, glandula lacrimalis.
  glándula mamaria mammary gland, lactiferous gland, milk gland, glandula mammaria.
  glándula parótida parotid gland, glandula parotidea, glandula parotis.
  glándula prostática prostate gland, glandula prostatica.

glándula salival salivary gland, glandulae salivariae.

glándula sexual sexual gland.

glándula sudorípara sudoriferous gland, sudoriparous gland, sweat gland, glandulae sudoriferae.

glandular *adj.* glandular.

glaucoma *m.* glaucoma.

glaucoma de ángulo abierto open-angle glaucoma.

glaucoma de ángulo cerrado angle-closure glaucoma.

glaucoma congénito congenital glaucoma.

glaucoma crónico chronic glaucoma.

glaucoma maligno malignant glaucoma.

glía *f.* glia.

glicemia *f.* glycemia, glykemia.

glicerina *f.* glycerin, glycerinum.

glicerol *m.* glycerol.

glicoproteína *f.* glycoprotein.

glioma *m.* glioma.

gliosis *f.* gliosis.

globo *m.* globus.

globo ocular, globo del ojo bulb, eyeball, globus of the eye.

globulina *f.* globulin.

globulina inmune contra la varicela zóster, globulina inmunitaria contra la varicela zóster varicella-zoster immune globulin (VZIG).

globulina séricas serum globulin.

globulinemia *f.* globulinemia.

glóbulo *m.* globule.

glóbulo rojo red blood cell.

glomerular *adj.* glomerular.

glomerulitis *f.* glomerulitis.

glomérulo *m.* glomerule, glomerulus.

glomerulonefritis *f.* glomerulonephritis.

glomerulonefropatía *f.* glomerulonephropathy.

glomerulopatía *f.* glomerulopathy.

glomo *m.* glomus.

glositis *f.* glossitis.

glótico, -ca *adj.* glottic.

glotis *f.* glottis.

glucagón *m.* glucagon.

glucagonoma *m.* glucagonoma.

glucemia *f.* glycemia, glykemia.

glúcido *m.* glucide.

glucógeno *m.* glucogen.

glucogenosis *f.* glycogenosis.

glucólisis *f.* glucolysis.

glucosa *f.* glucose.

glucosuria *f.* glucosuria, glycosuria.

gluten *m.* gluten.

glúteo, -a *adj.* gluteal.

gnosia *f.* gnosia.

goma *f.* gum.

gónada *f.* gonad.

gonadectomía *f.* gonadectomy.

gonartritis *f.* gonarthritis.

gonartrosis *f.* gonarthrosis.

gonorrea *f.* gonorrhea.

gota[1] *f.* drop.

gota para el oído ear drop.

gota ocular, gota para los ojos eye drop.

gota[2] *f.* gout, gutta.

gota articular articular gout.

gota tofácea tophaceous gout.

goteo *m.* drip.

goteo intravenoso intravenous drip.

goteo posnasal postnasal drip.

gotero *m.* dropper.

gradiente *m.* gradient.

grado[1] *m.* degree.

  grado de libertad degree of freedom.

grado[2] *m.* grade.

  grado tumoral de Gleason Gleason's tumor grade.

graduado, -da *adj.* graduated.

gráfica *f.* chart, graph.

gráfico *m.* chart, graph.

gramnegativo, -va *adj.* gram-negative.

grampositivo, -va *adj.* gram-positive.

grano *m.* grain, granum.

granulación *f.* granulation, granulatio.

granular *adj.* granular.

gránulo *m.* granule.

granulocitario, -ria *adj.* granulocytic.

granulocítico, -ca *adj.* granulocytic.

granulocito *m.* granulocyte.

  granulocito en banda band form granulocyte.

  granulocito inmaduro immature granulocyte.

  granulocito segmentado segmented granulocyte.

granulocitosis *f.* granulocytosis.

granuloma *m.* granuloma.

granulomatoso, -sa *adj.* granulomatous.

grapa *f.* clip.

grasa *f.* fat.

  grasa insaturada unsaturated fat.

  grasa poliinsaturada polyunsaturated fat.

graso, -sa *adj.* fatty.

grave *adj.* grave, gravis.

gravedad *f.* gravity.

grávida *f.* gravid, gravida.

gravidez *f.* gravidity, graviditas.

gripal *adj.* grippal.

gripe *f.* flu, influenza, grippe.

  gripe A swine flu.

  gripe aviar bird flu, avian flu.

  gripe endémica endemic flu.

  gripe porcina swine flu.

grupo *m.* group.

  grupo de control control group.

  grupo terapéutico therapeutic group.

guanidina *f.* guanidine.

guía *f.* guidance, guide, guideline.

gusano *m.* worm.

gustativo, -va *adj.* gustatory.

gusto *m.* taste.

H

habilidad *f.* ability, skill.

habla *f.* speech.

  habla confusa jumbled speech.

habón *m.* hive.

halitosis *f.* halitosis.

halo *m.* halo.

hambre *f.* hunger.

hapteno *m.* hapten, haptene.

haz *m.* beam.

  haz de rayos X X-ray beam.

hebra *f.* strand.

heces *f.* feces, stool.

  heces grasas fatty stool.

helminto *m.* helminth.

hemacromatosis *f.* hemachromatosis.

hemaglutinación *f.* hemagglutination.

hemaglutinina *f.* hemagglutinin.

hemangioma *m.* hemangioma.

hemapoyesis *f.* hemapoiesis.

hemapoyético, -ca *adj.* hemapoietic.

hemático, -ca *adj.* hematic.

hematíe *m.* red blood cell.

hematina *f.* hematin.

hematocito *m.* hematocyte.

hematocrito *m.* hematocrit, hematokrit.

hematoma *m.* hematoma.

  hematoma intracraneal intracranial hematoma.

  hematoma subdural subdural hematoma.

hematopoyesis *f.* hematopoiesis.

hematopoyético, -ca *adj.* hematopoietic.

hematuria *f.* hematuria.

  hematuria macroscópica macroscopic hematuria.

  hematuria microscópica microscopic hematuria.

  hematuria renal renal hematuria.

hembra *f.* female.

hemianopsia *f.* hemianopsia, hemianopia.

hemiartrosis *f.* hemiartrhosis.

hemicraneal *adj.* hemicranial.

hemiplejía *f.* hemiplegia.

hemipléjico, -ca *adj.* hemiplegic.

hemisferio *m.* hemispherium.

  hemisferio dominante dominant hemisphere.

hemocromatosis *f.* hemochromatosis, hemachromatosis.

hemodiálisis *f.* hemodialysis.

  hemodiálisis domiciliaria home hemodialysis.

  hemodiálisis hospitalaria hospital hemodialysis.

hemodializador *m.* hemodialyzer.

hemodinámica *f.* hemodynamics.

hemofilia *f.* hemophilia.

hemofílico *m.* hemophiliac.

hemofílico, -ca *adj.* hemophilic.

hemoglobina *f.* hemoglobin, hemiglobin.

hemoglobinemia *f.* hemoglobinemia.

hemoglobinuria *f.* hemoglobinuria.

hemograma *m.* hemogram.

hemólisis *f.* hemolysis.

hemolítico, -ca *adj.* hemolytic.

hemoptisis *f.* hemoptysis.

hemorragia *f.* bleeding, hemorrhage, haemorrhagia.

  hemorragia interna internal hemorrhage.

  hemorragia intracerebral intracerebral hemorrhage.

  hemorragia intestinal intestinal hemorrhage.

  hemorragia intracraneal intracranial hemorrhage.

  hemorragia masiva massive hemorrhage.

  hemorragia nasal nosebleed.

  hemorragia oculta occult bleeding.

  hemorragia posparto postpartum hemorrhage.

  hemorragia recidivante recurring hemorrhage.

hemorragia recurrente recurring hemorrhage.

hemorragia subaracnoidea HSA subarachnoid hemorrhage.

hemorragia subdural subdural hemorrhage.

hemorragia uterina uterine hemorrhage.

hemorragia uterina disfuncional (HUD) dysfunctional uterine hemorrhage (DUB).

hemorragia vaginal vaginal hemorrhage.

hemorrágico, -ca *adj.* hemorrhagic.

hemorroides *f.* hemorrhoids.

hemosiderosis *f.* hemosiderosis.

hemostasia *f.* hemostasia.

hemostático, -ca *adj.* hemostatic.

hemostasis *f.* hemostasia, hemostasis.

hendidura *f.* fissure, fissura.

heparina *f.* heparin.

  heparina cálcica heparin calcium.

  heparina sódica heparin sodium.

heparinización *f.* heparinization.

heparinizar *v.* heparinize.

hepático, -ca *adj.* hepatic.

hepatítico, -ca *adj.* hepatitic.

hepatitis *f.* hepatitis.

hepatobiliar *adj.* hepatobiliary.

hepatocito *m.* hepatocyte.

hepatoesplenomegalia *f.* hepatosplenomegaly.

hepatoma *m.* hepatoma.

hepatomegalia *f.* hepatomegalia, hepatomegaly.

hepatopatía *f.* hepatopathy.

hepatotoxicidad *f.* hepatotoxicity.

hereditario, -ria *adj.* hereditary.

herencia[1] *f.* heritability.

herencia[2] *f.* heredity, inheritance.

herencia autosómica autosomal heredity, autosomal inheritance.

herencia autosómica dominante autosomal dominant inheritance.

herencia autosómica recesiva autosomal recessive inheritance.

herencia cruzada crisscross inheritance.

herencia dominante ligada al cromosoma X X-linked dominant inheritance.

herencia ligada al sexo sex-linked heredity.

herencia ligada al cromosoma X X-linked heredity, X-linked inheritance.

herencia ligada al cromosoma Y Y-linked heredity.

herencia poligénica polygenic inheritance.

herencia recesiva recessive heredity.

herencia recesiva ligada al cromosoma X X-linked recessive inheritance.

herida *f.* wound.

herida abierta open wound.

herida no penetrante non-penetrating wound.

herida penetrante penetrating wound.

herida séptica septic wound.

herir *v.* wound.

hermafrodita *m. y adj.* hermaphrodite.

hermafroditismo *m.* hermaphroditism.

hernia *f.* hernia.

hernia abdominal abdominal hernia.

hernia diafragmática diaphragmatic hernia.

hernia discal, hernia de disco herniated disk.

hernia estrangulada strangulated hernia.

hernia incompleta incomplete hernia.

hernia inguinal inguinal hernia.

herniación *f.* herniation.

herniación cerebral cerebral herniation.

herniación de disco intervetebral herniation of the intervetebral disk.

herniado, -da *adj.* herniated.

herpes *m.* herpes.

herpes genital genital herpes, herpes genitalis.

herpes gestacional, herpes gravídico herpes gestationis.

herpes recidivante relapsing herpes.

herpes recurrente recurrent herpes, herpes recurrens.

herpes simple herpes simplex.

herpes zoster herpes zoster.

herpético, -ca *adj.* herpetic.

herpetiforme *adj.* herpetiform.

heterocigoto *m.* heterozygote.

heterogeneidad *f.* heterogeneity.

heterogeneidad genética genetic heterogeneity.

heterogéneo, -a *adj.* heterogeneous, heterogenous.

heterosexual *adj.* heterosexual.

heterosexualidad *f.* heterosexuality.

hialino, -na *adj.* hyaline.

hiato *m.* hiatus.

hibridación *f.* hybridization.

híbrido, -da *m. y adj.* hybrid.

hidradenitis *f.* hidradenitis.

hidratación *f.* hydration.

hidratado, -da *adj.* hydrous, hydrated.

hidrocefalia *f.* hydrocephalia.

hidrocefalia congénita congenital hydrocephalia.

hidrocefalia externa external hydrocephalia.

hidrocefalia interna internal hydrocephalia.

hidrocefalia normotensa normalpressure hydrocephalia.

hidrocefalia obstructiva obstructive hydrocephalia.

hidrocele *m.* hydrocele.

hidrofobia *f.* hydrophobia.

hidronefrosis *f.* hydronephrosis.

hidropesia *f.* dropsy, hydrops.

hidrosoluble *adj.* hydrosoluble.

hidroterapia *f.* hydrotherapy, hydrotherapeutics.

hierro *m.* iron, ferrum.

hígado *m.* liver, hepar.

hígado cirrótico cirrhotic liver.

hígado cirrótico biliar biliary cirrhotic liver.

hígado graso fatty liver.

higiene *f.* hygiene.

higiene dental dental hygiene.

higiénico, -ca *adj.* hygienic.

higroma *m.* hygroma, hydroma.

himen *m.* hymen.

himen imperforado imperforated hymen.

himen tabicado hymen septate.

himenal

himenal *adj.* hymenal.

hioideo, -a *adj.* hyoid.

hioides *m.* hyoid.

hiperactividad *f.* hyperactivity.

hiperactivo, -va *adj.* hyperactive.

hiperalgesia *f.* hyperalgesia.

hiperazoemia *f.* hyperazotemia, azotemia.

hiperbárico, -ca *adj.* hyperbaric.

hiperbetalipoproteinemia *f.* hyperbetalipoproteinemia.

hiperbilirrubinemia *f.* hyperbilirubinemia.

  hiperbilirrubinemia neonatal neonatal hyperbilirubinemia.

hipercalcemia *f.* hypercalcemia.

hipercalciuria *f.* hypercalciuria.

hipercaliemia *f.* hyperkalemia, hyperkaliemia.

hipercelularidad *f.* hypercellularity.

hipercinesia *f.* hyperkinesia, hyperkinesis.

hipercloremia *f.* hyperchloremia.

hiperclorhidria *f.* hyperchlorhydria.

hipercoagulabilidad *f.* hypercoagulability.

hipercolesterolemia *f.* hypercholesterolemia.

  hipercolesterolemia familiar familial hypercholesterolemia.

hipercolesterolémico, -ca *adj.* hypercholesterolemic.

hipercorticismo *m.* hypercorticism.

hiperecogenicidad *f.* hyperechogenicity.

hiperemesis *f.* hyperemesis.

  hiperemesis del embarazo, hiperemesis gravídica hyperemesis gravidarum.

hiperemia *f.* hyperemia.

hiperestesia *f.* hyperesthesia.

hiperextensión *f.* hyperextension.

hiperflexión *f.* hyperflexion.

hiperfosfatemia *f.* hyperphosphatemia.

hiperfosfaturia *f.* hyperphosphaturia.

hiperfunción *f.* hyperfunction.

hipergammaglobulinemia *f.* hypergammaglobulinemia.

  hipergammaglobulinemia monoclonal monoclonal hypergammaglobulinemia.

hiperglicemia *f.* hyperglycemia.

hiperglucemia *f.* hyperglycemia.

hipergonadismo *m.* hypergonadism.

hiperhidrosis *f.* hyperhidrosis.

hiperinsulinismo *m.* hyperinsulinism.

hiperlaxitud *f.* hyperlaxicity.

hiperlipemia *f.* hyperlipemia.

hiperlipidemia *f.* hyperlipidemia, hyperlipoidemia.

hiperlipoproteinemia *f.* hyperlipoproteinemia.

hipermenorrea *f.* hypermenorrhea.

hipermétrope *m.* hypermetrope.

hipermetropía *f.* hypermetropia, hypermetropy.

hipermotilidad *f.* hypermotility.

hipernatremia *f.* hypernatremia.

hiperostosis *f.* hyperostosis.

hiperparatiroidismo *m.* hyperparathyroidism.

hiperpigmentación *f.* hyperpigmentation.

hiperplasia *f.* hyperplasia.

hiperplasia prostática benigna (HBP) benign prostatic hyperplasia.

hiperplasia quística de la mama cystic hyperplasia of the breast.

hiperptialismo *m.* hyperptyalism.

hiperqueratinización *f.* hyperkeratinization.

hiperqueratosis *f.* hyperkeratosis.

hiperquilomicronemia *f.* hyperchylomicronemia.

hiperreflexia *f.* hyperreflexia.

hiperreactividad *f.* hyperreactivity.

hiperreactividad bronquial bronchial hyperreactivity.

hiperreactivo, -va *adj.* hyperreactive.

hipersalivación *f.* hypersalivation.

hipersecreción *f.* hypersecretion.

hipersensibilidad *f.* hypersensitivity.

hipersensibilidad por contacto contact hypersensitivity.

hipersensibilidad inmediata immediate hypersensitivity.

hipersensibilidad por inmunocomplejos immune complex hypersensitivity.

hipersensibilidad retardada (HR), de tipo retardado (HTR) delayed hypersensitivity (DH), delayed-type hypersensitivity (DTH).

hipersensibilidad tipo tuberculina tuberculin-type hypersensitivity.

hipersensibilización *f.* hypersensitization.

hipersístole *f.* hypersystole.

hipersistolia *f.* hypersystole.

hipersomnolencia *f.* hypersomnolence.

hipertelorismo *m.* hypertelorism.

hipertensión *f.* hypertension, high blood pressure.

hipertensión arterial arterial hypertension.

hipertensión arterial de bata blanca white coat arterial hypertension.

hipertensión arterial esencial essential arterial hypertension.

hipertensión arterial pulmonar pulmonary arterial hypertension.

hipertensión arterial secundaria secondary arterial hypertension.

hipertensión arterial sistémica systemic arterial hypertension.

hipertensión esencial essential hypertension.

hipertensión idiopática idiopathic hypertension.

hipertensión intracraneal intracranial hypertension.

hipertensión maligna malignant hypertension.

hipertensión ocular ocular hypertension.

hipertensión pulmonar pulmonary hypertension.

hipertensión renal renal hypertension.

hipertensión secundaria secondary hypertension.

hipertensión sintomática symptomatic hypertension.

hipertensión suprarrenal adrenal hypertension.

hipertensión vascular vascular hypertension.

hipertensivo, -va *adj.* hypertensive.

hipertenso, -sa *adj.* hypertensive.

hipertensor, -ra *adj.* hypertensor.

hipertermia *f.* hyperthermia.

hipertiroideo, -a *adj.* hyperthyroid.

hipertiroidismo *m.* hyperthyroidism.

hipertiroidismo oftálmico ophthalmic hyperthyroidism.

hipertiroidismo primario primary hyperthyroidism.

hipertiroidismo secundario secondary hyperthyroidism.

hipertonía *f.* hypertonia.

hipertonicidad *f.* hypertonicity.

hipertónico, -ca *adj.* hypertonic.

hipertricosis *f.* hypertrichosis.

hipertrigliceridemia *f.* hypertriglyceridemia.

hipertrofia *f.* hypertrophy.

hipertrofia prostática prostatic hypertrophy.

hipertrofia ventricular ventricular hypertrophy.

hipertrófico, -ca *adj.* hypertrophic.

hiperuricemia *f.* hyperuricemia.

hiperventilación *f.* hyperventilation.

hipervitaminosis *f.* hypervitaminosis.

hipervolemia *f.* hypervolemia.

hipervolémico, -ca *adj.* hypervolemic.

hipnosis *f.* hypnosis.

hipnótico, -ca *adj.* hypnotic.

hipo *m.* hiccough, hiccup.

hipoactividad *f.* hypoactivity.

hipoacusia *f.* hypoacusia, hypoacusis, hypacusia, hypacusis.

hipoalbuminemia *f.* hypoalbuminemia, hypalbuminemia.

hipoaldosteronemia *f.* hypoaldosteronemia.

hipoaldosteronismo *m.* hypoaldosteronism.

hipoalérgenico, -ca *adj.* hypoallergenic.

hipocalciuria *f.* hypocalciuria.

hipocalemia *f.* hypokalemia.

hipocaliemia *f.* hypokaliemia, hypokalemia.

hipocampo *m.* hippocampus.

hipocelular *adj.* hypocellular.

hipocondría *f.* hypochondria.

hipocondríaco, -ca[1] *m.*, *f.* hypochondriac.

hipocondríaco, -ca[2] *adj.* hypochondriacal.

hipocorticismo *m.* hypocorticoidism.

hipodinamia *f.* hypodinamia.

hipoecogenicidad *f.* hypoechogenicity.

hipoecogénico, -ca *adj.* hypoechogenic.

hipoestrogenismo *m.* hypoestrogenism.

hipofaringe *f.* hypopharynx.

hipofaríngeo, -a *adj.* hypopharyngeal.

hipófisis *f.* hypophysis, pituitary gland.

hipofosfatemia *f.* hypophosphatemia.

hipofosfaturia *f.* hypophosphaturia.

hipofunción *f.* hypofunction.

hipofuncionamiento *m.* hypofunction.

hipogammaglobulinemia *f.* hypogammaglobulinemia.

hipogammaglobulinemia fisiológica physiologic hypogammaglobulinemia.

hipogammaglobulinemia ligada a X, hipogammaglobulinemia infantil ligada a X linked-X hypogammaglobulinemia, X-linked infantile hypogammaglobulinemia.

hipogástrico, -ca *adj.* hypogastric.

hipogastrio *m.* hypogastrium.

hipoglucemia *f.* hypoglycemia.

hipoglucemia en ayunas fasting hypoglycemia.

hipoglucemia cetósica ketotic hypoglycemia.

hipoglucemiante *m.* hypoglycemic agent.

hipoglucémico, -ca *adj.* hypoglycemic.

hipogonadismo *m.* hypogonadism.

hipomanía *f.* hypomania.

hipomaníaco, -ca *m., f.* hypomaniac.

hiponatremia *f.* hyponatremia.

hipoparatiroidismo *m.* hypoparathyroidism.

hipoparatiroidismo familiar familial hypoparathyroidism.

hipoperfusión *f.* hypoperfusion.

hipopituitarismo *m.* hypopituitarism.

hipoplasia *f.* hypoplasia, hypoplasty.

hipoprolactinemia *f.* hypoprolactinemia.

hipoproteinemia *f.* hypoproteinemia.

hiposecreción *f.* hyposecretion.

hiposensibilidad *f.* hyposensitivity.

hiposensibilización *f.* hyposensitization.

hipospadia *m.* hypospadias.

hipotálamo *m.* hypothalamus.

hipotenar *m.* hypothenar.

hipotensión *f.* hypotension.

hipotensión arterial arterial hypotension.

hipotensión ortostática crónica, hipotensión ortostática idiopática crónica chronic orthostatic hypotension, chronic idiopathic orthostatic hypotension.

hipotensión postural postural hypotension.

hipotenso, -sa *adj.* hypotensive.

hipotensor, -ra *adj.* hypotensor.

hipótesis *f.* hypothesis.

hipotiroideo, -a *adj.* hypothyroid.

hipotiroidismo *m.* hypothyroidism.

hipotonía *f.* hypotonia, hypotony.

hipotónico, -ca *adj.* hypotonic.

hipovolemia *f.* hypovolemia.

hipovolémico, -ca *adj.* hypovolemic.

hipoxemia *f.* hypoxemia.

hipoxia *f.* hypoxia.

hipóxico, -ca *adj.* hypoxic.

hirsutismo *m.* hirsutism.

histamina *f.* histamine.

histerectomía *f.* hysterectomy.

histeria *f.* hysteria.

histérico, -ca *adj.* hysteric, hysterical.

histerosalpingografía *f.* hysterosalpingography.

histeroscopia *f.* hysteroscopy.

histeroscopio *m.* hysteroscope.

hístico, -ca *adj.* histic.

histiocitosis *f.* histiocytosis, histocytosis.

histocompatibilidad *f.* histocompatibility.

histocompatible *adj.* histocompatible.

histología *f.* histology.

histología normal normal histology.

histología patológica pathologic histology.

histoplasmosis *f.* histoplasmosis.

histoquímica *f.* histochemistry.

historia *f.* history.

historia clínica clinical history, health history.

historia familiar family history.

historia personal y familiar case history.

hombro *m.* shoulder.

homeópata *m., f.* homeopathist, homeopath.

homeopatía *f.* homeopathy.

homeopático, -ca *adj.* homeopathic.

homeostasia *f.* homeostasis.

homeostasis *f.* homeostasis.

homicidio *m.* homicide.

homocigosidad *f.* homozygosity.

homocigosis *f.* homozygosis.

homocigoto, -ta *adj.* homozygote.

homocistinemia *f.* homocystinemia.

homocistinuria *f.* homocystinuria.

homogenicidad *f.* homogenicity.

homónimo, -ma *adj.* homonymous.

homosexual *adj.* homosexual.

homosexualidad *f.* homosexuality.

hongo *m.* fungus.

hormona *f.* hormone.

hormonal *adj.* hormonal.

hospital *m.* hospital.

hospital general general hospital.

hospital geriátrico de día geriatric day care hospital.

hospital de maternidad, hospital materno maternity hospital.

hospital psiquiátrico psychiatric hospital.

hospitalización *f.* hospitalization.

hospitalizado, -da *adj.* inpatient.

hospitalizar *v.* institutionalize.

huella digital *f.* fingerprint.

huesecillo *m.* bonelet, ossicle.

hueso *m.* bone, os.

huésped *m.* host.

huevo *m.* ovum.

humectante *adj.* humectant.

humedad *f.* humidity.

húmero *m.* humerus.

humidificador *m.* humidifier.

humor *m.* humor.

humor vítreo humor vitreus, vitreous humor.

humoral *adj.* humoral.

huso *m.* spindle.

I

iatrogenia *f.* iatrogenia.

iatrogénico, -ca *adj.* iatrogenic.

ictericia *f.* jaundice, icterus.

ictericia acolúrica acholuric jaundice.

ictericia colestática cholestatic jaundice.

ictericia colérica choleric jaundice.

ictericia congénita congenital jaundice.

ictericia hemolítica congénita, icterus hemolítico congénito congenital hemolytic jaundice, congenital hemolytic icterus.

ictericia neonatal, icterus neonatal neonatal jaundice, icterus neonatorum.

ictericia del neonato icterus neonatorum.

ictericia no hemolítica non-hemolytic jaundice.

ictericia del recién nacido jaundice of the newborn.

ictérico, -ca *adj.* icteric.

ictiosis *f.* ichthyosis.

ictus *m.* ictus.

idiocia *f.* idiocy.

idiopático, -ca *adj.* idiopathic.

idiota *m., f. y adj.* idiot.

ileal *adj.* ileal.

ileectomía *f.* ileectomy.

ileítis *f.* ileitis.

íleo *m.* ileus.

íleon *m.* ileum.

ileostomía *f.* ileostomy.

ileostomía urinaria urinary ileostomy.

ileostomizado, -da *adj.* ileostomate.

ilíaco, -ca *adj.* iliac.

imagen *f.* image.

imagen corporal body image.

imagen visual visual image.

imaginación *f.* imagination.

impacción *f.* impaction.

impacto *m.* impact.

impermeabilidad *f.* impermeability.

impétigo *m.* impetigo.

implante *m.* implant.

implante dental dental implant.

impotencia *f.* impotence, impotency, impotentia.

impulsividad *f.* impulsivity, impulsiveness.

impulso *m.* drive.

impulso sexual sexual drive.

inactivación *f.* inactivation.

inadaptación *f.* maladjustment.

inanición¹ *f.* inanition.

inanición² *f.* starvation.

inapetencia *f.* inappetence.

incapacidad *f.* disability.

incapacidad mental mental disability.

incisión *f.* incision.

incisivo, -va *adj.* incisive.

inclinación *f.* inclination, incline, slant, inclinatio.

inclusión *f.* inclusion.

incompatibilidad *f.* incompatibility.

incompatibilidad HLA HLA mismatching.

incompatibilidad Rh Rh incompatibility.

incompatible *adj.* incompatible.

incompetencia *f.* incompetence, incompetency.

incompetente *adj.* incompetent.

inconsciencia *f.* unconsciousness.

inconsciente *m.* unconscious.

incontinencia *f.* incontinence, incontinentia.

incontinencia anal anal incontinence.

incontinencia fecal fecal incontinence.

incontinencia urinaria urinary incontinence, incontinence of urine, incontinentia urinae.

incremento *m.* increment.

index index.

indicación *f.* indication, indicatio.

indicador, -ra *m. y adj.* indicator.

índice *m.* rate, index.

índice metabólico metabolic rate.

índice de morbilidad morbidity rate.

índice de mortalidad mortality rate.

índice de saturación saturation index.

indiferencia *f.* indifference.

indigestión *f.* indigestion.

indirecto, -ta *adj.* indirect.

indoloro, -ra *adj.* indolent.

inducción *f.* induction.

inducido, -da *adj.* induced.

induración *f.* induration.

inercia *f.* inertia.

inervación *f.* innervation.

inespecífico, -ca *adj.* non-specific.

inestabilidad *f.* instability.

infancia *f.* babyhood, childhood, infancy.

infanticida *m., f.* infanticide.

infanticidio *m.* infanticide.

infantil *adj.* infantile.

infantilismo *m.* infantilism.

infarto *m.* infarct, infarction.

infarto cardíaco cardiac infarction.

infarto cerebral cerebral infarction.

infarto intestinal intestinal infarction.

infarto mesentérico mesenteric infarction.

infarto del miocardio (IM) myocardial infarction (MI).

infección *f.* infection.

infección adquirida en el hospital hospital-acquired infection.

infección cruzada cross infection.

infección iatrogénica iatrogenic infection.

infección nosocomial nosocomial infection.

infección oportunista opportunistic infection.

infección sistémica systemic infection.

infección transmitida por agua water-borne infection.

infección transmitida por el aire airborne infection.

infección transmitida por gotitas droplet infection.

infección transmitida por un vector vector-borne infection.

infección urinaria urinary infection.

infeccioso, -sa *adj.* infectious.

infectar *v.* infect.

inferior *adj.* inferior.

infertilidad *f.* infertility.

infiltración *f.* infiltration.

infiltrado *m.* infiltrate.

inflamación *f.* inflammation.

inflamatorio, -ria *adj.* inflammatory.

influenza *f.* influenza.

informe *m.* report.

infracción *f.* infraction.

infradiafragmático, -ca *adj.* infradiaphragmatic.

infrarrojo, -ja *adj.* infrared.

infusión *f.* infusion.

ingesta *f.* intake, ingesta.

  ingesta calórica caloric intake.

ingle *f.* groin, inguen.

ingravidez *f.* weightlessness.

ingreso *m.* intake.

inguinal *adj.* inguinal.

ingurgitación *f.* engorgement.

ingurgitado, -da *adj.* engorged.

inhalación *f.* inhalation.

inhalar *v.* inhale.

inhibición *f.* inhibition.

inhibidor *m.* inhibitor.

  inhibidor del apetito appetite inhibitor.

  inhibidor de la enzima de conversión de la angiotensina (ECA) angiotensin converting enzyme inhibitor (ACE).

inhibidor, -ra *adj.* inhibitive, inhibitory.

iniciación *f.* initiation.

inicial *adj.* initial.

injertar *v.* graft.

injerto *m.* graft.

  injerto autógeno autogenous graft.

  injerto autólogo autologous graft.

  injerto de cadáver cadaver graft.

  injerto corneal corneal graft.

  injerto cutáneo skin graft.

  injerto heterólogo heterologous graft.

  injerto homólogo homologous graft.

inmadurez *f.* immaturity.

inmaduro, -ra *adj.* immature.

inmediato, -ta *adj.* immediate.

inmovilidad *f.* immobility.

inmovilización *f.* immobilization.

inmovilizar *v.* immobilize.

inmune *adj.* immune.

inmunidad *f.* immunity.

  inmunidad activa active immunity.

  inmunidad adoptiva adoptive immunity.

  inmunidad adquirida acquired immunity.

  inmunidad celular cellular immunity.

  inmunidad cruzada cross immunity.

  inmunidad familiar familial immunity.

  inmunidad hereditaria inherited immunity.

  inmunidad humoral humoral immunity.

  inmunidad inespecífica non-specific immunity.

  inmunidad materna maternal immunity.

  inmunidad de mediación celular, inmunidad mediada por células (IMC), inmunidad mediada por células T (IMCT) cell-mediated immunity (CMI), T cell-mediated immunity (TCMI).

inmunización *f.* immunization.

  inmunización activa active immunization.

  inmunización pasiva passive immunization.

inmunizar *v.* immunize.

inmunocompetencia *f.* immunocompetence.

inmunocompetente *adj.* immunocompetent.

inmunocomplejo *m.* immunocomplex.

inmunocomprometido, -da *adj.* immunocompromised.

inmunodeficiencia *f.* immunodeficiency.

inmunodeficiente *adj.* immunodeficient.

inmunodepresión *f.* immunodepression.

inmunoensayo *m.* immunoassay.

inmunoestimulante *adj.* immunostimulant.

inmunofluorescencia *f.* immunofluorescence.

inmunoglobulina *f.* immunoglobulin.

inmunohistoquímica *f.* immunohistochemistry.

inmunología *f.* immunology.

inmunológico, -ca *adj.* immunologic, immunological.

inmunólogo, -ga *m., f.* immunologist.

inmunoperoxidasa *f.* immunoperoxidase.

inmunoproliferativo, -va *adj.* immunoproliferative.

inmunosupresión *f.* immunosuppression.

inmunosupresor *m.* immunosuppresant.

inmunoterapia *f.* immunotherapy.

innocuo, -cua *adj.* innocuous, innoxious.

inoculación *f.* inoculation.

inorgánico, -ca *adj.* inorganic.

inotrópico, -ca *adj.* inotropic.

inotrópico negativo negatively inotropic.

inotrópico positivo positively inotropic.

insalubre *adj.* insalubrious.

insano, -na *m., f.* insane.

insaturado, -da *adj.* unsaturated.

inscripción *f.* inscription, inscriptio.

inseminación *f.* insemination.

inseminación artificial artificial insemination.

insensibilidad *f.* insensibility.

inserción *f.* attachment, insert, insertion, insertio.

insolación *f.* insolation.

insoluble *adj.* insoluble.

insomne *adj.* insomniac, insomnic.

insomnio *m.* insomnia.

inspección *f.* inspection.

inspiración *f.* inspiration.

inspirar *v.* inspirate.

instilación *f.* instillation.

instilación de gotas óticas eardrop instillation.

instilación nasal de medicamentos nasal instillation of medication.

instinto *m.* instinct.

instrucción *f.* directive.

instrumentación *f.* instrumentation.

instrumental *adj.* instrumental.

instrumento *m.* instrument.

insuficiencia *f.* failure, insufficiency.

insuficiencia cardíaca cardiac insufficiency, heart failure.

insuficiencia cardíaca congestiva (ICC) congestive heart failure (CHF).

insuficiencia circulatoria circulatory insufficiency, circulatory failure.

insuficiencia coronaria* coronary insufficiency.

insuficiencia mitral* mitral failure, mitral insufficiency.

insuficiencia renal* renal insufficiency, renal failure.

insuficiencia respiratoria* respiratory insufficiency, respiratory failure.

insuflación *f.* insufflation.

insulina *f.* insulin.

insulina de acción corta* short-acting insulin.

insulina de acción intermedia* intermediate-acting insulin.

insulina de acción lenta* slow-acting insulin.

insulina de acción prolongada* long-acting insulin.

insulina de acción rápida* rapid-acting insulin.

insulina con cinc y globina, insulina cíncica globina* globin zinc insulin, globin zinc injection.

integración *f.* integration.

inteligencia *f.* intelligence.

intensidad *f.* intensity, strength.

interacción *f.* interaction.

interacción entre alimentos y fármacos* food and drug interaction.

interacción medicamentosa* drug-drug interaction.

intercambio *m.* exchange, interchange, intercourse.

interferón (IFN, INF) *m.* interferon (IFN, INF).

interleucina (IL) *f.* interleukin (IL).

interleuquina (IL) *f.* interleukin (IL).

internamiento *m.* commitment.

interno, -na *adj.* internal.

interno, -na *m., f.* intern, interne.

intervalo *m.* interval, gap.

intervención *f.* intervention, procedure.

intestinal *adj.* intestinal.

intestino *m.* gut, intestine, intestinum.

intestino ciego* blindgut, blind gut, blind intestine, intestinum caecum, intestinum cecum.

intestino delgado* small intestine, intestinum tenue.

intestino grueso* large intestine, intestinum crassum.

intestino íleon* ileum intestine, intestinum ileum.

intestino yeyuno* jejunum intestine, intestinum jejunum.

íntima *adj.* intima.

intolerancia *f.* intolerance.

intolerancia a fármacos* drug intolerance.

intolerancia al gluten* gluten intolerance.

intolerancia a la lactosa* lactose intolerance.

intoxación *f.* intoxation.

intoxicación *f.* intoxication, poisoning.

intoxicación alimentaria, intoxicación alimenticia* food poisoning.

intoxicación por cornezuelo del centeno* ergot poisoning.

intoxicación por setas* mushroom poisoning.

intraabdominal *adj.* intra-abdominal.

intracelular *adj.* intracellular.

intraescrotal *adj.* intrascrotal.

introito *m.* introitus.

introversión *f.* introversion.

intrusión *f.* intrusion.

intubación *f.* intubation.

  intubación intratraqueal intratracheal intubation.

  intubación nasal nasal intubation.

  intubación nasogástrica nasogastric intubation.

  intubación nasotraqueal nasotracheal intubation.

  intubación oral oral intubation.

  intubación orotraqueal orotracheal intubation.

intubar *v.* intubate.

invaginación *f.* invagination.

invalidez *f.* invalidism.

inválido, -da *adj.* invalid, handicapped.

invertebrado, -da *m., f.* invertebrate.

investigación *f.* investigation, research, searching.

  investigación clínica clinical investigation, clinical research.

inviable *adj.* non-viable.

involución *f.* involution.

  involución uterina, involución del útero uterine involution, involution of the uterus.

involuntario, -ria *adj.* involuntary.

inyección *f.* injection.

  inyección de insulina insulin injection.

  inyección intraarticular intraarticular injection.

  inyección intramuscular intramuscular injection.

  inyección intravascular intravascular injection.

  inyección intravenosa intravenous injection.

  inyección de recuerdo booster injection.

  inyección subcutánea subcutaneous injection.

inyectar *v.* inject.

iodo *m.* iodine.

ión *m.* ion.

ionización *f.* ionization.

ionoforesis *f.* ionophoresis.

ipsilateral *adj.* ipsilateral.

ipsolateral *adj.* ipsilateral.

ira *f.* anger, rage.

iridectomía *f.* iridectomy.

iridectomizar *v.* iridectomize.

iridoplejía *f.* iridoplegia.

iris *m.* iris.

irítico, -ca *adj.* iritic.

iritis *f.* iritis.

irradiación *f.* irradiation.

irradiado, -da *adj.* irradiate.

irradiar[1] *v.* irradiate.

irradiar[2] *v.* radiate.

irreal *adj.* dereistic.

irreducible *adj.* irreducible.

irregular *adj.* irregular.

irreversible *adj.* irreversible.

irrigación *f.* irrigation.

  irrigación vesical bladder irrigation.

irritabilidad *f.* irritability.

irritable *adj.* irritable.

irritación *f.* irritation.

irritante *m. y adj.* irritant.

islote *m.* islet.

  islote de Langerhans islet of Langerhans.

islote pancreático pancreatic islet.

isoalelismo *m.* isoallelism.

isoalelo *m.* isoallele.

isoanticuerpo *m.* isoantibody.

isoantígeno *m.* isoantigen.

isoenzima *f.* isoenzyme.

isoinmunización *f.* isoimmunization.

isoleucina *f.* isoleucine.

isosensibilización *f.* isosensitization.

isquemia *f.* ischemia.

isquemia cerebral cerebral ischemia.

isquemia intestinal crónica chronic intestinal ischemia.

isquemia del miocardio, isquemia miocárdica myocardial ischemia.

isquemia renal renal ischemia.

isquemia retiniana ischemia retinae.

isquemia subclínica silent ischemia.

isquémico, -ca *adj.* ischemic.

isquiático, -ca *adj.* ischiatic.

isquion *m.* ischium.

isquiotibial *adj.* ischiotibial.

istmo *m.* isthmus.

Ixodes Ixodes.

Ixodes bicornis Ixodes bicornis.

J

jabón *m.* soap, sapo.

jadear *v.* pant.

jadeo *m.* panting, wheeze.

jalea *f.* jelly.

jaqueca *f.* migraine.

jaqueca hemipléjica hemiplegic migraine.

jaqueca oftálmica ophthalmic migraine.

jaquecoso, -sa *adj.* migranoid, migranous.

jarabe *m.* syrup.

jeringa *f.* syringe.

jeringa de agua water syringe.

jeringa de aire air syringe.

jeringa de aspiración aspiration syringe.

jeringa hipodérmica hypodermic syringe.

jeringuilla *f.* syringe.

joroba *f.* hump, humpback.

juanete *m.* bunion.

jugo *m.* juice, succus.

jugo gástrico gastric juice, succus gastricus.

jugo intestinal intestinal juice, succus entericus.

jugo pancreático pancreatic juice, succus pancreaticus.

jugo prostático prostatic juice, succus prostaticus.

juramento *m.* oath, pledge.

juramento de Hipócrates, juramento hipocrático oath of Hippocrates, hippocratic oath.

K

keratectomía *f.* keratectomy.

kernicterus *m.* kernicterus.

kinesiología *f.* kinesiology.

L

laberintectomía f. labyrinthectomy.

laberintitis f. labyrinthitis.

laberinto m. labyrinth, labyrinthus.

laberintotomía f. labyrinthotomy.

labial adj. labial.

lábil adj. labile.

labilidad f. lability.

labio m. lip, labium.

labio fisurado cleft lip.

labio hendido cleft lip.

labio leporino harelip.

laboratorio m. laboratory.

laboratorio clínico clinical laboratory.

laceración f. laceration.

laceración cerebral brain laceration.

laceración del cuero cabelludo scalp laceration.

laceración vaginal vaginal laceration.

lacrimal adj. lachrymal, lacrimal.

lacrimonasal adj. lacrimonasal.

lactancia¹ f. lactation.

lactancia² f. infancy.

lactancia materna f. breast-feeding.

lactante m. infant, nursing infant.

lactar v. lactate.

lácteo, -a adj. lacteal.

láctico, -ca adj. lactic.

lactosa f. lactose.

lactosidosis f. lactosidosis.

ladilla f. crab, crablouse.

lado m. side.

lágrima f. tear.

lágrima artificial artificial tear.

lagrimal¹ m. lacrimal, lachrymal.

lagrimeo m. delacrimation, lacrimation, tearing.

lámina f. lamina.

laminectomía f. laminectomy.

lanceta f. lancet.

lanugo m. lanugo.

laparotomía f. laparotomy.

laparotomía de estadiaje staging laparotomy.

laparotomía exploradora exploration laparotomy.

lapsus m. lapsus.

laringe f. larynx.

laringe artificial artificial larynx.

laríngeo, -a adj. laryngeal.

laringitis f. laryngitis.

laringitis aguda acute catarrhal laryngitis.

laringitis catarral aguda acute catarrhal laryngitis.

laringitis catarral crónica chronic catarrhal laryngitis.

laringitis crupal, laringitis cruposa croupous laryngitis.

laringitis diftérica diphtheritic laryngitis.

laringitis espasmódica spasmodic laryngitis.

laringitis estridulosa laryngitis stridulosa.

laringofaringitis f. laryngopharyngitis.

laringoscopia f. laryngoscopy.

laringoscopia directa direct laryngoscopy.

laringoscopia de espejo indirect laryngoscopy.

laringoscopia indirecta indirect laryngoscopy.

laringoscopio *m.* laryngoscope.

laringospasmo *m.* laryngospasm.

laringotomía *f.* laryngotomy.

laringuectomía *f.* laryngectomy.

laringuectomizado, -da[1] *adj.* laryngectomized.

laringuectomizado, -da[2] *m., f.* laryngectomee.

láser *m.* laser.

latencia *f.* latency.

latenciación *f.* latenciation.

lateral *adj.* lateral.

lateralidad *f.* laterality.

latido *m.* beat.

latido cardíaco heart beat.

latido ectópico ectopic beat.

latido de escape escape beat, escaped beat.

latigazo *m.* whiplash.

latitud *f.* latitude.

lavado *m.* lavage.

lavado broncopulmonar bronchopulmonary lavage.

lavado bronquial bronchial lavage.

lavado del estómago gastric lavage.

lavado gástrico gastric lavage, gastrolavage.

lavado general blood lavage.

lavado peritoneal peritoneal lavage.

lavado pleural pleural lavage.

lavado quirúrgico surgical scrub.

lavado de la sangre, lavado sanguíneo blood lavage.

lavado vesical vesical lavage.

lavativa *f.* enema.

laxante *m.* laxative.

laxitud *f.* laxity.

laxo, -xa *adj.* lax.

leche *f.* milk.

lecho *m.* bed.

lecho capilar capillary bed.

lecho ungueal nail bed.

lectura *f.* reading.

lectura de labios, lectura del habla lip reading, speech reading.

legaña *f.* rheum.

legionelosis *f.* legionellosis.

legrado *m.* curettage.

legrado uterino curettage.

leiomioma *m.* leiomyoma.

leishmaniosis *f.* leishmaniosis, leishmaniasis.

lengua *f.* tongue, lingua.

lengua fisurada, lingua fissurata fissured tongue, lingua fissurata.

lengua saburral furred tongue.

lenguaje[1] *m.* language.

lenguaje corporal body language.

lenguaje sensitivo sensory-based language.

lenguaje de signos sign language.

lenguaje verbal verbal language.

lenguaje[2] *m.* speech.

lente *f.* lens.

lente bifocal bifocal lens.

lente de contacto contact lens.

lentilla *f.* contact lens.

lepra *f.* lepra, leprosy.

lepra cutánea cutaneous leprosy.

lepra lepromatosa lepromatous leprosy.

lepromatoso, -sa *adj.* lepromatous.

leprosería *f.* leprosary.

leproso, -sa *adj.* leper, leprose, leprous.

leptomeninges f. leptomeninges.
leptomeningitis f. leptomeningitis.
leptospirosis f. leptospirosis.
lesbiana adj. lesbian.
lesbianismo m. lesbianism.
lesión f. injury, lesion.
  lesión degenerativa degenerative lesion.
  lesión por desaceleración deceleration injury.
  lesión de descarga discharging lesion.
  lesión del disco intervertebral injury of the intervertebral disk.
  lesión por explosión blast injury.
  lesión histológica histologic lesion.
  lesión macroscópica gross lesion.
  lesión medular medullar lesion.
  lesión orgánica organic lesion.
  lesión vital vital injury.
letal adj. lethal.
letargo m. lethargy.
leucemia f. leukemia.
  leucemia aguda acute leukemia.
  leucemia aguda no linfocítica acute non-lymphocytic leukemia.
  leucemia aguda mieloblástica myeloblastic acute leukemia.
  leucemia granulocítica granulocytic leukemia.
  leucemia linfática lymphatic leukemia.
  leucemia linfoblástica lymphoblastic leukemia.
  leucemia linfoblástica aguda acute lymphoblastic leukemia.
  leucemia linfocítica lymphocytic leukemia.

leucemia linfocítica aguda acute lymphocytic leukemia.
leucemia linfocítica crónica (LLC) chronic lymphocytic leukemia (LLC).
leucemia linfoide lymphoid leukemia.
leucemia megacariocítica megakarycytic leukemia.
leucemia mieloblástica myeloblastic leukemia.
leucemia mielocítica myelocytic leukemia.
leucemia mieloide aguda acute myeloid leukemia.
leucemia mieloide crónica (LMC) chronic myelocytic leukemia.
leucemia mixta mixed leukemia.
leucemia monocítica monocytic leukemia.
leucemia plasmática plasmacytic leukemia.
leucemia prolinfocítica prolymphocytic.
leucémico, -ca adj. leukemic.
leucina f. leucine, leukina.
leucoblasto m. leukoblast.
leucocitario, -a adj. leukocytic, leukocytal.
leucocito m. leukocyte.
  leucocito basófilo basophilic leukocyte.
  leucocito cebado mast leukocyte.
  leucocito eosinófilo eosinophilic leukocyte.
  leucocito inmóvil non-motile leukocyte.
  leucocito linfoide lymphoid leukocyte.

leucocito multinuclear multinuclear leukocyte.

leucocito neutrófilo neutrophilic leukocyte.

leucocito polimorfonuclear polymorphonuclear leukocyte.

leucocito polinuclear polynuclear leukocyte.

leucocito segmentado segmented leukocyte.

leucocitólisis *f.* leukocytolysis.

leucocitosis *f.* leukocytosis.

leucocitosis absoluta absolute leukocytosis.

leucocitosis linfocítica lymphocytic leukocytosis.

leucocitosis monocítica monocytic leukocytosis.

leucocitosis mononuclear mononuclear leukocytosis.

leucocitosis del neonato leukocytosis of the newborn.

leucocitosis neutrófila neutrophilic leukocytosis.

leucocitosis patológica pathologic leukocytosis.

leucocituria *f.* leukocyturia.

leucodermia *f.* leukoderma, leukodermia.

leucodistrofia *f.* leukodystrophy.

leucoencefalitis *f.* leukencephalitis.

leucoencefalopatía *f.* leukoencephalopathy.

leucograma *m.* leukogram.

leucopenia *f.* leukopenia.

leucoplasia *f.* leukoplasia.

leucorrea *f.* leukorrhea.

leucosis *f.* leukosis.

levadura *f.* yeast.

leve¹ *adj.* laeve.

leve² *adj.* mild.

levocardia *f.* levocardia.

ley *f.* law.

ley de Mendel Mendel's law.

líbido *f.* libido.

libre elección de médico *f.* free choice of doctor.

lifting *m.* lifting.

lifting facial facial lifting.

ligado, -da *adj.* linked.

ligado al sexo sex-linked.

ligado a X X-linked.

ligado a Y Y-linked.

ligadura¹ *f.* ligation.

ligadura² *f.* ligature.

ligadura quirúrgica surgical ligature.

ligamento *m.* ligament, ligamentum.

lijado *m.* grinding.

lima *f.* file.

lima endodóntica endodontic file.

límbico, -ca *adj.* limbic.

limpieza *f.* cleaning, clearance.

linaje *m.* lineage.

linaje celular cell lineage.

línea *f.* line, linea.

línea celular cell line.

línea epifisaria epiphysial line.

lineal *adj.* linear.

linfa *f.* lymph.

linfadenitis *f.* lymphadenitis.

linfadenopatía *f.* lymphadenopathy.

linfangioma *m.* lymphangioma.

linfangitis *f.* lymphangitis.

linfático, -ca *adj.* lymphatic.

linfocítico, -ca *adj.* lymphocytic.

linfocito *m.* lymphocyte.
linfocito asesino killer lymphocyte.
linfocito B B lymphocyte.
linfocito T T lymphocyte.
linfocito T amplificador amplifier T lymphocyte.
linfocito T ayudador helper T lymphocyte.
linfocito T citotóxicos cytotoxic T lymphocyte.
linfocito transformado transformed lymphocyte.
linfocitosis *f.* lymphocitosis.
linfoide *adj.* lymphoid.
linfoma *m.* lymphoma.
linfoma de Hodgkin Hodgkin's lymphoma.
linfopatía *f.* lymphopathy, lymphopathia.
lingual *adj.* lingual, lingualis.
lipasa *f.* lipase.
lipemia *f.* lipemia.
lipídico, -ca *adj.* lipidic.
lípido *m.* lipid.
lipidosis *f.* lipidosis.
lipoatrofia *f.* lipoatrophia.
lipodistrofia *f.* lipodystrophy, lipodystrophia.
lipoide *adj.* lipoid.
lipoidosis *f.* lipoidosis.
lipoma *m.* lipoma.
lipomatosis *f.* lipomatosis.
lipoproteína *f.* lipoprotein.
liposoluble *adj.* liposoluble.
liposoma *m.* liposome.
liposucción *f.* liposuction.
lipotimia *f.* lipothymia.
liquen *m.* lichen.

liquen plano lichen planus.
líquido *m.* fluid, liquid, liquor.
líquido amniótico amniotic fluid.
líquido ascítico ascitic fluid.
líquido cefalorraquídeo cerebrospinal fluid, liquor cerebrospinalis.
líquido extravascular extravascular fluid.
líquido intersticial interstitial fluid.
líquido intracelular intracellular fluid.
líquido intraocular intraocular fluid.
líquido pericárdico pericardial fluid.
líquido peritoneal peritoneal fluid.
líquido pleural pleural fluid.
líquido prostático prostatic fluid.
líquido seminal seminal fluid.
líquido sinovial synovial fluid.
líquido tisular tissue fluid.
líquido, -da *adj.* liquid.
lisa *f.* lyssa, lyse.
lisado, -da *adj.* lysate.
lisosoma *m.* lysosome.
litiasis *f.* lithiasis.
litiasis pancreática pancreatic lithiasis.
litiasis urinaria urinary lithiasis.
litotomía *f.* lithotomy.
litotricia *f.* lithotrity.
lividez *f.* lividity.
lividez cadavérica livor mortis.
lividez postmortem postmortem lividity.
lívido, -da *adj.* livid.
llaga *f.* sore.
llaga por presión pressure sore.

lobotomía *f.* lobotomy.

lobulación *f.* lobulation, lobation.

lóbulo *m.* lobe, lobus.

local *adj.* local.

localización *f.* localization.

loción *f.* lotion, lotio.

loco, -ca *adj.* insane, mad.

logopeda *m.* speech-language pathologist.

logopedia *f.* logopedia, logopedics, speech pathology.

lombriz *f.* lumbricus.

longevidad *f.* longevity.

longitud *f.* length.

longitudinal *adj.* longitudinal, longitudinalis.

loquios *m.* lochia.

lordoescoliosis *f.* lordoscoliosis.

lordosis *f.* lordosis.

lucidez *f.* lucidity.

lúcido, -da *adj.* lucid.

ludopatía *f.* gambling.

ludoterapia *f.* play therapy.

lúes *f.* lues.

lugar *m.* site, locus.

lumbago *m.* lumbago.

lumbalgia *f.* low back pain.

lumbar *adj.* lumbar.

lupus *m.* lupus.

   lupus eritematoso sistémico (LES) systemic lupus erythematosus (SLE).

luteína *f.* lutein.

luteinización *f.* luteinization.

lúteo, -a *adj.* luteal.

luxación *f.* dislocation, luxation, luxatio.

   luxación de cadera dislocation of the hip.

   luxación de la clavícula dislocation of the clavicle.

   luxación completa complete dislocation.

   luxación complicada complicated luxation.

   luxación congénita congenital dislocation.

   luxación del cristalino dislocation of the lens.

   luxación dentaria dental luxation.

   luxación y fractura fractura dislocation.

   luxación del hombro dislocation of the shoulder.

   luxación incompleta incomplete dislocation.

   luxación recidivante habitual dislocation.

   luxación de la rodilla dislocation of the knee.

   luxación simple simple dislocation.

luxus luxus.

lux *f.* light, lux.

luz *f.* light, lux.

   luz infrarroja infrared light.

   luz ultravioleta ultraviolet light.

M

macerado *m.* macerate.

macerar *v.* macerate.

macroangiopatía *f.* macroangiopathy.

macrobiótico, -ca *adj.* macrobiotic.

macrobiótica *f.* macrobiotics.

macrocito *m.* macrocyte.

macrocitosis *f.* macrocytosis.

macrófago *m.* macrophage.

macroglobulina *f.* macroglobulin.

macroglobulinemia *f.* macroglobulinemia.

macroglosia *f.* macroglossia.

macrognatia *f.* macrognathia.

macrognatismo *m.* macrognathia.

macrólido *m.* macrolide.

macroscopia *f.* macroscopy.

macroscópico, -ca *adj.* macroscopic, macroscopical.

macrosigmoide *m.* macrosigmoid.

macrosis *f.* macrosis.

mácula, macula *f.* macula.

  mácula corneal macula corneae.

  mácula mongólica mongolian macula.

  mácula de la retina macula retinae.

maculopápula *f.* maculopapule.

madre *f. y adj.* mother.

  madre de alquiler surrogate mother.

maduración *f.* maturation.

  maduración cervical cervical maturation.

  maduración ósea bone maturation.

maduro, -ra *adj.* mature.

magma *m.* magma.

magnesio *m.* magnesium.

magnificación *f.* magnification.

mal *m.* mal.

  mal de altura mountain sickness.

  mal de los aviadores airsickness, aviator's disease.

  mal de las montañas mountain sickness.

  mal de Pott, mal vertebral de Pott Pott's disease.

  mal de riñones lumbago.

  mal venéreo syphilis.

malabsorción *f.* malabsorption.

  malabsorción congénita de lactosa congenital lactose malabsorption.

mala práctica *f.* malpractice.

maladaptado, -da *adj.* maladjusted.

maladaptación *f.* maladjustment.

maladigestión *f.* maldigestion.

malaerupción *f.* maleruption.

malar *adj.* malar.

malaria *f.* malaria.

malárico, -ca *adj.* malarious.

maldesarrollo *m.* maldevelopment.

maldigestión *f.* maldigestion.

malear *adj.* mallear.

maleolar *adj.* malleolar.

maléolo *m.* malleolus.

malestar *m.* malaise.

  malestar general malaise.

  malestar gravídico matutino morning sickness.

malformación *f.* malformation.

malignidad *f.* malignancy.

maligno, -na *adj.* malignant.

malla *f.* mesh.

malnutrición *f.* malnutrition.

  malnutrición proteicocalórica energy-protein malnutrition.

maloclusión *f.* malocclusion.

  maloclusión de mordida abierta open-bite malocclusion.

  maloclusión de mordida cerrada close-bite malocclusion.

malos tratos *m.* abuse.

  malos tratos a menores child abuse.

malos tratos al anciano abuse of the elderly, elder abuse.

malos tratos emocionales emotional abuse.

malos tratos físicos physical abuse.

malos tratos sexuales sexual abuse.

malpraxis *f.* malpraxis.

maltrato *m.* maltreatment.

mama *f.* breast, mamma.

mama accesorias (femeninas y masculinas) mammae accessoriae femininae et masculinae.

mama masculina mamma masculina.

mama supernumerarias supernumerary mammae.

mamalgia *f.* mamalgia.

mamaplastia *f.* mammaplasty.

mamilitis *f.* mamillitis, mammillitis.

mamitis *f.* mammitis.

mamografía *f.* mammography.

mamografía de barrido film screen mammography.

mamográfico, -ca *adj.* mammographic.

mamógrafo *m.* mammograph.

mamograma *m.* mammogram.

mamoplastia *f.* mammoplasty.

mamoplastia de aumento augmentation mammoplasty.

mamoplastia reconstructiva reconstructive mammoplasty.

mamoplastia de reducción reduction mammoplasty.

mancha *f.* dot, spot, tache.

mancha de café con leche café au lait spot.

mancha cerúlea macula caerulea.

mancha de color rojo de cereza cherry-red spot.

mancha de la córnea, mancha corneana corneal spot.

mancha de Fuchs Fuchs' spot.

mancha melánica pigmented nevus.

mancha mongólica Mongolian spot.

mancha rojo cereza cherry-red spot.

mancha en vino de Oporto Port wine spot.

manchado *m.* spotting.

manco, -ca *adj.* one-armed, armless.

mandíbula *f.* mandible.

mandíbula inferior lower mandible.

mandíbula superior upper mandible.

mandibular *adj.* mandibular.

mango *m.* handle.

manguito *m.* cuff.

manguito rotador del hombro rotator cuff.

manía *f.* mania.

manía megalomanía megalomania.

maníaco, -ca *adj.* maniac.

maniacodepresivo, -va *adj.* maniac-depressive.

manicomio *m.* mental hospital.

manifestación *f.* manifestation.

maniobra *f.* maneuver.

maniobra de aspiración aspirant maneuver.

maniobra de Valsalva Valsalva's maneuver.

manipulación *f.* manipulation.

manipulación genética genetic manipulation.

manipulación vertebral spinal manipulation.

mano *f.* hand, main, manus.

mano caída drop hand.

mano de cangrejo crab hand.

mano de comadrón accoucheur's hand, main d'accoucheur.

mano congelada frozen hand.

mano de escritor writing hand.

mano esquelética, mano de esqueleto skeleton hand, main en squelette.

mano extendida manus extensa.

mano en flexión manus flexa.

mano en garra claw hand.

mano muerta dead hand.

mano obstétrica obstetrical hand.

mano péndula drop hand.

mano vara manus vara.

mano zamba club hand.

manometría *f.* manometry.

manómetro *m.* manometer.

manómetro aneroide aneroid manometer.

manómetro de dial dial manometer.

manómetro diferencial differential manometer.

manómetro mercurial, manómetro de mercurio mercurial manometer.

manta *f.* blanket.

manta de baño bath blanket.

manta de hipotermia hypothermia blanket.

manual *adj.* manual.

mapa *m.* map.

mapa de actividad eléctrica cerebral (MAEC) brain electric activity map (BEAM).

mapa citológico cytologic map.

mapa cognitivo cognitive map.

mapa cromosómico chromosomal map.

mapa físico physical map.

mapa de ligadura, mapa de ligamiento linkage map.

mapa óseo bone map.

máquina *f.* machine, engine.

máquina cardiopulmonar heart-lung machine.

máquina corazón-púlmón heart-lung machine.

máquina quirúrgica surgical engine.

máquina renal kidney machine.

marasmo *m.* marasmus.

marca *f.* mark.

marca de fresa strawberry mark.

marca de nacimiento birth mark, birthmark.

marca registrada trademark.

marcador *m.* marker.

marcador bioquímico biochemical marker.

marcador celular de superficie cell-surface marker.

marcador genético genetic marker.

marcador radiactivo radioactive label.

marcador tumoral tumor marker.

marcador *m.* marker.

marcaje *m.* label.

marcaje radiactivo radioactive label.

marcapaso *m.* pacemaker.

marcapasos *m.* pacemaker.
  marcapaso cardíaco cardiac.
  marcapaso ectópico ectopic pacemaker.
  marcapaso errante wandering pacemaker.
  marcapaso externo external pacemaker.
marcha *f.* gait, walk.
  marcha antálgica antalgic gait.
  marcha atáxica ataxic gait.
  marcha cerebelosa cerebellar gait.
  marcha espástica spastic gait.
  marcha oscilante cerebellar gait.
  marcha de Trendelenburg Trendelenburg gait.
marea *f.* tide.
mareado, -da *adj.* sick.
mareo *m.* dizziness, giddiness.
margen *m.* margin, margo.
  margen anterior anterior margin.
  margen inferior inferior margin.
  margen lateral lateral.
  margen medial medial.
  margen posterior posterior.
  margen de seguridad margin of safety.
  margen superior superior margin.
marginación *f.* margination.
marginal *adj.* marginal.
marinoterapia *f.* medulla ossium rubra.
marmóreo, -a *adj.* marmoreal, marble.
masaje *m.* massage.
  masaje cardíaco cardiac massage, heart massage.
  masaje cardíaco externo external cardiac massage.

  masaje electrovibratorio electrovibratory massage.
  masaje gingival gingival massage.
  masaje prostático prostatic massage.
  masaje vibratorio vibratory massage.
masajista *m., f.* masseur.
masculinidad *f.* masculinity.
masculinización *f.* masculinization.
masculinizar *v.* masculinize.
masoterapia *f.* massotherapy.
mastadenitis *f.* mastadenitis.
mastalgia *f.* mastalgia.
mastectomía *f.* mastectomy.
  mastectomía lumpectomía mastectomy lumpectomy.
  mastectomía radical radical mastectomy.
  mastectomía radical ampliada extended radical mastectomy.
  mastectomía radical modificada modified radical mastectomy.
  mastectomía simple simple mastectomy.
  mastectomía subcutánea subcutaneous mastectomy.
  mastectomía total total mastectomy.
masticación *f.* mastication.
masticatorio, -ria *adj.* masticatory.
mastitis *f.* mastitis.
  mastitis aguda acute mastitis.
  mastitis neonatal mastitis neonatorum.
  mastitis quística cystic mastitis.
  mastitis del recién nacido mastitis neonatorum.
  mastitis retromamaria retromammary mastitis.

mastocito *m.* mastocyte, mast-cell.

mastocitoma *m.* mastocytoma.

mastocitosis *f.* mastocytosis.

mastodinia *f.* mastodynia.

mastografía *f.* mastography.

mastograma *m.* mastogram.

mastoidectomía *f.* mastoidectomy.

mastoideo, -a *adj.* mastoid.

mastoiditis *f.* mastoiditis.

mastopatía *f.* mastopathy.

  mastopatía fibroquística fibrocystic disease.

masturbación *f.* masturbation.

materia *f.* matter, materia.

material *m.* material.

  material dental dental material.

  material genético genetic material.

  material de sutura suture material.

maternal *adj.* maternal.

maternidad *f.* motherhood, maternity.

  maternidad de alquiler surrogate motherhood.

  maternidad genética genetic motherhood.

  maternidad gestacional gestational motherhood.

  maternidad legal legal motherhood.

  maternidad subrogada surrogate motherhood.

materno, -na *adj.* maternal.

matriz[1] *f.* matrix.

matriz[2] *f.* matrix.

  matriz de la uña nail matrix, matrix unguis.

  matriz ungueal nail matrix, matrix unguis.

matrona *f.* midwife.

maxilar[1] *m.* jaw, maxilla.

maxilar[2] *adj.* maxillary.

maxilodental *adj.* maxillodental.

máximo *m.* maximum.

meato *m.* meatus.

mecánica *f.* mechanics.

mecanismo *m.* mechanism.

  mecanismo de asociación association.

  mecanismo de defensa defense mechanism.

  mecanismo del dolor pain mechanism.

  mecanismo inmunológico immunological mechanism.

  mecanismo mental mental mechanism.

  mecanismo del parto mechanism of labor.

  mecanismo propioceptivo proprioceptive mechanism.

mecanorreceptor *m.* mechanoreceptor.

meconio *m.* meconium.

media *f.* mean.

  media aritmética arithmetic mean.

  error estándar de la media standard error of the mean.

  media muestral sample mean.

  media de la población population mean.

mediador *m.* mediator.

medial *adj.* medial, medialis.

mediana *f.* median.

mediano, -na *adj.* median.

mediastínico, -ca *adj.* mediastinal.

mediastinitis *f.* mediastinitis.

mediastino *m.* mediastinum.

medicable *adj.* medicable.

medicación *f.* medication.

medicación conservadora conservative medication.

medicación derivativa substitutive medication.

medicación hipodérmica hypodermic medication.

medicación intravenosa intravenous medication.

medicación iónica ionic medication.

medicación preanestésica preanesthetic medication.

medicación sublingual sublingual medication.

medicación sustitutiva substitutive medication.

medicación transduodenal transduodenal medication.

medicado, -da *adj.* medicated.

medicamento *m.* drug, medicine.

medicamento compuesto compound medicine.

medicamento patentado proprietary medicine.

medicamento sin receta patent medicine.

medicamentoso, -sa *adj.* medicamentous.

medicina *f.* medicine.

medicina alternativa alternative medicine.

medicina basada en la evidencia evidence based medicine.

medicina ciéntifica scientific medicine.

medicina clínica clinical medicine.

medicina comparada comparative medicine.

medicina comunitaria medicine community.

medicina del deporte, medicina deportiva sports medicine.

medicina experimental experimental medicine.

medicina de familia, medicina familiar family medicine.

medicina fetal fetal medicine.

medicina forense forensic medicine.

medicina geriátrica geriatric medicine.

medicina interna internal medicine.

medicina legal legal medicine.

medicina neonatal neonatal medicine.

medicina osteopática osteopathic medicine.

medicina pediátrica pediatric medicine.

medicina perinatal perinatal medicine.

medicina preventiva preventive medicine.

medicina psicosomática psychosomatic medicine.

medicina del trabajo occupational medicine.

medicina tropical tropical medicine.

medicina de urgencia emergency medicine.

medición *f.* measurement.

médico, -ca *m., f.* physician.

médico de atención primaria primary care physician.

médico de cabecera general practitioner.

médico de urgencia emergency physician.

médico especialista specialist.

médico de familia family physician.

médico generalista general practitioner.

médico osteópata osteopathic physician.

médico residente resident physician.

médico, -ca *adj.* medical.

medida *f.* measure.

medidor *m.* meter.

medio *m.* average, medium.

medio de contraste contrast medium.

medio de contraste radiactivo radioactive contrast medium.

medio de cultivo culture medium.

medio externo external medium, milieu extérieur.

medio interno milieu intérieur.

médula *f.* marrow, medulla.

megacariocito *m.* megakaryocyte.

megacolon *m.* megacolon.

mejilla *f.* cheek.

mejoría *f.* amelioration.

melanina *f.* melanin.

melanocito *m.* melanocyte.

melanocitoma *m.* melanocytoma.

melanoma *m.* melanoma.

melanoma cutáneo primario primary cutaneous melanoma.

melanoma juvenil, melanoma juvenil benigno juvenile melanoma, benign juvenile melanoma.

melanoma maligno malignant melanoma.

melanoma maligno in situ in situ malignant melanoma.

melanoma nodular nodular melanoma.

melanoma de úvea choroidal melanoma.

melanosis *f.* melanosis.

melasma *m.* melasma.

melasma gravídico, melasma uterino melasma gravidarum.

melasma suprarrenal melasma suprarenale.

melatonina *f.* melatonin.

melena *f.* melena.

melena neonatal, melena del recién nacido melena neonatorum.

melena verdadera melena vera.

mellizo *m.* sibling.

membrana *f.* membrane, membrana.

membrana aracnoidea arachnoid membrane.

membrana celular cell membrane.

membrana diftérica diphtheritic membrane.

membrana embrionaria embryonic membrane.

membrana hialina hyaline membrane.

membrana del huevo egg membrane.

membrana nuclear nuclear membrane.

membrana placentaria placental membrane.

membrana plasmática plasma membrane.

membrana vitelina viteline membrane.

membranoso, -sa *adj.* webbed, membranous.

memoria *f.* memory.

memoria anterógrada anterograde memory.

memoria a corto plazo (MCP) short-term memory (STM).

memoria inmunológica inmunologic memory.

memoria a largo plazo (MLP) long term memory (LTM).

memoria retrógrada retrograde memory.

memoria selectiva selective memory.

memoria senil senile memory.

memoria visual visual memory.

menarca *f.* menarche.

menarquia *f.* menar-che.

mendeliano, -na *adj.* Mendelian.

meninge *f.* meninx.

meníngeo, -a *adj.* meningeal.

meninginitis *f.* meninginitis.

meningioma *m.* meningioma, meningeoma, meningoma.

meningismo *m.* meningism.

meningítico, -ca *adj.* meningitic.

meningitis *f.* meningitis.

meningitis aséptica, meningitis aséptica aguda aseptic meningitis, acute aseptic meningitis.

meningitis bacteriana bacterial meningitis.

meningitis cefalorraquídea cerebrospinal meningitis.

meningitis cerebral cerebral meningitis.

meningitis cerebroespinal cerebrospinal meningitis.

meningitis meningocócica meningococcal meningitis.

meningitis neoplásica neoplastic meningitis.

meningitis neumocócica pneumococcal meningitis.

meningitis serosa circunscrita, meningitis serosa circunscrita quística meningitis serosa circumscripta.

meningitis traumática traumatic meningitis.

meningitis viral, meningitis virásica viral meningitis.

meningocele *m.* meningocele.

meningocicemia *f.* meningococcemia.

meningocicemia fulminante aguda acute fulminating meningococcemia.

meningococia *f.* meningococcemia.

meningococo *m.* meningococci.

meningoencefalitis *f.* meningoencephalitis.

meniscal *adj.* meniscal.

meniscectomía *f.* meniscectomy.

meniscitis *f.* meniscitis.

menisco *m.* meniscus.

menopausia *f.* menopause.

menopausia artificial artificial menopause.

menopausia masculina male menopause.

menopausia precoz, menopausia prematura menopause praecox.

menopausia quirúrgica surgical menopause.

menopáusico, -ca *adj.* menopausal.

menorrea *f.* menorrhea.

menorreico, -ca *adj.* menorrheal.

mensajero *m.* messenger.

segundo mensajero second messenger.

menstruación *f.* menstruation.

menstruación anovular, menstruación anovulatoria anovular menstruation, anovulatory menstruation.

menstruación no ovulatoria nonovulational menstruation.

menstruación retrasada delayed menstruation.

menstruación retrógrada regurgitant menstruation, retrograde menstruation.

menstruación sin ovulación nonovulational menstruation.

menstruación suprimida suppressed menstruation.

menstruación sustitutiva vicarious menstruation.

menstrual *adj.* menstrual.

menstruar *v.* menstruate.

menstruo *m.* menstruum.

mental *adj.* mental.

mentalidad *f.* mentality.

mente *f.* mind.

mentón *m.* chin, menton, mentum.

mentoplastia *f.* mentoplasty.

meralgia *f.* meralgia.

mercurio *m.* mercury.

mesa *f.* table.

mesa basculante tilt table.

mesa de examen examining table.

mesa inclinada tilt table.

mesa de laparotomía lap-board.

mesa de operaciones operating table.

mesangial *adj.* mesangial.

mesangio *m.* mesangium.

mesencefalitis *f.* mesencephalitis.

mesencéfalo *m.* mesencephalon.

mesénquima *m.* mesenchyma.

mesenquimatoso, -sa *adj.* mesenchymal.

mesenquimoma *m.* mesenchymoma.

mesentérico, -ca *adj.* mesenteric.

mesenterio *m.* mesentery, mesenterium.

meseta *m.* plateau.

mesial *adj.* mesial, mesially.

mesocardio *m.* mesocardium.

mesodermo *m.* mesoderm.

mesodermo intraembrionario intraembryonic mesoderm.

mesotelial *adj.* mesothelial.

mesotelio *m.* mesothelium.

mesotelioma *m.* mesothelioma.

mestizo, -za *adj.* half-caste.

meta *f.* goal.

metaalbúmina *f.* metalbumin.

metabólico, -ca *adj.* metabolic.

metabolismo *m.* metabolism.

metabolismo acidobásico acid-base metabolism.

metabolismo anaeróbico anaerobic metabolism.

metabolismo basal basal metabolism.

metabolismo de carbohidratos carbohydrate metabolism.

metabolismo del colesterol cholesterol metabolism.

metabolismo de los electrólitos electrolyte metabolism.

metabolismo endógeno endogenous metabolism.

metabolismo energético energy metabolism.

metabolismo exógeno exogenous metabolism.

metabolismo farmacológico drug metabolism.

metabolismo de las grasas, metabolismo graso fat metabolism.

metabolismo de los hidratos de carbono carbohydrate metabolism.

metabolismo del hierro iron metabolism.

metabolismo intermediario intermediary metabolism.

metabolismo proteico, metabolismo de las proteínas protein metabolism.

metabolismo renal renal metabolism.

metabolismo respiratorio respiratory metabolism.

metabolito *m.* metabolite.

metabolizable *adj.* metabolizable.

metabolizar *v.* metabolize.

metacarpiano, -na *adj.* metacarpal.

metacarpo *m.* metacarpus.

metacarpofalángico, -ca *adj.* metacarpophalangeal.

metadona *f.* methadone.

metafase *f.* metaphase.

metafisario, -ria *adj.* metaphyseal, metaphysial.

metáfisis *f.* metaphysis.

metafisitis *f.* metaphysitis.

metahemoglobina *f.* methemoglobin.

metahemoglobinemia *f.* methemoglobinemia.

metal *m.* metal.

metálico, -ca *adj.* metallic.

metamorfosis *f.* metamorphosis.

metaplasia *f.* metaplasia.

metaplásico, -ca *adj.* metaplastic.

metastásico, -ca *adj.* metastatic.

metástasis *f.* metastasis.

metástasis bioquímica biochemical metastasis.

metástasis calcárea calcareous metastasis.

metástasis de contacto contact metastasis.

metástasis cruzada crossed metastasis.

metástasis directa direct metastasis.

metástasis paradójica paradoxical metastasis.

metástasis pulsátil pulsating metastasis.

metástasis retrógrada retrograde metastasis.

metástasis satélite satellite metastasis.

metastático, -ca *adj.* metastatic.

metatarsalgia *f.* metatarsalgia.

metatarsectomía *f.* metatarsectomy.

metatarsiano, -na *adj.* metatarsal.

metatarso *m.* metatarsus.

metilación *f.* methylation.

metilado, -da *adj.* methylated.

metilcelulosa *f.* methylcellulose.

método *m.* method.

método del calendario de planificación familiar calendar method of family planning.

método comparativo comparative.

método contraceptivo contraceptive method.

método *correlativo* correlational method.

método de cortes transversales cross-sectional method.

método de difusión diffusion method.

método directo direct method.

método empírico trial and error method.

método experimental experimental method.

método natural natural method.

método de la ovulación para planificación familiar ovulation method of family planning.

método de planificación familiar del moco cervical cervical mucus method of family planning.

método de planificación familiar mediante la temperatura basal basal body temperature method of family planning.

método de planificación familiar natural natural family planning method.

método de la retirada withdrawal method.

método del ritmo rhythm method.

método de temperatura basal basal temperature method.

metodología *f.* methodology.

metritis *f.* metritis.

metro *m.* meter.

metrorrea *f.* metrorrhea.

mezcla *f.* mixture.

mialgia *f.* myalgia.

mialgia abdominal myalgia abdominis.

mialgia cefálica myalgia capitis.

mialgia cervical myalgia cervicalis.

mialgia craneal myalgia capitis.

mialgia epidémica epidemic myalgia.

mialgia lumbar lumbar myalgia.

mialgia térmica myalgia thermica.

miastenia *f.* myasthenia.

miastenia grave, miastenia grave seudoparalítica myasthenia gravis, myasthenia gravis pseudoparalytica.

miastenia neonatal neonatal myasthenia.

miasténico, -ca *adj.* myasthenic.

micción *f.* miction, urination.

micción en dos tiempos pis en deux temps.

micción involuntaria enuresis.

micción precipitante precipitant urination.

micción refleja enuresis.

micción tartamuda, micción tartamudeante stuttering urination.

micela *f.* micella, micelle.

micelio *m.* mycelium.

micelio aéreo aerial mycelium.

micobacteria *f.* mycobacteria.

micología *f.* mycology.

micólogo, -ga *m.* mycologist.

micosis *f.* mycosis.

micosis cutánea tinea.

micosis crónica mycosis chronica.

micosis fungoides mycosis fungoides.

micosis interdigital athlete's foot.

micosis intestinal, micosis intestinalis mycosis intestinalis.

micótico, -ca *adj.* mycotic.

microabsceso *m.* microabscess.

microadenoma *m.* microadenoma

microadenopatía *f.* microadenopathy.

microalbuminuria *f.* microalbuminuria.

microanatomía *f.* micranatomy.

microanatomista *m., f.* microanatomist.

microbicida[1] *m.* microbicide.

microbicida[2] *adj.* microbicidal.

microbio *m.* microbe.

microbiología *f.* microbiology.

microbiológico, -ca *adj.* microbiological.

microbiólogo, -ga *m., f.* microbiologist.

microcefalia *f.* microcephalia, microcephaly.

microcefálico, -ca *adj.* microcephalic, microcephalous.

microcéfalo *m.* microcephalus.

microcirculación *f.* microcirculation.

microcirugía *f.* microsurgery.

microcítico, -ca *adj.* microcytic.

micrófono *m.* microphone.

microftalmo *m.* microphthalmus.

microftalmos *m.* microphthalmos.

micrognatia *f.* micrognathia.

microinfarto *m.* microinfarct.

microinjerto *m.* micrograft.

micromanipulación *f.* micromanipulation.

microquiste *m.* microcyst.

microscopía *f.* microscopy.

microscopía clínica clinical microscopy.

microscopía electrónica electron microscopy.

microscopía electrónica de barrido scanning electron microscopy.

microscopía electrónica de barrido de transmisión (MEBT) transmission scanning electron microscopy (TSEM).

microscopía de fluorescencia, microscopía fluorescente fluorescence microscopy.

microscopía de fondo, microscopía fúndica fundus microscopy.

microscopía de inmersión immersion microscopy.

microscopía inmunoelectrónica immune electron microscopy.

microscopía de inmunofluorescencia, microscopía inmunofluorescente immunofluorescence microscopy.

microscopía ultravioleta ultraviolet microscopy.

microscópico, -ca *adj.* microscopic, microscopical.

microscopio *m.* microscope.

microscopio de barrido scanning microscope.

microscopio de campo oscuro dark-field microscope.

microscopio compuesto compound microscope.

microscopio electrónico electron microscope.

microscopio electrónico de barrido (MEG) scanning electron microscope (SEM).

microscopio electrónico de barrido de transmisión transmission scanning electron microscope.

microscopio de lámpara de hendidura slit lamp microscope.

microscopio láser laser microscope.

microscopio de luz light microscope.

microscopio de luz polarizada polarizing microscope.

microscopio de operaciones, microscopio operatorio operating microscope.

microscopio quirúrgico operating microscope.

microscopista *m., f.* microscopist.

microsección *f.* microsection.

microsutura *f.* microsuture.

microtomo *m.* microtome.

midriasis *f.* mydriasis.

midriasis alternante alternating mydriasis.

midriasis amaurótica amaurotic mydriasis.

midriasis artificial pharmacologic mydriasis.

midriasis espasmódica spasmodic mydriasis.

midriasis espástica spastic mydriasis.

midriasis espinal spinal mydriasis.

midriasis farmacológica pharmacologic mydriasis.

midriasis paralítica paralytic mydriasis.

midriático, -ca *adj.* mydriatic.

miedo *m.* fear.

miel *f.* honey.

mielina *f.* myelin.

mielínico, -ca *adj.* myelinic.

mielinización *f.* myelinization.

mielinizado, -da *adj.* myelinated.

mielitis *f.* myelitis.

mielitis aguda acute myelitis.

mielitis ascendente, mielitis ascendente aguda ascending myelitis, acute ascending myelitis.

mielitis bulbar bulbar myelitis.

mielitis central central myelitis.

mielitis por compresión compression myelitis.

mielitis por conmoción concussion myelitis.

mielitis crónica chronic myelitis.

mielitis descendente descending myelitis.

mielitis difusa diffuse myelitis.

mielitis diseminada disseminated myelitis.

mielitis hemorrágica hemorrhagic myelitis.

mielitis neuroóptica neuro-optic myelitis.

mielitis transversa, mielitis transversal transverse myelitis.

mielitis transversa aguda, mielitis transversal aguda acute transverse myelitis.

mielitis traumática traumatic myelitis.

mielitis por vacuna postvaccinal myelitis, myelitis vaccinia.

mieloblasto *m.* myeloblast.

mielocito *m.* myelocyte.

mieloide *adj.* myeloid.

mieloma *m.* myeloma.

mieloma de células plasmática plasma cell myeloma.

mieloma múltiple multiple myeloma.

mielopatía *f.* myelopathy.

mielopoyético, -ca *adj.* myelopoietic.

mieloproliferativo, -va *adj.* myeloproliferative.

mielosis *f.* myelosis.

mielosupresión *f.* myelosuppression.

mielosupresor, -ra *adj.* myelosuppressive.

miembro *f.* limb, member, membrum.

miembro fantasma phantom member.

miembro inferior inferior limb, lower limb, membrum inferius.

miembro de la mujer membrum muliebre.

miembro superior superior limb, upper limb, membrum superius.

miembro torácico thoracic limb.

miembro viril virile member, membrum virile.

migración *f.* migration.

migraña *f.* migraine.

migraña acompañada accompanied migraine.

migraña con aura migraine with aura.

migraña sin aura migraine without aura.

migraña clásica classic migraine.

migraña común common migraine.

migraña fulgurante fulgurating migraine.

migraña hemipléjica hemiplegic migraine.

migraña oftálmica ophthalmic migraine.

migraña oftalmopléjica ophthalmoplegic migraine.

migrañoso, -sa *adj.* migrainous.

miliar *adj.* miliary.

mimetismo *m.* mimicry.

mímica *f.* mimic.

mineral *m.* mineral.

mineralcorticoide *m.* mineralcorticoid.

mineralocorticoide *m.* mineralcorticoid.

mineralización *f.* mineralization.

mineralizado, -da *adj.* mineralized.

mini examen del estado mental *m.* mini mental state examination.

minilaparatomía *f.* minilaparatomy.

mínima *f.* minim.

minimización *f.* minimization.

mínimo *m.* minimum.

mínimo audible minimum audibile.

mínimo cognoscible minimum cognoscibile.

mínimo legible minimum legibile.

mínimo de luz light minimum.

mínimo separable minimum separabile.

mínimo visible visibile minimum.

minusvalía mental *f.* mental handicap.

minusválido, -da *adj.* handicapped.

mioblasto *m.* myoblast.

miocárdico, -ca *adj.* myocardiac, myocardial.

miocardio *m.* myocardium.

miocardiopatía *f.* myocardiopathy.

miocardiopatía alcohólica alcoholic myocardiopathy.

miocardiopatía congestiva congestive myocardiopathy.

miocardiopatía constrictiva constrictive myocardiopathy.

miocardiopatía diabética diabetic myocardiopathy.

miocardiopatía dilatada dilated myocardiopathy.

miocardiopatía hipertrófica hypertrophic myocardiopathy.

miocardiopatía hipertrófica obstructiva hypertrophic obstructive myocardiopathy.

miocardiopatía idiopática idiopathic myocardiopathy.

miocardiopatía infiltrante infiltrative myocardiopathy.

miocardiopatía periparto peripartum myocardiopathy.

miocardiopatía posparto post partum myocardiopathy.

miocardiopatía primaria primary myocardiopathy.

miocardiopatía restrictiva restrictive myocardiopathy.

miocardiopatía secundaria secondary myocardiopathy.

miocarditis *f.* myocarditis.

miocarditis crónica chronic myocarditis.

miocarditis fibrosa fibrous myocarditis.

miocarditis idiopática idiopathic myocarditis.

miocarditis intersticial interstitial myocarditis.

miocarditis reumática rheumatic myocarditis.

miocarditis séptica aguda acute septic myocarditis.

miocarditis tóxica toxic myocarditis.

miocarditis tuberculosa tuberculous myocarditis.

miocito *m.* myocyte.

mioclonía *f.* myoclonia.

mioclonía cortical cortical myoclonia.

mioclonía epiléptica myoclonia epileptica.

mioclonía espinal spinal myoclonia.

mioclonía fibrilar fibrillary myoclonia.

mioclonía focal focal myoclonia.

mioclonía generalizada disseminated myoclonia.

mioclonía múltiple multiplex myoclonia.

mioclonía sensible a los estímulos stimulus sensitive myoclonia.

mioclónico, -ca *adj.* myoclonic.

mioclono *m.* myoclonus.

mioclono nocturno nocturnal myoclonus.

miodistrofia *f.* myodystrophy, myodystrophia.

mioglobina *f.* myoglobin.

mioglobinuria *f.* myoglobinuria.

mioglobulina *f.* myoglobulin.

mioglobulinuria *f.* myoglobulinuria.

miograma *m.* myogram.

mioma *m.* myoma.

miopatía *f.* myopathy.

miopatía alcohólica alcoholic myopathy.

miopatía cardiaca myopathy cordis.

miopatía mitocondrial mitochondrial myopathy.

miopatía ocular ocular myopathy.

miopatía tirotóxica thyrotoxic myopathy.

miope *adj.* myope.

miopericarditis *f.* myopericarditis.

miopía *f.* myopia.

  miopía cromática chromatic myopia.

  miopía de curvatura curvature myopia.

  miopía degenerativa degenerative myopia.

  miopía espacial space myopia.

  miopía maligna malignant myopia.

  miopía nocturna night myopia.

  miopía patológica pathologic myopia.

  miopía prematura premature myopia.

  miopía primaria primary myopia.

  miopía progresiva progressive myopia.

  miopía simple simple myopia.

  miopía transitoria transient myopia.

miorrelajante *adj.* lissive.

miosis *f.* miosis, myosis.

miositis *f.* myositis.

miringitis *f.* myringitis.

miringoplastia *f.* myringoplasty.

miringotomía *f.* myringotomy.

misoginia *f.* misogyny.

mitigar *v.* mitigate.

mitocondria *f.* mitochondria.

mitocondrial *adj.* mitochondrial.

mitomanía *f.* mythomania.

mitosis *f.* mitosis.

  mitosis patológica pathologic mitosis.

mitral *adj.* mitral.

mixedema *m.* myxedema.

  mixedema pretibial pretibial myxedema.

mixoma *m.* myxoma.

  mixoma auricular atrial myxoma.

mixto, -ta *adj.* mixed.

mnemotecnia *f.* mnemotechnics.

moco *m.* mucus.

modalidad *f.* modality.

modelo *m.* cast.

  modelo de diagnóstico diagnostic cast.

  modelo de estudio study cast.

  modelo patrón master cast.

  modelo preoperatorio preoperative cast.

modelo *m.* model.

  modelo médico medical model.

modificación *f.* modification.

  modificación de conducta behavior modification.

moho *m.* mold.

mola *f.* mole.

  mola hidatídica, mole hidatiforme hydatid mole, hydatidiform mole.

  mola maligna malignant mole.

  mola vesicular vesicular mole.

molar *adj.* molar.

molar *m. y adj.* molar.

  molar de los doce años twelfth-year molar.

  primer molar first molar.

  segundo molar second molar.

  molar de los seis años, molar del sexto años sixth-year molar.

  tercer molar third molar, molaris tertius.

  molar supernumerario supernumerary.

molaridad *f.* molarity.

molde *m.* cast.

molécula *f.* molecule.

molécula de adhesión adhesion molecule.

molecular *adj.* molecular.

molusco *m.* molluscum.

molusco contagioso molluscum contagiosum.

mongolismo *m.* mongolism.

mongolismo por traslocación translocation mongolism.

monitor *m.* monitor.

monitor cardíaco cardiac monitor.

monitor fetal electrónico electronic fetal monitor.

monitor Holter Holter monitor.

monitor de presión arterial blood pressure monitor.

monitor de presión venosa central central venous pressure monitor.

monitor de PVC CVP monitor.

monitorizar *v.* monitor.

monoarticular *adj.* monoarticular.

monoartritis *f.* monarthritis.

monocapa *f.* monolayer.

monocigótico, -ca *adj.* monozygotic.

monocigoto, -ta *adj.* monozygous.

monocito *m.* monocyte.

monocitopenia *f.* monocytopenia.

monoclonal *adj.* monoclonal.

monocromático, -ca *adj.* monochromatic.

mononuclear *adj.* mononuclear.

mononucleosis *f.* mononucleosis.

mononucleosis por citomegalovirus cytomegalovirus mononucleosis.

mononucleosis infecciosa infectious mononucleosis.

mononucleótido *m.* mononucleotide.

monóxido *m.* monoxide.

monoxigenasa *f.* monoxygenase.

monstruo *m.* monster, monstrum.

monstruosidad *f.* monstrosity.

monte *m.* mount, mons.

monte de venus mount of venus, mons veneris.

morbididad *f.* morbidity.

mórbido, -da *adj.* morbid.

morbilidad *f.* morbility.

morbosidad *f.* morbidity.

morboso, -sa *adj.* morbid.

mordedura *f.* bite.

mordida *f.* bite.

mordida abierta open bite.

mordida cerrada closed bite.

mordida cruzada cross bite.

mordida normal normal bite.

morfea *f.* morphea.

morfina *f.* morphine.

morfología *f.* morphology.

morfológico, -ca *adj.* morphological.

morgue *f.* morgue.

moribundo, -da *adj.* moribund, dying.

morir *v.* die.

mortalidad *f.* mortality.

mortalidad fetal fetal mortality.

mortalidad infantil infant mortality.

mortalidad maternal maternal mortality.

mortalidad neonatal neonatal mortality.

mortalidad perinatal perinatal mortality.

mortalidad prenatal prenatal mortality.

mortandad *f.* toll.
mortífero, -ra *adj.* deadly.
mortinato, -ta *adj.* stillborn.
mortuorio *m.* mortuary.
mórula *f.* morula.
morulación *f.* morulation.
mosaicismo *m.* mosaicism.
  mosaicismo celular cellular mosaicism.
  mosaicismo cromosómico chromosome mosaicism.
  mosaicismo de genes gene mosaicism.
mosaico *m.* mosaic.
  mosaico cervical colposcopic mosaic.
  mosaico de cromosomas sexuales sex chromosomic mosaic.
  mosaico sexual sex mosaic.
motilidad *f.* motility.
motivación *f.* motivation.
motivo *adj.* motive.
motoneurona *f.* motoneuron.
motricidad *f.* motoricity.
movible *adj.* motile.
movilidad *f.* mobility.
móvil *adj.* motile.
movilización *f.* mobilization.
movilizar *v.* mobilize.
movimiento *m.* movement.
  movimiento activo active movement.
  movimiento asociado associated movement.
  movimiento automático automatic movement.
  movimiento en bisagra hinge movement.
  movimiento ciliar ciliary movement.

movimiento circular circus movement.
movimiento conjugado de los ojos conjugate movement of the eyes.
movimiento no conjugado de los ojos disconjugate movement of the eyes.
movimiento contralateral asociado contralateral associated movement.
movimiento coreico, movimiento coreiforme choreic movement.
movimiento corporal body movement.
movimiento de decorticación decorticated movement, decorticated posturing movement.
movimiento distónico dystonic movement.
movimiento espontáneo spontaneous movement.
movimiento fetal fetal movement.
movimiento de flujo streaming movement.
movimiento forzado forced movement.
movimiento lateral lateral movement.
movimiento mandibular jaw movement, mandibular movement.
movimiento masticatorio masticatory movement.
movimiento del maxilar inferior jaw movement, mandibular movement.
movimiento muscular muscular movement.
movimiento ocular de fijación fixational ocular movement.

movimiento ocular no rápido non-rapid eye movement.

movimiento ocular rápido rapid eye movement (REM).

movimiento paradójico de los párpados paradoxical movement of the eyelids.

movimiento pasivo passive movement.

movimiento pendular pendular movement.

movimiento precordial precordial movement.

movimiento reflejo reflex movement.

movimiento resistido, movimiento de resistencia resistive movement.

movimiento traslatorio, movimiento de traslación translatory movement.

mucina *f.* mucin.

mucinoide *adj.* mucinoid.

mucinosis *f.* mucinosis.

mucocele *m.* mucocele.

mucoide *adj.* mucoid.

mucolítico, -ca *adj.* mucolytic.

mucopurulento, -ta *adj.* mucopurulent.

mucosa *f.* mucosa.

mucosidad *f.* mucus.

mucositis *f.* mucositis.

mucoso, -sa *adj.* mucous.

muda *f.* moulting.

mudo, -da *adj.* dumb, mute.

muela *f.* molar, tooth.

   muela del juicio wisdom tooth.

muermo *m.* glanders, farcy.

muerte *f.* death.

   muerte accidental accidental death.

muerte aparente, mors putativa apparent death.

muerte asistida assisted death.

muerte cardíaca súbita sudden cardiac death.

muerte celular cell death.

muerte cerebral cerebral death.

muerte encefálica brain death.

muerte fetal fetal death.

muerte infantil infant death.

muerte materna maternal death.

muerte natural natural death.

muerte neonatal neonatal death.

muerte neocortical neocortical death.

muerte perinatal perinatal death.

muerte súbita, mors subitanea sudden death unexpected death.

muerte violenta violent death.

muerto, -ta *adj.* dead.

muesca *f.* notch.

muesca *f.* nick.

muestra *f.* sample.

   muestra al azar random sample.

   muestra sesgada biased sample.

muestra *f.* specimen.

   muestra citológica cytologic specimen.

   muestra de esputo sputum specimen.

   muestra miccional aleatoria random voided specimen.

   muestra no contaminada clean-catch specimen.

   muestra de orina de mitad de micción midstream-catch urine specimen.

muestreo *m.* sampling.

   muestreo aleatorio random sampling.

muguet *m.* thrush.

mujer gestante *f.* pregnant woman.

mulato, -ta *m., f. y adj.* mulatto.

muleta *f.* crutch.

multiarticular *adj.* multiarticular.

multicelular *adj.* multicellular.

multifactorial *adj.* multifactorial.

multifocal *adj.* multifocal.

multigrávida *adj.* multigravida.

multilobular *adj.* multilobar.

multilobulillar *adj.* multilobular.

multípara *adj.* multipara.

multiparidad *f.* multiparity.

multíparo, -ra *adj.* multiparous.

múltiple *adj.* multiple.

multiplicación *f.* multiplication.
  multiplicación bacteriana bacterial growth.

multisensibilidad *f.* multisensitivity.

muñeca *f.* wrist.
  muñeca caída wristdrop.
  muñeca de tenis tennis wrist.

muñón *m.* stump.
  muñón cónico conical stump.
  muñón duodenal duodenal stump.
  muñón gástrico gastric stump.
  muñón rectal rectal stump.

murmullo *m.* murmur.
  murmullo venoso venous hum.
  murmullo vesicular vesicular breath sound.

muscarina *f.* muscarinique.

muscarínico, -ca *adj.* muscarinic.

muscular *adj.* muscular.

musculatura *f.* musculature.

músculo *m.* muscle, musculus.
  músculo agonista agonistic muscle.

músculo antagonista antogonistic muscle.

músculo antigravitatorio antigravity muscle.

músculo articular articular muscle.

músculo estriado striated muscle, striped muscle.

músculo extrínseco extrinsic muscle.

músculo de fibra estriada striated muscle, strimped muscle.

músculo de fibra lisa smooth muscle, nonstriated muscle.

músculo intrafusal intrafusal muscle.

músculo intrínseco intrinsic muscle.

músculo involuntario involuntary muscle.

músculo isométrico isometric muscle.

músculo liso smooth muscle, nonstriated muscle.

músculo miotómico myotomic muscle.

músculo principal prime muscle.

músculo voluntario voluntary muscle.

músculo sinérgico synergitic muscle.

musculoaponeurótico, -ca *adj.* musculoaponeurotic.

musculocutáneo, -a *adj.* musculocutaneous.

musculoesquelético, -ca *adj.* musculoskeletal.

musculotendinoso, -sa *adj.* musculotendinous.

musicoterapia *f.* musicotherapy.

muslo *m.* thigh.

mutación *f.* mutation.

mutación alélica allelic mutation.

mutación constitutiva constitutive mutation.

mutación corregida reverse mutation.

mutación cromosómica chromosomal mutation.

mutación espontánea spontaneous mutation.

mutación inducida induced mutation.

mutación por inserción-deleción addition-deletion mutation.

mutación inversa reverse mutation.

mutación letal lethal mutation.

mutación mortal lethal mutation.

mutación natural natural mutation.

mutación neutra neutral mutation.

mutación retrógrada back mutation.

mutación silente silent mutation.

mutación somática somatic mutation.

mutación supresora supressor mutation.

mutación visible visible mutation.

mutagénesis *f.* mutagenesis.

mutagénico, -ca *adj.* mutagenic.

mutágeno *m.* mutagen.

mutante *m. y adj.* mutant.

mutilación *f.* mutilation.

mutilar *v.* maim.

mutismo *m.* mutism.

mutualista *adj.* mutualist.

N

nacarado, -da *adj.* nacreous.

nacido, -da sin asepsia *adj.* born out of asepsis.

nacido, -da vivo, -va *adj.* liveborn.

nacimiento *m.* birth.

nacimiento completo complete birth.

nacimiento múltiple multiple birth.

nacimiento natural natural childbirth.

nacimiento prematuro preterm birth.

nacimiento pretérmino preterm birth.

nacimiento con producto muerto dead birth.

nacimiento tardío post-term birth.

nacimiento transversal cross birth.

nacimiento de vértice head birth.

nada por boca nothing per os (NPO).

nanismo *m.* nanism.

naranja *f.* orange.

narcisismo *m.* narcissism.

narcisista *adj.* narcissistic.

narcolepsia *f.* narcolepsia, narcolepsy.

narcoléptico, -ca *adj.* narcoleptic.

narcosis *f.* narcosis.

narcótico, -ca *adj.* narcotic.

narcótico hipnótico narcotic hypnoytic.

narcótico sedante narcotic sedative.

narcotizar *v.* narcotize.

nariz *f.* nose, nasus.

   nariz de bebedor toper's nose.

   nariz en dorso de silla de montar saddle-back nose.

   nariz en martillo hammer nose.

   nariz respingona upturned nose.

   nariz en silla de montar saddle nose.

nasal *adj.* nasal, nasalis.

nasalidad *f.* nasonnement.

nasalización *f.* snuffling.

nasobucal *adj.* naso-oral.

nasofaringe *f.* nasopharynx.

nasofaríngeo, -a *adj.* nasopharyngeal.

nasofaringitis *f.* nasopharyngitis.

nasolabial *adj.* nasolabial.

nasolacrimal *adj.* nasolacrimal.

natal *adj.* natal.

natalidad *f.* natality.

nativo, -va *adj.* native.

natremia *f.* natremia, natriemia.

natriuresis *f.* natriuresis.

natruresis *f.* natruresis, natriuresis.

natriurético, -ca *adj.* natruretic, natriuretic.

natural *adj.* natural.

naturaleza *f.* nature.

naturópata *m., f.* naturopath.

naturopatía *f.* naturopathy.

naturopático, -ca *adj.* naturopathic.

náusea *f.* nausea.

   náusea gravídica nausea gravidarum.

   náusea marítima nausea marina.

   náusea naval nausea marina.

nauseabundo, -da *adj.* nauseant.

nebulización *f.* spray, nebulization.

nebulizador *m.* nebulizer.

nebulizar *v.* nebulize.

necesidad *f.* necessity, need.

   necesidad básica basic human necessity.

   necesidad diaria mínima (NMD) minimum daily requirement (MDR).

necrobiosis *f.* necrobiosis.

necrofilia *f.* necrophily, necrophilia.

necrófilo *m.* necrophile.

necrófilo, -la *adj.* necrophilous.

necrología *f.* necrology.

necrosante *adj.* necrotizing.

necrosis *f.* necrosis.

   necrosis caseosa cheesy necrosis, caseous necrosis, caseation necrosis.

   necrosis gangrenosa gangrenous necrosis.

   necrosis periférica peripheral necrosis.

   necrosis por presión pressure necrosis.

   necrosis total total necrosis.

necrotizante *adj.* necrotizing.

nefrectomía *f.* nephrectomy.

nefrectomizar *v.* nephrectomize.

néfrico, -ca *adj.* nephric.

nefritis *f.* nephritis.

   nefritis aguda acute nephritis.

   nefritis por analgésicos analgesic nephritis.

   nefritis antimembrana basal antibasement membrane nephritis.

   nefritis arteriosclerótica arteriosclerotic nephritis.

   nefritis bacteriana bacterial nephritis.

   nefritis capsular capsular nephritis.

nefritis caseosa cheesy nephritis, nephritis caseosa, caseous nephritis.

nefritis congénita congenital nephritis.

nefritis crónica chronic nephritis.

nefritis crónica por pérdida de potasio potassium-losing nephritis.

nefritis del embarazo nephritis of pregnancy.

nefritis focal focal nephritis.

nefritis glomerular glomerular nephritis.

nefritis glomerulocapsular glomerulocapsular nephritis.

nefritis hemorrágica hemorrhagic nephritis.

nefritis hereditaria hereditary nephritis.

nefritis hiperazoémica azotemic nephritis.

nefritis por inmunocomplejos immune complex nephritis.

nefritis intersticial interstitial nephritis.

nefritis intersticial aguda acute interstitial nephritis.

nefritis lúpica, nefritis del lupus lupus nephritis.

nefritis mesangial mesangial nephritis.

nefritis parenquimatosa parenchymatous nephritis.

nefritis tubular tubular nephritis, tubal nephritis.

nefritis tubulointersticial tubulointerstitial nephritis.

nefritis tubulointersticial aguda acute tubulointerstitial nephritis.

nefritis tubulointersticial infec- *ciosa* infective tubulointerstitial nephritis.

nefroesclerosis *f.* nephrosclerosis, nephroscleria.

nefroesclerótico, -ca *adj.* nephrosclerotic.

nefrogénico, -ca *adj.* nephrogenetic.

nefrolitotomía *f.* nephrolithotomy.

nefrología *f.* nephrology.

nefrólogo, -ga *m., f.* nephrologist.

nefrona *f.* nephron.

nefropatía *f.* nephropathy, nephropathia.

nefropatía por analgésicos analgesic nephropathy.

nefropatía crónica chronic nephropathy.

nefropatía gravídica toxemia of pregnancy.

nefropatía hipopotasémica hypokalemic nephropathy.

nefropatía por IgA IgA nephropathy.

nefropatía por IgM IgM nephropathy.

nefropatía con pérdida de potasio potassium-losing nephropathy.

nefropatía con pérdida de sal salt-losing nephropathy.

nefropatía postransfusional transfusion nephropathy.

nefropatía de reflujo, nefropatía por reflujo reflux nephropathy.

nefrosclerosis *f.* nephrosclerosis.

nefroscopia *f.* nephroscopy.

nefrosis *f.* nephrosis.

nefrostomía *f.* nephrostomy.

nefrótico, -ca *adj.* nephrotic.

nefrotoxicidad *f.* nephrotoxicity.

nefrotóxico, -ca *adj.* nephrotoxic.

negación *f.* negation, denial.

negatividad *f.* negativity.

negativismo *m.* negativism.

negativo, -va *adj.* negative.

negligencia *f.* negligence.

neissérico, -ca *adj.* neisserial.

neoformación *f.* neoformation.

neonatal *adj.* neonatal.

neonato *m.* baby, neonate.

  neonato azul blue baby.

  neonato malformado malformed neonate.

  neonato prematuro, neonato pretérmino premature infant, preterm infant.

neonatología *f.* neonatology.

neonatólogo, -ga *m., f.* neonatologist.

neoplasia *f.* neoplasia.

  neoplasia benigna benign neoplasia.

  neoplasia endocrina múltiple multiple endocrine neoplasia.

  neoplasia endocrina múltiple, tipo I type I neoplasia.

  neoplasia endocrina múltiple, tipo II type II neoplasia.

  neoplasia endocrina múltiple, tipo III type III neoplasia.

  neoplasia maligna malignant neoplasia.

  neoplasia mixta mixed neoplasia.

neoplásico, -ca *adj.* neoplastic.

nerviosismo *m.* nervosism, nervousness.

nervioso, -sa *adj.* nervous.

nervus nervus.

neumoartrosis *f.* pneumarthrosis.

neumocito *m.* pneumocyte.

neumología *f.* pneumology.

neumonía *f.* pneumonia.

  neumonía aguda acute pneumonia.

  neumonía alérgica extrínseca extrinsic allergic pneumonia.

  neumonía por aspiración aspiration pneumonia.

  neumonía por aspiración congénita congenital aspiration pneumonia.

  neumonía atípica, neumonía atípica primaria atypical pneumonia, primary atypical pneumonia.

  neumonía bacteriana bacterial pneumonia.

  neumonía caseosa caseous pneumonia, cheesy pneumonia.

  neumonía estafilocócica staphylococcal pneumonia.

  neumonía estreptocócica streptococcal pneumonia.

  neumonía por inhalación inhalation pneumonia.

  neumonía intersticial interstitial pneumonia.

  neumonía metastásica metastatic pneumonia.

  neumonía no resuelta unresolved pneumonia.

  neumonía parenquimatosa parenchymatous pneumonia.

  neumonía secundaria secondary pneumonia.

  neumonía séptica septic pneumonia.

  neumonía terminal terminal pneumonia.

neumonía tuberculosa tuberculous pneumonia.

neumonía por varicela varicella pneumonia.

neumonía viral, neumonía vírica viral pneumonia.

neumonía por virus de la gripe influenzal pneumonia, influenza virus pneumonia.

neumonitis *f.* pneumonitis.

neumopatía *f.* pneumopathy.

neumopericardio *m.* pneumopericardium.

neumoperitoneal *adj.* pneumoperitoneal.

neumoterapia *f.* pneumotherapy.

neumotórax *m.* pneumothorax.

neumotórax espontáneo spontaneous pneumothorax.

neumotórax a presión pressure pneumothorax.

neumotórax a tensión tension pneumothorax.

neumotórax valvular valvular pneumothorax.

neural *adj.* neural.

neuralgia *f.* neuralgia.

neuralgia ciática sciatic neuralgia.

neuralgia craneal cranial neuralgia.

neuralgia del trigémino trigeminal neuralgia.

neurálgico, -ca *adj.* neuralgic.

neurastenia *f.* neurasthenia.

neurasténico, -ca *adj.* neurasthenic.

neurectomía *f.* neurectomy, neurectomy.

neurinoma *m.* neurinoma.

neurinoma acústico acoustic neurinoma.

neurinoma del trigémino trigeminal neurinoma.

neurita *f.* neurite, neurit.

neurítico, -ca *adj.* neuritic.

neuritis *f.* neuritis.

neuritis axial, neuritis axonal axial neuritis.

neuritis central central neuritis.

neuritis diseminada disseminated neuritis.

neuritis facial facial neuritis.

neuritis intersticial interstitial neuritis.

neuritis intraocular intraocular neuritis.

neuritis óptica optic neuritis.

neuritis retrobulbar retrobulbar neuritis.

neuroanastomosis *f.* neuroanastomosis.

neuroanatomía *f.* neuroanatomy.

neurobiología *f.* neurobiology.

neurobiólogo, -ga *m., f.* neurobiologist.

neurociencias *f.* neurosciences.

neurocientífico, -ca *m., f. y adj.* neuroscientist.

neurocirugía *f.* neurosurgery.

neurocirujano *m.* neurosurgeon.

neurodermatitis *f.* neurodermatitis.

neuroestimulación *f.* neurostimulation.

neuroestimulador *m.* neurostimulator.

neuroestimulante *m.* central nervous system stimulant.

neurofisiología *f.* neurophysiology.

neurofisiólogo, -ga *m., f.* neurophysiologist.

neuroglía *m.* neuroglia.

neurohipofisario, -a *adj.* neurohypophyseal.

neurohipófisis *f.* neurohypophysis.

neurohormona *f.* neurohormone.

neurohormonal *adj.* neurohormonal.

neurología *f.* neurology.

neurológico, -ca *adj.* neurologic.

neurólogo, -ga *m., f.* neurologist.

neuroma *m.* neuroma.

neuromuscular *adj.* neuromuscular.

neurona *f.* neuron, neurone.

  neurona aferente afferent neuron.

  neurona eferente efferent neuron.

  neurona motora motor neuron.

  neurona posganglionar postganglionic neuron.

  neurona preganglionar preganglionic neuron.

  neurona sensitiva, neurona sensorial sensory neuron.

neuronal *adj.* neuronal.

neuroncología *f.* neuroncology.

neuropatía *f.* neuropathy.

  neuropatía diabética diabetic neuropathy.

neuropsicología *f.* neuropsychology.

neuropsiquiatría *f.* neuropsychiatry.

neurosífilis *f.* neurosyphilis.

neurosis *f.* neurosis.

neurótico, -ca *adj.* neurotic.

neurotoxicidad *f.* neurotoxicity.

neurotóxico, -ca *adj.* neurotoxic.

neurotransmisión *f.* neurotransmission.

neurotransmisor *m.* neurotransmitter.

neutral *adj.* neutral.

neutralización *f.* neutralization.

  neutralización viral viral neutralization.

neutralizar *v.* neutralize.

neutro, -tra *adj.* neutral.

neutrofilia *f.* neutrophilia.

neutrófilo *m.* neutrophil.

  neutrófilo en banda band neutrophil.

  neutrófilo hipersegmentado hypersegmented neutrophil.

  neutrófilo inmaduro immature neutrophil.

  neutrófilo maduro mature neutrophil.

  neutrófilo segmentado segmented neutrophil.

neutropenia *f.* neutropenia.

  neutropenia congénita congenital neutropenia.

  neutropenia periódica periodic neutropenia.

nevo *m.* nevus, naevus.

  nevo adquirido acquired nevus.

  nevo en araña spider nevus.

  nevo azul blue nevus.

  nevo de Becker Becker's nevus.

  nevo capilar capillary nevus.

  nevo cavernoso naevus cavernosus.

  nevo congénito congenital nevus.

  nevo epidérmico epidermal nevus.

  nevo gigante congénito pigmentado giant congenital pigmented nevus.

  nevo pigmentado, nevo pigmentario, nevo pigmentoso pigmented nevus, naevus pigmentosus.

  nevo plano naevus spilus.

nevus nevus.

nexo *m.* nexus.

nicotina *f.* nicotine.

nicotinamida *f.* nicotinamide.

nido *m.* nest, nidus.

niñez *f.* childhood.

niño, -ña *m., f.* child.

nistagmo *m.* nystagmus.

  nistagmo central central nystagmus.

  nistagmo congénito congenital nystagmus, congenital hereditary nystagmus.

  nistagmo conjugado conjugate nystagmus.

  nistagmo convergente convergence nystagmus.

  nistagmo disociado dissociated nystagmus.

  nistagmo lateral lateral nystagmus.

  nistagmo ocular ocular nystagmus.

nitrogenado, -da *adj.* nitrogenous.

nitrógeno *m.* nitrogen.

nivel *m.* level.

  nivel auditivo hearing level.

  nivel de consciencia level of consciousness.

  nivel de creatinina en suero serum creatinine level.

  nivel operativo operant level.

  nivel sanguíneo blood level.

  nivel sanguíneo de glucosa blood level of glucose.

no adherente *adj.* non-adherent.

no antigénico, -ca *adj.* non-antigenic.

no enfermedad *f.* non-disease.

no fisiológico, -ca *adj.* unphysiologic.

no infeccioso, -sa *adj.* non-infectious.

no inmune *adj.* non-immune.

no intentar la reanimación (NIR) do not attempt resuscitation (DNAR).

no invasivo, -va *adj.* non-invasive.

no neoplásico, -ca *adj.* non-neoplastic.

no respuesta (NR) *f.* no response (NR).

no vascular *adj.* non-vascular.

no viable *adj.* non-viable.

nocardiosis *f.* nocardiosis.

nocicepción *f.* nociception.

nociceptivo, -va *adj.* nociceptive.

nociceptor *m.* nociceptor.

nocivo, -va *adj.* noxious.

noctambulismo *m.* noctambulism.

noctámbulo, -la *adj.* noctambulic.

nocturia *f.* nocturia.

nocturno, -na *adj.* nocturnal.

nodal *adj.* nodal.

nodulación *f.* nodulation.

nodulado, -da *adj.* nodulate, nodulated.

nodular *adj.* nodular.

nodulitis *f.* nodulitis.

nódulo¹ *m.* nodule, nodulus.

nódulo² *m.* node.

  nódulo auriculoventricular atrioventricular node.

  nódulo de cantante singer's node.

  nódulo sifilítica syphilitic node.

  nódulo sinoauricular sinoatrial node, sinoauricular node.

  nódulo sinusal sinoatrial node, sinoauricular node.

nodulosis *f.* nodulosis.

nombre *m.* name.

  nombre genérico generic name.

nombre patentado proprietary name.

nombre no patentado non-proprietary name.

nombre registrado proprietary name.

nombre no registrado non-proprietary name.

nombre sistemático systematic name.

nombre trivial trivial name.

nombre vulgar trivial name.

nomenclatura *f.* nomenclature.

norma[1] *f.* rule.

norma[2] *f.* norma.

normal *adj.* normal.

normalidad *f.* normality.

normalización *f.* normalization.

normalizar *v.* normalize.

normoblasto *m.* normoblast.

normocromía *f.* normochromia.

normocrómico, -ca *adj.* normochromic.

nosocomial *adj.* nosocomial.

nosología *f.* nosology.

notocorda *m.* notochord.

noxa *f.* noxa.

nuca *f.* nape, nucha.

nucal *adj.* nuchal.

nucleación *f.* nucleation.

nucleado, -da *adj.* nucleated.

nuclear *adj.* nuclear.

núcleo *m.* nucleus.

nucléolo *m.* nucleolus.

nucleótido *m.* nucleotide.

nudo *m.* knot, node, nodus.

nudo de cirujano surgeon's knot.

nudo quirúrgico surgical knot.

nudo sincitial syncytial node.

nuligrávida *f.* nulligravida.

nulípara *f.* nullipara.

nuliparidad *f.* nulliparity.

numeración *f.* count.

numérico, -ca *adj.* numerical.

número *m.* number.

nutrición *f.* nutrition.

nutrición adecuada adequate nutrition.

nutrición parenteral parenteral nutrition.

nutrición parenteral total (npt) total parenteral nutrition (tpn).

nutricional *adj.* nutritional.

nutriente *m.* nutrient.

O

obesidad *f.* obesity.

obesidad cushingoide cushingoid obesity.

obesidad mórbida morbid obesity.

obesidad troncular truncal obesity.

obeso, -sa *adj.* obese.

óbito *m.* decease.

objetivo *m.* objective.

objeto *m.* object.

oblicuidad *f.* obliquity.

obligado, -da *adj.* obligate.

oblongada *adj.* oblongata.

observador *m.* observer.

obsesión *f.* obsession.

obsesivo, -va *adj.* obsessive.

obsesivo-compulsivo, -va *adj.* obsessive-compulsive.

obstetra *m.* obstetrician.

obstetricia *f.* obstetrics.

obstétrico, -ca *adj.* obstetric, obstetrical.

obstrucción *f.* obstruction.

obstrucción de la arteria central de la retina retinal central arterial obstruction.

obstrucción biliar biliary obstruction.

obstrucción crónica de las vías respiratorias chronic airway obstruction.

obstrucción por cuerpo extraño foreign body obstruction.

obstrucción intestinal intestinal obstruction.

obstrucción nasal nasal obstruction.

obstrucción de la vía aérea airway obstruction.

obstrucción de las vías respiratorias superiores (OVRS) upper airway obstruction (UAO).

obstructivo, -va *adj.* obstructive.

obturación¹ *f.* filling.

obturación² *f.* obturation.

obturación de un canal, obturación de un conducto canal obturation.

occipital *adj.* occipital, occipitalis.

ocelo *m.* ocellus.

ocena *f.* ozena.

ocluido, -da *adj.* occluded.

ocluir *v.* occlude.

oclusal *adj.* occlusal.

oclusión *f.* occlusion.

oclusión anatómica anatomic occlusion.

oclusión anormal abnormal occlusion.

oclusión fisiológica physiologic occlusion, physiological occlusion.

ocular¹ *adj.* ocular.

ocular² *m.* eyepiece, ocular.

oculista *m., f.* oculist.

ocupación *f.* occupancy.

odinofagia *f.* odynophagia, odynphagia.

odinofobia *f.* odynophobia.

odinofonía *f.* odynophonia.

odinólisis *f.* odynolysis.

odontalgia *f.* odontalgia.

odontoides *adj.* odontoid.

odontología *f.* dentistry, odontology.

odontólogo, -ga *m.* odontologist.

Oestridae Oestridae.

oficial *adj.* official.

oftalmía *f.* ophthalmia.

oftálmico, -ca *adj.* ophthalmic.

oftalmodinamómetro *m.* ophthalmodynamometer.

oftalmología *f.* ophthalmology.

oftalmológico, -ca *adj.* ophthalmologic, ophthalmological.

oftalmólogo, -ga *m., f.* ophthalmologist.

oftalmopatía *f.* ophthalmopathy.

oftalmoplejía *f.* ophthalmoplegia.

oftalmopléjico, -ca *adj.* ophthalmoplegic.

oftalmoscopia *f.* ophthalmoscopy.

oftalmoscopio *m.* ophthalmoscope.

ofuscación *f.* obfuscation.

oído *m.* ear, auris.

oído externo, auris externa external ear, outer ear, auris externa.

oído interno, auris interna internal ear, inner ear, auris interna.

oído medio, auris media middle ear, auris media.

oído de nadador swimmer's ear.

oír *v.* hear.

ojo *m.* eye, oculus.

ojo afáquico aphakic eye.

ojo artificial artificial eye.

banco de ojo bank eye.

ojo bizco squinting eye.

ojo de cíclope cyclopean eye, cyclopian eye.

ojo desviado deviating eye.

ojo dominante dominant eye.

ojo errante following eye.

ojo escotópico scotopic eye.

ojo esquemático schematic eye.

ojo estrábico squinting eye.

ojo legañoso bleary eye.

oleaginoso, -sa *adj.* oleaginous.

olécranon *m.* olecranon.

oleoso, -sa *adj.* oily, oleosus.

oler *v.* smell.

olfato *m.* olfact, olfactus.

oligoamnios *m.* oligoamnios.

oligodendrocito *m.* oligodendrocyte.

oligofrenia *f.* oligophrenia.

oligofrénico, -ca *adj.* oligophrenic.

oligonefrónico, -ca *adj.* oligonephronic.

oligosacárido *m.* oligosaccharide.

oliguria *f.* oliguria.

oligúrico, -ca *adj.* oliguric.

olor *m.* odor.

olor corporal body odor.

olor mínimo identificable minimal identifiable odor.

oloroso, -sa *adj.* odorous.

olvido *m.* forgetting.

ombligo *m.* navel, umbilicus.

omentitis *f.* omentitis.

omento *m.* omentum.

omisión *f.* omission.

oncogén *m.* oncogene.

oncogénesis *f.* oncogenesis.

oncogénico, -ca *adj.* oncogenic.

oncología *f.* oncology.

oncología radioterápica radiation oncology.

oncólogo, -ga *m.* oncologist.

oncólogo radioterapeuta radiation oncologist.

onda *f.* wave.

onda electroencefalográfica electroencephalographic wave.

onda P P wave.

onda de pulso, onda del pulso pulse wave.

onda Q Q wave.

onda R R wave.

onda S S wave.

onda T T wave.

onicomicosis *f.* onychomycosis.

oniquia *f.* onychia.

onírico, -ca *adj.* oneiric.

oocito *m.* oocyte.

oocito de primer orden primary oocyte.

oocito primario primary oocyte.

oocito secundario secondary oocyte.

oocito de segundo orden secondary oocyte.

ooforectomía *f.* oophorectomy.

ooforitis *f.* oophoritis.

opacificación *f.* opacification.

opacificado, -da *adj.* opacified.

opaco, -ca *adj.* opaque.

operable *adj.* operable.

operación *f.* operation.

  operación abdominal abdominal section.

  operación abierta open operation.

  operación cesárea cesarean operation.

  operación de Juvara Juvara's operation.

  operación menor minor operation.

  operación de Trendelenburg Trendelenburg's operation.

operar *v.* operate.

opiáceo, -a *adj.* opiate.

opio *m.* opium.

opioide *m.* opioid.

opistótonos *m.* opisthotonos, opisthotonus.

oponente *adj.* opposing, opponens.

oportunista *adj.* opportunistic.

opresión *f.* suffocation.

opsonina *f.* opsonin.

óptico, -ca¹ *adj.* optic, optical.

óptico, -ca² *m., f.* optician, opticist, optist.

optimismo *m.* optimism.

óptimo, -ma *adj.* optimal.

óptimo *m.* optimum.

optometría *f.* optometry.

optometrista *m.* optometrist.

oral¹ *adj.* oral.

oral² *m.* orale.

orbicular¹ *adj.* orbicular.

orbicular² *m.* orbicularis.

órbita *f.* orbit, orbita.

orbitario, -ria *adj.* orbitalis.

orden¹ *m.* order.

orden² *f.* order.

  orden de no reanimación, orden de no resucitar do-not-resuscitate order, DNR order.

  orden de no reanimación sin consentimiento do-not-resuscitate-without-consent order.

ordenada *f.* ordinate.

ordenador *m.* computer.

oreja *f.* ear.

  oreja caída lop ear.

organela *f.* organelle, organella.

orgánico, -ca *adj.* organic.

organismo *m.* organism.

organización *f.* organization.

  Organización Mundial de la Salud (OMS) World Health Organization (WHO).

organizador, -ra *m., f.* organizer.

órgano *m.* organ, organon, organum.

  órgano accesorio accessory organ.

  órgano acústico acoustic organ.

  órgano de la audición organ of hearing.

  órgano auditivo organum auditus.

  órgano de Corti Corti's organ, organ of Corti.

  órgano diana target organ.

  órgano digestivo digestive organ, apparatus digestorius.

  órgano errante wandering organ.

  órgano extraperitoneal extraperitoneal organ, organum extraperitoneale.

  órgano flotante floating organ.

  órgano genital organa genitalia.

  órgano genital externo external genital organ, genitalia externa.

  órgano genital femenino female

genital organ.

órgano genital femenino externo organa genitalia femenina externa.

órgano genital femenino interno organa genitalia femenina interna.

órgano genital interno internal genital organ, organa genitalia interna.

órgano genital masculino male genital organ.

órgano genital masculino externo organa genitalia masculina externa.

órgano genital masculino interno organa genitalia masculina interna.

órgano gustativo, órgano gustatorio, órgano del gusto gustatory organ, taste organ, organ of taste, organon gustus, organum gustatorium, organum gustus.

órgano linfático lymphatic organ.

órgano linfoide lymphoid organ.

órgano olfatorio, órgano del olfato olfactory organ, organ of smell, organon olfactus, organum olfactus, organum olfactorium.

órgano ptótico ptotic organ.

órgano reproductor reproductive organ.

órgano reproductor femenino female reproductive organ.

órgano reproductor del varón male reproductive organ.

órgano retroperitoneal retroperitoneal organ, organum retroperitoneale.

órgano sensorial, órgano de los sentidos sense organ, sensory organ, organa sensoria, organa sensuum.

órgano del tacto organ of touch.

órgano terminal end organ, terminal organ.

órgano urinario urinary organ, organa urinaria.

órgano vestibular vestibular organ.

órgano vestibulococlear vestibulocochlear organ, organum vestibulocochleare.

órgano vestigial vestigial organ.

órgano de la visión, órgano visual organ of vision, visual organ, organum visuale, organum visus.

organoespecífico, -ca adj. organ-specific.

organogénesis f. organogenesis.

organoterapia f. organotherapy.

orgásmico, -ca adj. orgasmic.

orgasmo m. orgasm.

orientación f. orientation.

orientación sexual sexual orientation.

orientar v. orient.

orificio m. orifice, orificium.

origen m. origin.

orina f. urine, urina.

orina en jarabe de arce maple syrup urine.

orina turbia cloudy urine.

orinal m. urinal.

orinar v. urinate.

ornitina f. ornithine.

oro m. gold.

orofaringe f. oropharynx.

orofaríngeo, -a adj. oropharyngeal.

orquectomía f. orchectomy.

orquialgia f. orchialgia.

orquidectomía f. orchidectomy.

orquiditis f. orchiditis.

orquiectomía *f.* orchiectomy.
orquiepididimitis *f.* orchiepididymitis.
orquioepididimitis *f.* orchiepididymitis.
orquitis *f.* orchitis.
ortesis *f.* orthesis.
ortiga *f.* nettle.
ortodoncia *f.* orthodontia, orthodontics, denturism.
  ortodoncia correctiva corrective orthodontics.
  ortodoncia preventiva preventive orthodontics, prophylactic orthodontics.
  ortodoncia quirúrgica surgical orthodontics.
ortodoncista *adj.* orthodontist, denturist.
ortognática *f.* orthognathics.
ortopeda *m.* orthopod.
ortopedia *f.* orthopedics.
ortopédico, -ca *adj.* orthopedic.
ortostático, -ca *adj.* orthostatic.
ortostatismo *m.* orthostatism.
orzuelo *m.* sty, stye, hordeolum.
  orzuelo externo external sty, hordeolum externum.
  orzuelo interno internal sty, hordeolum internum.
os os.
osamenta *f.* ossature.
oscilación *f.* oscillation.
oscilatorio, -ria *adj.* oscillatory.
oscuro, -ra *adj.* dark.
óseo, -a *adj.* osseous, bony.
oseocartilaginoso, -sa *adj.* osseocartilaginous.
osificación *f.* ossification.

osificar *v.* ossify.
osmolalidad *f.* osmolality.
osmolar *adj.* osmolar.
osmolaridad *f.* osmolarity.
  osmolaridad de la orina, osmolaridad urinaria urine osmolarity.
  osmolaridad sanguínea blood osmolarity.
  osmolaridad del suero, osmolaridad sérica serum osmolarity.
osmosidad *f.* osmosity.
osmosis, ósmosis *f.* osmosis.
osteartritis *f.* ostearthritis.
osteítis *f.* osteitis.
  osteítis deformante osteitis deformans.
osteoarticular *adj.* osteoarticular.
osteoartritis *f.* osteoarthritis.
osteoartrosis *f.* osteoarthrosis.
osteoblasto *m.* osteoblast.
osteocito *m.* osteocyte.
osteocondritis *f.* osteochondritis.
osteocondrosis *f.* osteochondrosis.
osteodistrofia *f.* osteodystrophy, osteodystrophia.
osteoesclerosis *f.* osteosclerosis.
osteófito *m.* osteophyte.
osteoma *m.* osteoma.
osteomalacia *f.* osteomalacia.
osteomielitis *f.* osteomyelitis.
osteópata *m.* osteopath.
osteopatía *f.* osteopathy, osteopathia.
osteopenia *f.* osteopenia.
osteoporosis *f.* osteoporosis.
  osteoporosis posmenopáusica postmenopausal osteoporosis.
  osteoporosis senil senile osteoporosis.

osteoporótico, -ca *adj.* osteoporotic.

osteosarcoma *m.* osteosarcoma.

osteosíntesis *f.* osteosynthesis.

osteosis *f.* osteosis.

osteotomía *f.* osteotomy.

ostomía *f.* ostomy.

ostomizado, -da *adj.* ostomate.

otalgia *f.* otalgia.

ótico, -ca *adj.* otic, otor.

otítico, -ca *adj.* otitic.

otitis *f.* otitis.

   otitis externa external otitis, otitis externa.

   otitis interna otitis interna.

   otitis media otitis media.

   otitis micótica otitis mycotica.

otorragia *f.* otorrhagia.

otorrea *f.* otorrhea.

otorrinolaringología *f.* otorhinolaryngology.

otorrinolaringólogo, -ga *m., f.* otorhinolaryngologist.

otoscopio *m.* otoscope.

oval *adj.* oval.

ovalado, -da *adj.* oval.

ovalbúmina *f.* ovalbumin.

ovárico, -ca *adj.* ovarian.

ovariectomía *f.* ovariectomy.

ovario *m.* ovary, ovarium.

   ovario poliquístico polycystic ovary.

ovicida[1] *adj.* ovicide.

ovicida[2] *adj.* ovicidal.

ovocito *m.* ovocyte.

ovogenesia *f.* ovogenesis.

ovulación *f.* ovulation.

   ovulación amenstrual amenstrual ovulation.

ovulatorio, -ria *adj.* ovulatory.

óvulo, -m. ovule, ovum.

   óvulo fecundado fertilized ovum.

   óvulo fertilizado fertilized ovum.

   óvulo de Graaf Graafian ovule.

   óvulo primordial primordial ovule, primordial ovum.

   óvulo vaginal vaginal ovum.

oxidación *f.* oxidation.

   oxidación de ácidos grasos fatty acid oxidation.

oxidado, -da *adj.* oxidized.

óxido *m.* oxide.

oxigenación *f.* oxygenation.

   oxigenación extracorpórea extracorporeal oxygenation.

oxigenado, -da *adj.* oxygenated.

oxigenar *v.* oxygenate.

oxígeno *m.* oxygen.

oxigenoterapia *f.* oxygentherapy, oxygen therapy.

   oxigenoterapia hiperbárica hyperbaric oxygen therapy.

oxihemoglobina *f.* oxyhemoglobin.

oxitócico, -ca *adj.* oxytocic.

oxitocina (OXT) *f.* oxytocin (OXT).

ozena *f.* ozena.

ozono *m.* ozone.

P

pabellón *m.* pavilion.

paciente *m., f.* patient.

padrastro *m.* hangnail.

paidofilia *f.* pedophilia.

paladar *m.* palate, palatum.

   paladar caído falling palate.

   paladar fisurado cleft palate.

   paladar hendido cleft palate.

palanca *f.* lever.
palatino, -na *adj.* palatine.
paliar *v.* palliate.
paliativo, -va *adj.* palliative.
palidez *f.* pallor.
palma *f.* palm.
  palma de la mano palma manus.
palmar *adj.* palmar.
palpable *adj.* palpable.
palpación *f.* palpation.
  palpación bimanual bimanual palpation.
palpebral *adj.* palpebral.
palpebritis *f.* palpebritis.
palpitación *f.* palpitation.
palúdico, -ca *adj.* paludal.
paludismo *m.* malaria.
panarteritis *f.* panarteritis.
panartritis *f.* panarthritis.
pancitopenia *f.* pancytopenia.
páncreas *m.* pancreas.
pancreatitis *f.* pancreatitis.
  pancreatitis aguda acute pancreatitis.
pandemia *f.* pandemia.
pandémico, -ca *adj.* pandemic.
panencefalitis *f.* panencephalitis.
pánico *m.* panic.
paniculitis *f.* panniculitis.
pantalla *f.* screen.
paño *m.* pannus.
paperas *f.* mumps.
papila *f.* papilla.
papilar *adj.* papillary, papillate.
papiledema *m.* papilledema.
papilitis *f.* papillitis.
papiloma *m.* papilloma.
  papiloma acuminado papilloma acuminatum.

  papiloma venéreo papilloma venereum.
pápula *f.* papule.
paquimeninge *f.* pachymeninx.
paquimeningitis *f.* pachymeningitis.
paracentesis *f.* paracentesis.
  paracentesis abdominal abdominal paracentesis.
  paracentesis ocular paracentesis oculi.
  paracentesis timpánica tympanic paracentesis.
paracusia *f.* paracusia, paracusis.
paradoja *f.* paradox.
paraesternal *adj.* parasternal.
parálisis *f.* paralysis.
  parálisis bulbar bulbar paralysis.
  parálisis central central paralysis.
  parálisis centrocortical centrocortical paralysis.
  parálisis cerebral cerebral paralysis.
  parálisis emocional emotional paralysis.
  parálisis incompleta incomplete paralysis.
  parálisis infantil infantile paralysis.
  parálisis obstétrica obstetrical paralysis.
  parálisis ocular ocular paralysis.
paralizador, -ra *m. y adj.* paralyzant.
paralizante *m. y adj.* paralyzant.
parametrio *m.* parametrium.
parametritis *f.* parametritis.
parámetro *m.* parameter.
paranoia *f.* paranoia.
paranoico, -ca *adj.* paranoiac.

paranoide *adj.* paranoid.

paranormal *adj.* paranormal.

paraparesia *f.* paraparesis.

paraplejia *f.* paraplegia.

  paraplejia atáxica ataxic paraplegia.

  paraplejia cerebral cerebral paraplegia.

  paraplejia espástica spastic paraplegia.

parapléjico, -ca *adj.* paraplectic, paraplegic.

parasimpático, -ca *adj.* parasympathetic.

parasimpaticolítico, -ca *adj.* parasympatholytic.

parasimpaticomimético, -ca *adj.* parasympathomimetic.

parasitario, -ria *adj.* parasitic.

parasitemia *f.* parasitemia.

parasiticida[1] *m.* parasiticide.

parasiticida[2] *adj.* parasiticidal.

parásito *m.* parasite.

  parásito obligado obligate parasite.

parasitología *f.* parasitology.

parasitólogo, -ga *m., f.* parasitologist.

parasitosis *f.* parasitosis.

paratiroideo, -a *adj.* parathyroid.

paratiroides *f.* parathyroid.

paravertebral *adj.* paravertebral.

pared *f.* wall.

  pared celular cell wall.

parénquima *m.* parenchyma.

parental *adj.* parental.

parenteral *adj.* parenteral.

paresia *f.* paresis.

parestesia *f.* paresthesia.

paridad *f.* parity.

parietal *adj.* parietal.

parodontitis *f.* parodontitis.

parótida *f.* parotid.

parotidectomía *f.* parotidectomy.

parotídeo, -a *adj.* parotid.

parotiditis *f.* parotiditis.

párpado *m.* eyelid, palpebra.

parte *f.* part, pars.

partícula *f.* particle.

parto *m.* delivery, labor, partus.

  parto abdominal abdominal delivery.

  parto artificial artificial labor.

  parto complicado complicated labor.

  parto espontáneo spontaneous delivery.

  parto eutócico spontaneous delivery.

  parto inducido induced labor.

  parto instrumental instrumental labor.

  parto múltiple multiple labor.

  parto prematuro premature delivery.

  parto prolongado prolonged labor.

  parto provocado induced labor.

  parto vaginal vaginal delivery.

parturienta *adj.* parturient.

párvulo, -la *adj.* parvule.

pasión *f.* passion.

pasivo, -va *adj.* passive.

paso[1] *m.* step.

paso[2] *m.* passage.

pasta *f.* paste.

pasteurización *f.* pasteurization.

patela *f.* patella.

patelar *adj.* patellar.

paternalismo *m.* paternalism.

paternidad *f.* fatherhood.

patético, -ca *adj.* pathetic.

patogénesis *f.* pathogeny.

patogenia *f.* pathogeny.

patogenicidad *f.* pathogenicity.

patógeno *m.* pathogen.

patógeno, -na *adj.* pathogenic.

patología *f.* pathology.

　patología celular cellular pathology.

　patología clínica clinical pathology.

　patología comparada comparative pathology.

　patología dental dental pathology.

　patología experimental experimental pathology.

　patología externa external pathology.

　patología funcional functional pathology.

　patología general general pathology.

　patología interna internal pathology.

　patología médica medical pathology.

　patología mental mental pathology.

　patología quirúrgica surgical pathology.

patológico, -ca *adj.* pathologic, pathological.

patólogo, -ga *m., f.* pathologist.

patrón *m.* pattern.

pausa *f.* pause.

pavor *m.* pavor.

peca *f.* freckle.

pectoral *adj.* pectoral.

pecho *m.* chest, pectus.

pediatra *m., f.* pediatrician.

pediatría *f.* pediatrics.

pediátrico, -ca *adj.* pediatric.

pediculado, -da *adj.* pediculate.

pedículo *m.* pedicle, pediculus.

pediculosis *f.* pediculosis.

pedofilia *f.* pedophilia.

pedofílico, -ca *adj.* pedophilic.

pedófilo, -la[1] *adj.* pedophilic.

pedófilo, -la[2] *m., f.* pedophile.

pedunculado, -da *adj.* pedunculated.

pedúnculo *m.* peduncle, pedunculus.

pelagra *f.* pellagra.

película[1] *f.* pellicle.

　película lagrimal tear pellicle.

película[2] *f.* film.

　película dental dental film.

pelirrojo, -ja *adj.* ginger, red-haired, red-headed.

pelo *m.* hair.

　pelo invaginado ingrown hair.

pelúcido, -da *adj.* pellucid.

peludo, -da *adj.* hairy.

pelviano, -na *adj.* pelvic.

pélvico, -ca *adj.* pelvic.

pelvigrafía *f.* pelviography.

pelvimetría *f.* pelvimetry.

pelvis *f.* pelvis.

pena *f.* grief.

pendiente *f.* slant.

pendular *adj.* pendular.

pene *m.* penis.

penetrabilidad *f.* penetrability.

penetración *f.* penetration.

penetrancia *f.* penetrance.

penetrante *adj.* penetrating.

pénfigo *m.* pemphigus.

penfigoide *m.* pemphigoid.

pensamiento *m.* thinking, thought.

  pensamiento abstracto abstract thinking.

  pensamiento autista autistic thinking.

  pensamiento creativo creative thinking.

pentosa *f.* pentose.

pentosuria *f.* pentosuria.

péptico, -ca *adj.* peptic.

pequeño mal *m.* petit mal.

percepción *f.* perception.

  percepción consciente conscious perception.

  percepción extrasensorial (PES) extrasensory perception (ESP).

perceptivo, -va *adj.* perceptive.

percusión *f.* percussion.

  percusión bimanual bimanual percussion.

  percusión digital finger percussion.

  percusión directa direct percussion.

  percusión profunda deep percussion.

pérdida *f.* deletion.

perenne *adj.* perennial.

perfeccionismo *m.* perfectionism.

perfil *m.* profile.

  perfil antigénico antigenic profile.

  perfil bioquímico biochemical profile.

  perfil de la personalidad personality profile.

  perfil de pruebas test profile.

perforación *f.* perforation.

perforado, -da *adj.* perforated.

perforante *adj.* perforans.

perforar *v.* drill.

perfundido, -da *adj.* perfusate.

perfundir *v.* perfuse.

perfusión *f.* perfusion.

perianal *adj.* perianal.

periapical *adj.* periapical.

pericardíaco, -ca *adj.* pericardiac, pericardial.

pericárdico, -ca *adj.* pericardiac, pericardial.

pericardio *m.* pericardium.

pericarditis *f.* pericarditis.

pericondritis *f.* perichondritis.

peridural *adj.* peridural.

periferia *f.* periphery.

periférico, -ca *adj.* peripheral.

perifoliculitis *f.* perifolliculitis.

perimetral *adj.* perimetric.

perímetro *m.* perimeter.

perinatal *adj.* perinatal.

perinatología *f.* perinatology.

periné *m.* perineum.

perineal *adj.* perineal.

perineo *m.* perineum.

periodicidad *f.* periodicity.

periódico, -ca *adj.* periodic.

período *m.* period.

  período fértil fertile period.

  período de incubación incubative period.

  período menstrual menstrual period.

  período puerperal puerperal period.

periodoncia *f.* periodontics.

periodoncista *m.* periodontist.

periodontal *adj.* periodontal.

periodontitis *f.* periodontitis.

periorbitario, -ria *adj.* periorbital.

periostio *m.* periosteum.

periostitis *f.* periostitis.

peristáltico, -ca *adj.* peristaltic.

peristaltismo *m.* peristalsis.

peritoneal *adj.* peritoneal.

peritoneo *m.* peritoneum.

peritonitis *f.* peritonitis.

periumbilical *adj.* periumbilical.

perivascular *adj.* perivascular.

perivertebral *adj.* perivertebral.

permeabilidad *f.* permeability.

permeable *adj.* permeable.

pernicioso, -sa *adj.* pernicious.

peroné *m.* fibula.

peroneo, -a *adj.* peroneal.

per os *adv.* per os.

persistencia *f.* persistence.

persona *f.* persona.

personalidad *f.* personality.

  personalidad escindida split personality.

persuasión *f.* persuasion.

perversión *f.* perversion.

  perversión sexual sexual perversion.

pervertido, -da *adj.* perverted.

pesadilla *f.* nightmare.

pesario *m.* pessary.

pesimismo *m.* pessimism.

pestaña *f.* eyelash.

peste *f.* plague, pestis.

  peste bubónica bubonic plague.

  peste negra black plague.

pestilencia *f.* pestilence.

pestilente *adj.* pestilential.

petequia *f.* petechia.

petequial *adj.* petechial.

pétreo, -a *adj.* petrous.

pezón *m.* nipple.

piamadre *f.* pia mater.

pica *f.* pica.

picadura *f.* sting.

picazón *f.* itching.

pie *m.* foot, pes.

  pie de atleta athlete's foot.

  pie caído drop foot.

  pie cavo, pes cavus clawfoot, pes cavus.

  pie equino pes equinus.

  pie equinovalgo, pes equinovalgus pes equinovalgus.

  pie equinovaro, pes equinovarus pes equinovarus.

  pie plano, pes planus flat foot, pes planus.

  pie valgo, pes valgus pes valgus.

  pie varo, pes varus pes varus.

  pie zambo club foot, skewfoot.

piedra *f.* piedra.

piel *f.* skin.

  piel bronceada bronzed skin.

  piel laxa loose skin.

  piel de naranja peau d'orange.

pielitis *f.* pyelitis.

pielografía *f.* pyelography.

pielonefritis *f.* pyelonephritis.

pielonefrosis *f.* pyelonephrosis.

pieloplastia *f.* pyeloplasty.

pierna *f.* leg.

pieza *f.* piece.

pigmentación *f.* pigmentation.

pigmentado, -da *adj.* pigmented.

pigmento *m.* pigment.

  pigmento biliar bile pigment.

  pigmento visual visual pigment.

píldora *f.* pill.

piloerección *f.* piloerection.
piloritis *f.* pyloritis.
píloro *m.* pylorus.
piloroespasmo *m.* pylorospasm.
piloroplastia *f.* pyloroplasty.
pilosebáceo, -a *adj.* pilosebaceous.
piloso, -sa *adj.* pilose.
pineal *adj.* pineal.
pinealocito *m.* pinealocyte.
pinzas *f.* forceps.
  pinzas para biopsias cup biopsy
  forceps.
  pinzas para cortar cutting forceps.
piogénico, -ca *adj.* pyogenic.
piógeno *m.* pyogen.
piojo *m.* louse, pediculus.
piorrea *f.* piorrea.
pipeta *f.* pipette, pipet.
piramidal *adj.* pyramidal.
pirámide *f.* pyramid.
pirético, -ca *adj.* pyrectic, pyretic.
pirógeno *m.* pyrogen.
pirosis *f.* pyrosis.
pitiriasis *f.* pityriasis.
  pitiriasis capitis pityriasis capitis.
  pitiriasis rosácea, pitiriasis rosa-
  da pityriasis rosea.
  pitiriasis versicolor pityriasis versicolor.
pituitaria *f.* pituitarium.
pituitario, -ria *adj.* pituitary.
pituitarismo *m.* pituitarism.
piuria *f.* pyuria.
placa¹ *f.* patch.
  placa mucosa mucous patch.
placa² *f.* plaque.
  placa bacteriana bacterial plaque.
  placa dentaria dental plaque.
  placa senil senile plaque.

placa³ *f.* plate.
  placa neural neural plate.
  placa ósea bone plate.
placebo *m.* placebo.
placenta *f.* placenta.
  placenta fetal fetal placenta, placenta fetalis.
  placenta materna maternal placenta.
  placenta previa placenta previa.
placer *m.* pleasure.
plano *m.* plane, planum.
plantar *adj.* plantar.
plantilla *f.* template.
plaqueta *f.* platelet.
plaquetaféresis *f.* plateletpheresis.
plasma *m.* plasma.
  plasma sanguíneo blood plasma.
plasmaféresis *f.* plasmapheresis.
plásmido *m.* plasmid.
plástia *f.* plasty.
plástico, -ca *adj.* plastic.
pleura *f.* pleura.
pleuresía *f.* pleurisy.
pleuritis *f.* pleuritis.
pleurodinia *f.* pleurodynia.
plexo *m.* plexus.
pliegue *m.* fold.
pluripotencial *adj.* pluripotential.
podagra *f.* podagra.
podálico, -ca *adj.* podalic.
poder *m.* power.
podología *f.* podology.
podólogo, -ga *m., f.* podologist.
polaquiuria *f.* pollakiuria.
polar *f.* polar.
polaridad *f.* polarity.
polarización *f.* polarization.
poliadenitis *f.* polyadenitis.

poliarticular *adj.* polyarticular.

poliartritis *f.* polyarthritis.

policitemia *f.* polycythemia.

policitemia verdadera, policitemia vera polycythemia vera.

policlínica *f.* polyclinic.

polidactilia *f.* polydactylia, polydactyly.

polidipsia *f.* polydipsia.

polifármacia *f.* polypharmacy.

polímero *m.* polymer.

polineuritis *f.* polyneuritis.

polinucleado, -da *adj.* polynucleate, polynucleated.

polinuclear *adj.* polynuclear.

polio *f.* polio.

poliomielitis *f.* poliomyelitis.

poliomieloencefalitis *f.* poliomyeloencephalitis.

poliopía *f.* polyopia.

polipéptido *m.* polypeptide.

pólipo *m.* polyp.

pólipo bronquial bronchial polyp.

pólipo fibroso fibrous polyp.

pólipo juvenil juvenile polyp.

pólipo laríngeo laryngeal polyp.

pólipo nasal nasal polyp.

pólipo vascular vascular polyp.

polisacárido *m.* polysaccharide.

polivalente *adj.* polyvalent.

polo *m.* pole.

pomada *f.* ointment.

ponderable *adj.* ponderable.

ponderal *adj.* ponderal.

pontocerebeloso, -sa *adj.* pontocerebellar.

poplíteo, -a *adj.* popliteal.

porción *f.* portion.

porfiria *f.* porphyria.

porfobilinógeno *m.* porphobilinogen.

poro *m.* pore.

porta *m.* porta.

portaagujas *m.* needle-carrier, needle-driver, needle-holder.

portador, - ra *m., f.* carrier.

posición *f.* position.

posición anatómica anatomical position.

posición de decúbito dorsal dorsal recumbent position.

posición de decúbito lateral lateral recumbent position.

posición de decúbito prono prone position.

posición de decúbito supino dorsal recumbent position.

posición dorsal dorsal position.

posición fetal fetal position.

posición frontal transversa, posición frontotransversa frontotransverse position.

posición de litotomía lithotomy position.

posición obstétrica obstetric position.

posición prona prone position.

posición supina supine position.

posición de Trendelenburg Trendelenburg's position.

positivo, -va *adj.* positive.

posmenopáusico, -ca *adj.* postmenopausal.

posnatal *adj.* postnatal.

posología *f.* posology.

posoperatorio, -ria *adj.* postoperative.

posparto *m.* post partum.

posprandial *adj.* postprandial.

posterior, -ra *adj.* posterior.

posteroanterior *adj.* posteroanterior.

posteroinferior *adj.* posteroinferior.

posterointerno, -na *adj.* posterointernal.

posterolateral *adj.* posterolateral.

posteromediano, -na *adj.* posteromedian.

posteroparietal *adj.* posteroparietal.

posterosuperior, -ra *adj.* posterosuperior.

post mortem post mortem.

post partum post partum.

postraumático, -ca *adj.* post-traumatic.

postulado *m.* postulate.

póstumo, -ma *adj.* posthumous.

postura *f.* posture.

postural *adj.* postural.

potable *adj.* potable.

potasemia *f.* potassemia.

potasio *m.* potassium.

potencia *f.* potency.

potenciación *f.* potentiation.

potencial *m. y adj.* potential.

práctica *f.* practice.

prandial *adj.* prandial.

praxis *f.* praxis.

precanceroso, -sa *adj.* precancerous.

precipitación *f.* precipitation.

precipitado *m. y adj.* precipitate.

precisión *f.* accuracy.

preclínico, -ca *adj.* preclinical.

precocidad *f.* precocity.

precoz *adj.* precocious.

precursor, -ra *adj.* precursor.

preeclampsia *f.* pre-eclampsia.

premaligno, -na *adj.* premalignant.

prematuro, -ra *m. y adj.* premature.

premenstrual *adj.* premenstrual.

prenatal *adj.* prenatal.

preneoplásico, -ca *adj.* preneoplastic.

prensa *f.* torcula.

prensión *f.* prehension.

preóptico, -ca *adj.* preoptic.

preparación *f.* preparation.

preperforativo, -va *adj.* preperforative.

prepucio *m.* preputium.

presbiacusia *f.* presbyacusia.

presbicia *f.* presbyopia.

presbiopia *f.* presbyopia.

presenil *adj.* presenile.

presentación *f.* presentation.

presentación anormal malpresentation.

presentación de cara face presentation.

presentación cefálica cephalic presentation.

presentación doble de nalgas double breech presentation.

presentación facial face presentation.

presentación de frente brow presentation.

presentación de hombros shoulder presentation.

presentación mentoanterior anterior presentation.

presentación mentoposterior posterior presentation.

presentación de nalgas breech presentation.

presentación de nalgas completa breech complete presentation.

presentación oblicua oblique presentation.

presentación pelviana, presentación pélvica pelvic presentation.

presentación de la placenta placental presentation.

presentación podálica footing presentation.

presentación de rodillas knee presentation.

presentación transversa transverse presentation.

presentación de tronco trunk presentation.

presentación de vértice vertex presentation.

preservativo *m.* condom.

presináptico *m.* presynaptic.

presión *f.* pressure.

presión arterial blood pressure.

presión arterial diastólica diastolic blood pressure.

presión atmosférica atmospheric pressure.

presión capilar capillary pressure.

presión cefalorraquídea cerebrospinal pressure.

presión crítica critical pressure.

presión de enclavamiento wedge pressure.

presión estática static pressure.

presión hidrostática hydrostatic pressure.

presión intraabdominal intra-abdominal pressure.

presión intracraneal intracranial pressure.

presión intraocular intraocular pressure.

presión intraventricular intraventricular pressure.

presión de llenado filling pressure.

presión negativa negative pressure.

presión osmótica osmotic pressure.

presión de perfusión cerebral (PPC) cerebral perfusion pressure (CPP).

presión pleural pleural pressure.

presión positive positive pressure.

presión pulmonar pulmonary pressure.

presión del pulso pulse pressure.

presión retrógrada back pressure.

presión sistólica systolic pressure.

presión venosa venous pressure.

presión venosa central (PVC) central venous pressure (CVP).

presístole *f.* presystole.

presor, -ra *adj.* pressor.

prevalencia *f.* prevalence.

prevención *f.* prevention.

prevención primaria primary prevention.

prevención secundaria secondary prevention.

prevención terciaria tertiary prevention.

preventivo, -va *adj.* preventive.

previo, -via *adj.* previous.

priapismo *m.* priapism.

primario, -ria *adj.* primary.

primigrávida *f.* primigravida.

primípara *f.* primipara.

primitivo, -va *adj.* primitive.

primordial *adj.* primordial.

principio *m.* principle.

principio de abstinencia abstinence principle.

principio activo active principle.

prión *m.* prion.

privación *f.* deprivation.

probeta *f.* test tube.

probiótico, -ca *adj.* probiotic.

procariota *m.* prokaryote.

procedimiento *m.* procedure.

procedimiento invasivo invasive procedure.

procesamiento de la información *f.* information processing.

proceso *m.* process.

procrear *m.* procreate.

proctología *f.* proctology.

proctólogo, -ga *m., f.* proctologist.

prodrómico, -ca *adj.* prodromic, prodomous.

pródromo *m.* prodrome.

productivo, -va *adj.* productive.

producto *m.* product.

proenzima *f.* proenzyme.

profase *f.* prophase.

profiláctico, -ca *adj.* prophylactic.

profilaxis *f.* prophylaxis.

profilaxis activa active prophylaxis.

profilaxis pasiva passive prophylaxis.

profilaxis química chemical prophylaxis.

profundidad *f.* depth.

profundo, -da *adj.* deep.

progenie *f.* progeny.

progenitor, -ra *m., f.* progenitor.

progeria *f.* progeria.

progestacional *adj.* progestational.

progestágeno *m.* progestogen.

progesterona *f.* progesterone.

progestógeno *m.* progestogen.

prognatismo *m.* prognathism.

progresión *f.* progression.

progresivo, -va *adj.* progressive.

progreso *m.* progress.

prohormona *f.* prohormone.

prolactina *f.* prolactin.

prolapso *m.* prolapse.

prolapso del cordón umbilical prolapse of the umbilical cord.

prolapso de la válvula mitral mitral valve prolapse.

proliferación *f.* proliferation.

proliferativo, -va *adj.* proliferative.

prolongación *f.* prolongation.

prominencia *f.* prominence, prominentia.

prominente *adj.* prominent.

pronación *f.* pronation.

pronación del antebrazo pronation of the forearm.

pronación del pie pronation of the foot.

pronador, -ra *adj.* pronator.

prono *m.* prone.

propagación *f.* propagation.

propagar *v.* propagate.

propiocepción *f.* proprioception.

proporción *f.* ratio.

propósito *m.* propositus.

propulsión *f.* propulsion.

próstata *f.* prostate.

prostatectomía *f.* prostatectomy.

prostático, -ca *adj.* prostatic.

prostatitis *f.* prostatitis.

protamina *f.* protamine.

proteico, -ca *adj.* protean.

proteína *f.* protein.

proteináceo, -a *adj.* proteinaceous.

proteinograma *m.* proteinogram.

proteinuria *f.* proteinuria.

  proteinuria gestacional gestational proteinuria.

  proteinuria transitoria transient proteinuria.

  proteinuria verdadera true proteinuria.

protésico, -ca *adj.* prosthetic.

prótesis *f.* prosthesis.

  prótesis coclear cochlear prosthesis.

  prótesis dental, dentaria dental prosthesis.

  prótesis de implante implant prosthesis.

  prótesis ocular ocular prosthesis.

  prótesis parcial partial prosthesis.

  prótesis parcial fija fixed partial prosthesis.

  prótesis parcial removible removable partial prosthesis.

  prótesis provisional provisional prosthesis.

  prótesis de prueba trial prosthesis.

  prótesis superpuesta overlay prosthesis.

  prótesis temporal temporary prosthesis.

  prótesis total full prosthesis.

  prótesis transitoria transitional prosthesis.

  prótesis de válvula cardíaca cardiac valve prosthesis.

prototipo *m.* prototype.

protozoario, -ria *adj.* protozoal.

protozoo *m.* protozoon.

protrusión *f.* protrusion.

protuberancia *f.* protuberance.

proximal *adj.* proximal.

proyección *f.* projection.

  proyección visual visual projection.

prueba *f.* test.

pruriginoso, -sa *adj.* pruriginous.

prurigo *m.* prurigo.

prurito *m.* itch, pruritus.

  prurito anal o ani pruritus ani.

  prurito generalizado essential pruritus.

  prurito vulvar pruritus vulvae.

psicoanálisis *m.* psycho-analysis.

psicoanalista *m., f.* psychoanalyst.

psicoestimulante *m.* psychostimulant.

psicofármaco *m.* psychopharmaceutical.

psicología *f.* psychology.

  psicología de la educación, psicología educacional educational psychology.

psicólogo, -ga *m., f.* psychologist.

psicópata *m., f.* psychopath.

psicopatía *f.* psychopathy.

psicopatología *f.* psychopathology.

psicosis *f.* psychosis.

psicosocial *adj.* psychosocial.

psicosomático, -ca *adj.* psychosomatic.

psicoterapeuta *m., f.* psychotherapist.

psicoterapia *f.* psychotherapy.

psicótico, -ca *adj.* psychotic.

psique *f.* psyche.

psiquiatra *m., f.* psychiatrist.

psiquiatría *f.* psychiatry.

psíquico, -ca *adj.* psychic.

punzada

psoriasis *f.* psoriasis.

ptiriasis *f.* phthiriasis.

ptosis *f.* ptosis.

pubarquia *f.* pubarche.

pubertad *f.* puberty.

  pubertad precoz precocious puberty.

pubis *m.* pubis.

puente[1] *m.* pons.

puente[2] *m.* bridge.

puericultura *f.* puericulture.

puerperal *adj.* puerperal.

puerperio *m.* puerperium.

pulgar *m.* thumb.

pulido *m.* polishing.

pulmón *m.* lung.

  pulmón de granjero farmer's lung.

  pulmón de los mineros del carbón coalminer's lung.

  pulmón en panal, pulmón en panal de abeja honeycomb lung.

pulmonía *f.* pulmonitis.

pulpa *f.* pulp, pulpa.

  pulpa del dedo, pulpa digital pulp of the finger, digital pulp.

  pulpa dental dental pulp.

  pulpa desvitalizada devitalized pulp.

  pulpa no vital non-vital pulp.

  pulpa radicular radicular pulp.

pulpalgia *f.* pulpalgia.

pulpectomía *f.* pulpectomy.

pulpitis *f.* pulpitis.

pulsación *f.* pulsation.

pulsador *m.* pulsator.

pulsátil *adj.* pulsatile.

pulsión[1] *m.* drive, instinct.

  pulsión agresiva aggressive drive, aggressive instinct.

pulsión[2] *m.* pulsion.

pulso *m.* pulse, pulsus.

  pulso abdominal abdominal pulse, pulsus abdominalis.

  pulso acelerado pulsus celer.

  pulso alternante pulsus alternans.

  pulso anacrótico, pulso anacroto anacrotic pulse.

  pulso bigémino bigeminal pulse, pulsus bigeminus.

  pulso celer celer pulse.

  pulso desigual pulsus inaequalis.

  pulso filiforme filiform pulse.

  pulso intermitente intermittent pulse.

  pulso irregular irregular pulse.

  pulso ondulante undulating pulse.

  pulso paradójico, pulso paradójico de Kussmaul paradoxical pulse, Kussmaul's paradoxical pulse.

  pulso periférico peripheral pulse.

  pulso poplíteo popliteal pulse.

  pulso rápido rapid pulse.

  pulso yugular jugular pulse.

pulverización *f.* pulverization.

pulverizar *v.* pulverize.

punción *f.* puncture.

  punción digital finger stick.

  punción lumbar (PL) lumbar puncture (LP).

punta *f.* point.

punteado *m.* stippling.

puntiforme *adj.* punctiform.

punto *m.* point.

  punto doloroso painful point, point dolorosum.

  punto de osificación point of ossification.

  punto de presión pressure point.

punzada *f.* twinge.

pupila *f.* pupil, pupilla.
  pupila fija fixed pupil.
  pupila puntiforme pinhole pupil.
  pupila tónica tonic pupil.
purgante *adj.* purgative.
púrpura[1] purple.
púrpura[2] *f.* purpura.
  púrpura alérgica allergic purpura.
  púrpura hemorrágica hemorrhagic purpura.
  púrpura de Henoch-Schönlein Henoch-Schönlein purpura.
  púrpura trombocitopénica thrombocytopenic purpura.
purulento, -ta *adj.* purulent.
pus *m.* pus.
pústula *f.* pustule.
pustulosis *f.* pustulosis.
pustuloso, -sa *adj.* pustular.
putrefacción *f.* putrefaction.
putrescencia *f.* putrefaction.
pútrido, -da *adj.* putrid.

Q

queilitis *f.* cheilitis.
quejido *m.* grunting.
quelante *m.* chelating agent.
quelar *v.* chelate.
queloide *m.* cheloid, keloid.
queloides *m.* cheloid, keloid.
quemadura *f.* burn.
  quemadura eléctrica electric burn, electrical burn.
  quemadura química chemical burn.
  quemadura por radiación radiation burn.
  quemadura por rayos X X-ray burn.
  quemadura de segundo grado second degree burn.
  quemadura solar solar burn, sun burn, sunburn.
  quemadura superficial superficial burn.
  quemadura de tercer grado third degree burn.
  quemadura térmica thermal burn.
quemazón *f.* burning.
quemosis *f.* chemosis.
  quemosis conjuntival conjunctival chemosis.
queratán-sulfato *m.* keratan sulfate.
queratina *f.* ceratin, keratin.
queratinización *f.* keratinization.
queratinizado, -da *adj.* keratinized.
queratinizar *v.* keratinize.
queratinocito *m.* keratinocyte.
queratitis *f.* keratitis.
queratoacantoma *m.* keratoacanthoma.
queratocito *m.* keratocyte.
queratoconjuntivitis *f.* keratoconjunctivitis.
queratocono *m.* keratoconus.
queratodermia *f.* keratoderma.
queratoiditis *f.* keratoiditis.
queratopatía *f.* keratopathy.
queratoplasia *f.* keratoplasia.
queratosis *f.* keratosis.
  queratosis actínica actinic keratosis.
  queratosis palmar y plantar keratosis palmaris et plantaris.
  queratosis seborreica seborrheic keratosis, keratosis seborrheica.

queratosis senil senile keratosis, keratosis senilis.

queratosis solar solar keratosis.

querubismo *m.* cherubism.

quiasma *m.* chiasm, chiasma.

quiasma óptico optic chiasm, chiasma opticum.

quiasmático, -ca *adj.* chiasmatic.

quiescente *adj.* quiescent.

quijada *f.* jaw.

quilo *m.* chyle.

quilomicrón *m.* chylomicron.

quilosis¹ *f.* chilosis.

quilosis² *f.* chylosis.

quilosis³ *f.* kyllosis.

quiloso, -sa *adj.* chylous.

quiluria *f.* chyluria.

quimera *f.* chimera, chimaera, chiomera.

química *f.* chemistry.

químico, -ca¹ *m., f.* chemist.

químico, -ca² *adj.* chemical.

quimioabrasión *f.* chemabrasion.

quimioprevención *f.* chemoprevention.

quimioprofilaxis *f.* chemoprophylaxis.

quimiorreceptor *m.* chemoreceptor.

quimiotaxis *f.* chemotaxis.

quimioterapia *f.* chemotherapy.

quimioterapia adyuvante adjuvant chemotherapy.

quimioterapia combinada combination chemotherapy.

quimioterapia de consolidación consolidation chemotherapy.

quimioterapia intraarterial, quimioterapia I.A. intraarterial chemotherapy.

quimioterapia de inducción induction chemotherapy.

quimioterapia de intensificación intensification chemotherapy.

quimioterapia radioactiva chemotherapy (unsealed radioactive).

quimioterápico, -ca *adj.* chemotherapeutic.

quimo *m.* chyme.

quintillizo, -za *adj.* quintuplet.

quintípara *f.* quintipara.

quiropráctico, -ca *m., f.*, chiropractor.

quirúrgico, -ca *adj.* chirurgic, surgical.

quiste *m.* cyst.

quiste de Bartholin, quiste de Bartolino Bartholin's cyst.

quiste congénito congenital cyst.

quiste hepático hepatic cyst, cyst of the liver.

quiste hidatídico hydatid cyst.

quiste renal renal cyst.

quiste vocal intracordal cyst.

quístico, -ca¹ *adj.* cystic.

quístico, -ca² *adj.* cystose, cystous.

R

rabia *f.* rabies.

rabieta *f.* tantrum.

racial *adj.* racial.

ración *f.* ration.

racional *adj.* rational.

radiación *f.* radiation, radiato.

radiación ultravioleta ultraviolet radiation.

radiación X X-radiation.

radioactividad *f.* radioactivity.

radiactivo, -va *adj.* radioactive.

radicular *adj.* radicular.

radiculitis *f.* radiculitis.

radiculopatía *f.* radiculopathy.

radio¹ *m.* radium.

radio² *m.* radius.

radiografía¹ *f.* radiography.

radiografía dental dental radiograph.

radiografía digital digital radiography.

radiografía² *f.* radiogram.

radiografía panorámica panoramic radiogram.

radioinmunoanálisis (RIA) *m.* radioimmunoassay (RIA).

radiología *f.* radiology.

radiólogo, -ga *m., f.* radiologist.

radiopaco, -ca *adj.* radiopaque.

radiosensibilidad *f.* radiosensibility, radiosensitiveness, radiosensitivity.

radiosensible *adj.* radiosensitive, radiosensible.

radioterapia *f.* radiation therapy, radiotherapy, X-ray therapy.

radioterapia externa external radiation therapy.

radioterapia intracavitaria intracavitary radiotherapy.

raíz *f.* root, radix.

rama¹ *f.* branch, ramus.

rama² *f.* branch.

ramificación *f.* ramification.

ramificado, -da *adj.* branching, ramified.

ramificar *v.* ramify.

rampa *f.* scala.

rango *m.* range.

rango de movimiento range of motion.

rapto *m.* raptus.

raquialgia *f.* rachialgia.

raquianalgesia *f.* rachianalgesia.

raquianestesia *f.* rachianesthesia, spinal anesthesia.

raquídeo, -a *adj.* rachidial.

raquítico, -ca *adj.* rachitic, rickety.

raquitis *f.* rachitis.

raquitismo *m.* rachitis, rickets.

raquitismo vitaminorresistente resistant rachitis.

rasgado, -da *adj.* lacerated.

rasgo *m.* trait.

rasgo adquirido acquired trait.

rasgo del carácter, rasgo caracterial character trait.

rasgo codominante codominant trait.

rasgo condicionado por el sexo sex-conditioned trait.

rasgo cromosómico chromosomal trait.

rasgo dependiente dependent trait.

rasgo dominante dominant trait.

rasgo hereditario hereditary trait.

rasgo influido por el sexo sex-influenced trait.

rasgo intermedio intermediate trait.

rasgo ligado al sexo sex-linked trait.

rasgo limitado por el sexo sex-limited trait.

rasgo no penetrante non-penetrant trait.

rasgo de la personalidad personality trait.

rash *m.* rash.

rash del pañal diaper rash.

rash de erisipela wildfire rash.

rash en mariposa butterfly rash.

rash por ortigas nettle rash.

rash por orugas caterpillar rash.

rash de verano summer rash.

raspado *m.* strip, curettage.

rastreo *m.* scan.

  rastreo genético genetic screening.

  rastreo isotópico isotopic scan.

rata *f.* rat, rattus.

raticida *m.* raticide, mort-aux-rats.

ratón *m.* mouse.

  ratón nu/nu nu/nu mouse.

raya *f.* streak.

rayo *m.* ray.

  rayo ultravioleta ultraviolet ray.

  rayo X x-ray.

raza *f.* race.

razón¹ *f.* rational faculty.

razón² *f.* ratio.

reabsorber *v.* reabsorb.

reabsorbible *adj.* reabsorbable.

reabsorción *f.* reabsorption.

  reabsorción gingival gingival reabsorption.

  reabsorción ósea bone reabsorption.

  reabsorción tubular tubular reabsorption.

reacción *f.* reaction.

  reacción adversa adverse reaction.

  reacción adversa a un fármaco adverse drug reaction.

  reacción alérgica allergic reaction.

  reacción anafiláctica anaphylactic reaction.

  reacción anestésica local local anesthetic reaction.

  reacción antígeno-anticuerpo antigen-antibody reaction.

  reacción ante cuerpos extraños, reacción de cuerpo extraño foreign body reaction.

  reacción cutánea cutaneous reaction.

  reacción dolorosa, reacción de dolor pain reaction.

  reacción de duelo grief reaction.

  reacción a estrés stress reaction.

  reacción focal focal reaction.

  reacción de hipersensibilidad hypersensivity reaction.

  reacción inmune immune reaction.

  reacción irreversible irreversible reaction.

  reacción local local reaction.

  reacción de Mantoux Mantoux's reaction.

  reacción positiva falsa false-positive reaction.

  reacción primaria primary reaction.

  reacción pupilar indirecta indirect pupillary reaction.

  reacción retrasada delayed reaction.

  reacción de roncha y pápula, reacción de roncha y eritema wheal-and-erythema reaction.

  reacción de tipo reflejo reflex type reaction.

  reacción transfusional transfusion reaction.

  reacción por transfusión sanguínea incompatible incompatible blood transfusion response.

reacción de la tuberculina tuberculin reaction.

reacción vital vital reaction.

reaccionar v. react.

reactivación f. reactivation.

reactivo m. reagent.

real adj. real, true.

realidad f. reality.

reamputación f. reamputation.

reanimación f. resuscitation.

reanimación boca a boca mouth-to-mouth resuscitation.

reanimación cardiopulmonar cardiopulmonary resuscitation.

reblandecimiento m. softening.

recaída f. relapse.

recalcificación f. recalcification.

recanalización f. recanalization.

recanalizar v. recanalize.

receptor, -ra m., f. y adj. receptor.

receptor alfa-adrenérgico alpha-adrenergic receptor.

receptor beta-adrenérgico beta-adrenergic receptor.

receptor colinérgico cholinergic receptor.

receptor de dopamina dopamine receptor.

receptor de estrógenos estrogen receptor.

receptor hormonal hormone receptor.

receptor de insulina insulin receptor.

receptor de lipoproteínas de baja densidad (LDL) LDL receptor.

receptor para opiáceo opiate receptor.

receptor de dolor pain receptor.

receptor de presión pressure receptor.

receptor de progesterona progesterone receptor.

receptor químico chemical receptor.

receptor sensitivo sensory receptor.

receptor táctiles touch receptor.

receptor de transfusión receiver of transfusion.

receptor de trasplante receiver of transplant.

receptor universal universal recipient.

receptor de volumen volume receptor.

recesión f. recession.

recesivo, -va adj. recessive.

receta f. prescription, recipe.

rechazo m. rejection.

rechazo agudo acute rejection.

rechazo humoral humoral rejection.

rechazo de órgano organ rejection.

rechazo m. rebound.

recidiva f. recidivation, relapse.

recidiva de los tumores tumor relapse.

recién nacido m. newborn.

reclutamiento m. recruitment.

recombinación f. recombination.

recombinante adj. recombinant.

recompensa f. reward.

reconocimiento m. recognition.

reconstitución f. reconstitution.

reconstituyente m. restorative.

reconstrucción f. reconstruction.

recrudecimiento m. recrudescence.

rectal *adj.* rectal.

rectalgia *f.* rectalgia.

rectificación *f.* rectification.

rectificar *v.* rectify.

rectitis *f.* rectitis.

recto *m.* rectum.

recto, -ta *adj.* straight.

rectoabdominal *adj.* rectoabdominal.

rectovaginal *adj.* rectovaginal.

rectovesical *adj.* rectovesical.

rectovulvar *adj.* rectovulvar.

recuento *m.* count.

  recuento sanguíneo completo complete blood count.

  recuento sanguíneo diferencial de glóbulos blancos differential white blood count.

recuerdo *m.* recall.

recuperación¹ *f.* recuperation.

recuperación² *f.* recovery.

  recuperación espontánea spontaneous recovery.

  recuperación posoperatoria postoperatory recovery.

recuperarse *v.* recuperate.

recurrencia *f.* recurrence.

recurrente¹ *adj.* recurrent.

recurrente² *adj.* relapsing.

red *f.* net, rete.

reducción *f.* reduction.

  reducción abierta open reduction.

  reducción abierta de fractura open reduction of fracture.

  reducción cerrada de fractura closed reduction of fracture.

  reducción cerrada closed reduction.

  reducción de fractura reduction of fracture.

  reducción de la mama, reducción mamaria breast reduction, mammaplasty reduction.

  reducción de peso weight reduction.

reducible *adj.* reducible.

reducir *v.* reduce.

reductor *m.* reductant.

referencia *f.* reference.

refinar *v.* refine.

reflejado, -da *adj.* reflected.

reflejar *v.* reflect.

reflejo, -ja *m. y adj.* reflex.

  reflejo de acomodación accommodation reflex.

  reflejo adquirido acquired reflex.

  reflejo anal anal reflex.

  reflejo de atención de la pupila attention reflex of the pupil.

  reflejo condicionado conditional reflex, conditioned reflex, trained reflex.

  reflejo de defensa defense reflex.

  reflejo estático, reflejo estatocinético static reflex, statokinetic reflex.

  reflejo del llanto cry reflex.

  reflejo muscular muscular reflex.

  reflejo ocular eye reflex.

  reflejo patelar knee-jerk reflex.

  reflejo patológico pathologic reflex.

  reflejo plantar sole reflex, plantar reflex.

  reflejo plantar en hiperflexión Guillain-Barré reflex.

  reflejo postural postural reflex.

  reflejo pupilar pupillary reflex.

  reflejo de la rodilla knee reflex.

reflejo rotuliano* patellar reflex.
reflejo tendinoso* tendon reflex.
reflejo tendinoso de Aquiles, reflejo del tendón de Aquiles* Achilles tendon reflex.
reflejo del tendón rotuliano* patellar tendon reflex.
reflexionar *v.* reflect.
reflujo *m.* reflux.
reflujo gastroesofágico* gastroesophageal reflux.
reforzamiento *m.* reinforcement.
refracción *f.* refraction.
refrescar *v.* refresh.
refrigeración *f.* refrigeration.
refringente *adj.* refringent.
refuerzo *m.* reinforcement.
refuerzo positivo* positive reinforcement.
regeneración *f.* regeneration.
regenerar *v.* regenerate.
régimen *m.* regimen, diet.
región *f.* region.
registro *m.* record.
registro electrocardiográfico* electrocardiographic record.
registro electroencefalográfico* electroencefalographic record.
registro hospitalario* hospital record.
registro hospitalario de pacientes* patient's hospital record.
registro médico* medical record.
regla[1] *f.* period.
regla[2] *f.* rule.
regresión *f.* regression.
regulación *f.* regulation.
regulador, -ra *adj.* regulatory.
regular *adj.* regular.

regularidad *f.* regularity.
regurgitación *f.* regurgitation.
regurgitación valvular* valvular regurgitation.
regurgitante *adj.* regurgitant.
regurgitar *v.* regurgitate.
rehidratación *f.* rehydratation.
rehidratar *v.* rehydrate.
rehospitalizar *v.* rehospitalize.
reimplantación *f.* reimplantation.
reimplante *m.* replant.
reintubación *f.* reintubation.
rejuvenecimiento *m.* rejuvenescence.
relación *f.* relation, relationship.
relajación *f.* relaxation.
relajante *m. y adj.* relaxant.
relajante muscular* muscular relaxant.
relajar *v.* relax.
relativo, -va *adj.* relative.
remanente *m. y adj.* remanent.
remedio *m.* remedy.
remineralización *f.* remineralization.
remisión *f.* remission.
remisión espontánea* spontaneous remission.
remitir *v.* remit.
renal *adj.* renal.
reparación *f.* reparation, repair.
reparador, -ra *adj.* reparative, restorative.
repelente *adj.* repellent.
replicación *f.* replication.
repolarización *f.* repolarization.
reposición *f.* repositioning.
reposo *m.* rest.
reproducción *f.* reproduction.

reproducción sexual sexual reproduction.

reproductivo, -va *adj.* reproductive.

reproductor, -ra *adj.* reproductive.

rescisión *f.* excision.

resecable *adj.* resectable.

resecar *v.* resect.

resección *f.* resection.

reserva *f.* reserve.

reservorio *m.* reservoir.

reservorio de infección reservoir of infection.

resfriado *m.* cold.

residual *adj.* residual.

residuo *m.* residue.

resistencia *f.* resistance.

resistencia a la insulina insulin resistance.

resolver *v.* resolve.

resonancia *f.* resonance.

respirable *adj.* respirable.

respiración *f.* breathing, respiration.

respiración abdominal abdominal respiration.

respiración aeróbica aerobic respiration.

respiración anaeróbica anaerobic respiration.

respiración artificial artificial respiration.

respiración asistida assisted respiration.

respiración boca a boca mouth-to-mouth respiration.

respiración costal costal respiration.

respiración cutánea cutaneous respiration.

respiración diafragmática diaphragmatic respiration.

respiración entrecortada interrupted respiration.

respiración estertorosa stertorous respiration.

respiración interrumpida interrupted respiration.

respiración paradójica paradoxical respiration.

respiración superficial shallow breathing.

respiración torácica thoracic respiration.

respirador *m.* respirator.

respirar *v.* respire.

respiratorio, -ria *adj.* respiratory.

respuesta *f.* response.

respuesta inmune immune response.

restablecimiento *m.* recovery.

restauración *f.* restoration.

resto *m.* residue.

resto embrionario embryonic residue.

restricción *f.* restraint.

resucitación *f.* resuscitation.

resucitador *m.* resuscitator.

resultado *m.* result.

resurrección *f.* resuscitation.

retardado *m.* retardate.

retención *f.* retention.

retención de orina urine retention, retention of urine.

retención placentaria retention of placenta, retention of placental fragments.

retención protésica denture retention.

retención de la respiración breath-holding.

reticulado, -da *adj.* reticulated.

retículo *m.* reticulum.

reticulosis *f.* reticulosis.

retina *f.* retina.

retina desprendida detached retina.

retinal *adj.* retinal.

retiniano, -na *adj.* retinal.

retinitis *f.* retinitis.

retinoblastoma *m.* retinoblastoma.

retinocoroiditis *f.* retinochoroiditis.

retinopapilitis *f.* retinopapillitis.

retinopatía *f.* retinopathy.

retinopatía hipertensiva hypertensive retinopathy.

retinopatía macular macular retinopathy.

retinopatía de los prematuros retinopathy of prematurity.

retinopatía proliferativa proliferative retinopathy.

retinoscopia *f.* retinoscopy.

retinoscopio *m.* retinoscope.

retinosis *f.* retinosis.

retorno *m.* return.

retorno venoso venous return.

retortijón *m.* gripe, stomach cramp.

retracción *f.* retraction.

retracción del útero uterine muscle retraction.

retráctil *adj.* retractile.

retrasado, -da *adj.* retardate.

retraso *m.* retardation.

retraso mental mental retardation.

retraso mental leve mild mental retardation.

retraso mental moderado moderate mental retardation.

retraso mental grave severe mental retardation.

retraso mental profundo profound mental retardation.

retraso psicomotor psychomotor retardation.

retroalimentación *f.* feedback.

retroceso *m.* retrocession.

retrognatia *f.* retrognathia.

retroperitoneal *adj.* retroperitoneal.

retroperitonitis *f.* retroperitonitis.

retroplacentario, -ria *adj.* retroplacental.

retrorrectal *adj.* retrorectal.

retrospección *f.* retrospection.

retrospectivo, -va *adj.* retrospective.

retrosternal *adj.* retrosternal.

retroversión *f.* retroversion.

retrovirus *m.* retrovirus.

reuma, reúma *m., f.* rheum, rheuma.

reumático, -ca *adj.* rheumatic, rheumatismal.

reumatismo *m.* rheumatism.

reumatología *f.* rheumatology.

reumatólogo, -ga *f.* rheumatologist.

reunión *f.* union.

revacunación *f.* revaccination.

revascularización *f.* revascularization.

reversible *adj.* reversible.

reversión *f.* reversion.

revestimiento *m.* lining.

ribonucleótido *m.* ribonucleotide.

ribosoma *m.* ribosome.

rictus *m.* rictus.

riesgo *m.* risk.

rigidez *f.* rigidity.

  rigidez cadavérica cadaveric rigidity.

  rigidez catatónica catatonic rigidity.

  rigidez post mortem postmortem rigidity.

  rigidez en rueda dentada cogwheel rigidity.

rigor *m.* rigor.

  rigor mortis rigor mortis.

rinitis *f.* rhinitis.

  rinitis alérgica allergic rhinitis.

  rinitis analfiláctica anaphylactic rhinitis.

rinofaringe *f.* rhinopharynx.

rinofaríngeo, -a *adj.* rhinopharyngeal.

rinofaringitis *f.* rhinopharyngitis.

rinolaringitis *f.* rhinolaryngitis.

rinoplastia *f.* rhinoplasty.

rinorrea *f.* rhinorrhea.

rinovirus *m.* rhinovirus.

riñón *m.* kidney.

  riñón ectópico floating kidney.

  riñón en herradura horseshoe kidney.

  riñón pielonefrítico pyelonephritic kidney.

  riñón poliquístico polycystic kidney.

risa *f.* laugh, risus.

rítmico, -ca *adj.* rhythmical.

ritmo *m.* rhythm.

  ritmo fetal fetal rhythm.

  ritmo de galope cantering rhythm.

  ritmo nodal nodal rhythm.

  ritmo nodal auriculoventricular atrioventricular nodal rhythm.

  ritmo rápido fast rhythm.

  ritmo sinusal sinus rhythm.

  ritmo sinusal coronario coronary sinus rhythm.

  ritmo ventricular ventricular rhythm.

ritual *m.* ritual.

roce *m.* rubbing.

  roce pericárdico pericardial rubbing.

  roce pleurítico pleuritic rubbing.

rodilla *f.* knee, genu.

  rodilla bloqueada locked knee.

rodillera *f.* kneeguard.

rojo *m.* red.

rojo, -ja *adj.* red.

rol *m.* role.

roncha *f.* wheal.

ronco, -ca *adj.* hoarse.

ronquera *f.* hoarseness.

ronquido *m.* snore.

rosa *f.* rose.

rosácea *f.* rosacea.

roséola *f.* roseola.

rotación *f.* rotation.

  rotación intestinal intestinal rotation.

rotatorio, -ria *adj.* rotator.

rótula *f.* rotula, patella.

rotura *f.* rhexis, rupture.

rozadura *f.* gall.

rubefacción *f.* erubescence, rubefaction.

rubefaciente *adj.* rubefacient.

rubéola *f.* rubella, rubeola.

rubor *m.* flush, redness, rubor.

rudimentario, -ria *adj.* rudimentary.

rueda *f.* wheel.
  rueda dentada cogwheel rigidity.
rugosidad *f.* rugosity.
rugoso, -sa *adj.* rugous, rugose, wrinkled.
ruido *m.* noise, sound, bruit, sonitus.
  ruido ambiental ambient noise.
  ruido auscultatorio auscultatory sound.
  ruido cardíaco cardiac sound.
  ruido intestinal bowel sound.
  ruido de Korotkoff Korotkoff sound.
  ruido respiratorio respiratory sound.
ruptura *f.* break, rupture.
rutina¹ *f.* habit.
rutina² *f.* rutin.

S

sabañón *m.* chilblain.
sabor *m.* flavor.
sacarina *f.* saccharin.
sacarosa *f.* sucrose.
saco *m.* sac, saccus.
sacral *adj.* sacral.
sacro *m.* sacrum.
sacrococcígeo, -a *adj.* sacrococcygeal.
sacrocóccix *m.* sacrococcyx.
sacudida *f.* jerk, saccade.
sacudidas *f.* shakes.
sacular *adj.* saccular.
saculococlear *adj.* sacculocochlear.
sádico, -ca *m., f.* sadist.
sadismo *m.* sadism.

sadomasoquismo *m.* sadomasochism.
sadomasoquista *adj.* sadomasochistic.
sagital *adj.* sagittal.
sal *f.* salt, sal.
sala *f.* room, ward.
  sala de cuidados intensivos intensive therapy room.
  sala de operaciones (SO) operating room (OR).
  sala de partos, paritorio delivery room.
  sala posparto postdelivery room.
  sala de reanimación recovery room (RR).
  sala de recuperación recovery room.
  sala de urgencias (SU) emergency room (ER).
salida *f.* outlet.
salidas *f.* output.
salino, -na *adj.* saline.
saliva *f.* saliva.
salivación *f.* salivation.
salival *adj.* salivary.
salpingectomía *f.* salpingectomy.
salpingitis *f.* salpingitis.
salubre *adj.* salubrious.
salubridad *f.* salubrity.
salud *f.* health.
  salud familiar family health.
  salud laboral industrial health.
  salud medioambiental environmental health.
  salud mental mental health.
  salud mental comunitaria community mental health.
  salud profesional occupational health.

salud sexual sexual health.

saludable *adj.* salutary.

sanatorio *m.* sanatorium.

saneamiento *m.* sanitation.

sanear *v.* sanitize.

sangrado *m.* bleeding.

sangrado uterino disfuncional dysfunctional uterine bleeding.

sangramiento *m.* bleeding.

sangrar *v.* bleed.

sangre *f.* blood.

sangre arterial arterial blood.

sangre central central blood.

sangre circulante circulating bloodstream.

sangre del cordón cord blood.

sangre estancada sludged blood.

sangre oculta occult blood.

sangre periférica peripheral blood.

sangre total whole blood.

sangre venosa venous blood.

sangre venosa mixta mixed venous blood.

sangría *f.* bloodletting.

sanguíneo, -a *adj.* sanguine, sanguineous.

sanguinolento, -ta *adj.* sanguinolent.

sanidad *f.* sanitation, sanity.

sanitario, -ria *adj.* sanitary.

sanitas health.

sano, -na *adj.* healthy.

sarampión *m.* measles.

sarcoidosis *f.* sarcoidosis.

sarcoma *m.* sarcoma.

sarcómero *m.* sarcomere.

sarna *f.* scabies.

sarnoso, -sa *adj.* scabietic.

sarpullido *m.* tetter.

sarpullido por calor prickly heat tetter.

sarpullido costroso crusted tetter.

sarro *m.* tartar.

satélite *m.* satellite.

saturación *f.* saturation.

saturación de oxígeno oxygen saturation.

saturación de oxígeno en la hemoglobina hemoglobin oxygen saturation.

saturado, -da *adj.* saturated.

saturnismo *m.* saturnism.

sebáceo, -a *adj.* sebaceous, sebaceus.

sebo *m.* sebum.

seborrea *f.* seborrhea.

seborreico, -ca *adj.* seborrheic.

sebum *m.* sebum.

sección *f.* section, sectio.

sección cesárea cesarean section.

sección frontal frontal section.

sección lateral sectio lateralis.

sección mediana sectio mediana.

sección perineal perineal section.

sección sagital sagittal section, sagittal sectio.

sección suprapúbica sectio alta.

seco, -ca *adj.* dry.

secreción *f.* secretion.

secreción apocrina apocrine secretion.

secreción autocrina autocrine secretion.

secreción bronquial bronchial secretion.

secreción externa external secretion.

secreción holocrina holocrine secretion.

secreción interna internal secretion.

secreción merocrina merocrine secretion.

secreción paracrina paracrine secretion.

secreción paralítica paralytic secretion.

secreción del pezón nipple discharge.

secretar *v.* secrete.

secretor, -ra *adj.* secretory.

sectario, -ria *adj.* sectarian.

sector *m.* sector.

secuela *f.* sequela.

secuencia *f.* sequence.

secuestrar *v.* sequester.

secuestro *m.* sequestration, sequestrum.

secuestro subclavio subclavian sequestration.

secundario, -ria *m. y adj.* secondary.

secundípara *f.* secundipara.

secundiparidad *f.* secundiparity.

sed *f.* thirst.

seda *f.* silk.

seda dental dental floss.

seda quirúrgica surgical silk.

sedación *f.* sedation.

sedante *m. y adj.* sedative, sedativus.

sedante nervioso nervous sedative.

sedante respiratorio respiratory sedative.

sedentario, -ria *adj.* sedentary.

sedimento *m.* sediment.

segmentación *f.* cleavage, segmentation.

segmentario, -ria *adj.* segmental.

segmento *m.* segment, segmentum.

segregación *f.* segregation.

segregar *v.* secrete.

selección *f.* selection.

selección aleatoria random selection.

selección múltiple multiple selection.

selección natural natural selection.

selección sesgada truncate selection.

selectividad *f.* selectivity.

selectivo, -va *adj.* selective.

sellado *m.* seal.

semen *m.* semen.

seminal *adj.* seminal.

seminoma *m.* seminoma.

semivida *f.* half-life.

senectud *f.* senium.

senil *adj.* senile.

senilidad *f.* senility.

seno *m.* sinus.

senografía *f.* senography.

sensación *f.* sensation.

sensación de calor sensation of warmth.

sensación cutánea skin sensation.

sensación dérmica dermal sensation.

sensación de impotencia powerlessness.

sensación subjetiva subjective sensation.

sensibilidad *f.* sensibility, sensitivity.

sensibilidad de contraste contrast sensitivity.

sensibilidad cruzada cross sensitivity.

sensibilidad cutánea cutaneous sensation.

sensibilidad fototóxica phototoxic sensitivity.

sensibilización *f.* sensitization.

sensibilización cruzada cross sensitization.

sensibilización Rh Rh sensitization.

sensibilizado, -da *adj.* sensitized.

sensible *adj.* sensitive.

sensitivo, -va *adj.* sensory.

sensitivomotor, -ra *adj.* sensorimotor.

sensor, -ra *m. y adj.* sensor.

sensorial *adj.* sensorial.

sensual *adj.* sensual.

sensualidad *f.* sensualism.

sentido *m.* sense.

sentido del equilibrio sense of equilibrium.

sentimiento *m.* sentiment, feeling.

sentimiento de culpabilidad feeling of guilt.

sentimiento de inferioridad feeling of inferiority.

señal *f.* signal, cue.

separación *f.* separation.

separador[1] *m.* retractor.

separador[2] *m.* separator.

sepsis *f.* sepsis.

sepsis puerperal puerperal sepsis.

septado, -da *adj.* septate.

septicemia *f.* septicemia.

septicémico, -ca *adj.* septicemic.

séptico, -ca *adj.* septic.

septo *m.* septum.

seriado, -da *adj.* serial.

sérico, -ca *adj.* serumal.

serie *f.* series.

serie leucocítica leukocytic series.

seroalbúmina *f.* seralbumin.

seroconversión *f.* seroconversion.

seroconvertir *v.* seroconvert.

serocultivo *m.* seroculture.

serogrupo *m.* serogroup.

serología *f.* serology.

serología diagnóstica diagnostic serology.

serológico, -ca *adj.* serologic, serological.

seroma *m.* seroma.

seronegatividad *f.* seronegativity.

seronegativo, -va *adj.* seronegative.

seropositivo, -va *adj.* seropositive.

serotipificar *v.* serotype.

serotipo *m.* serotype.

serotonina *f.* serotonin.

serotoninérgico, -ca *adj.* serotoninergic.

serpiente *f.* snake.

serpiginoso, -sa *adj.* serpiginous.

serrado, -da *adj.* serrated, serratus.

serum *m.* serum.

servicio *m.* department, service.

servicio básico de salud basic health service.

servicio de hospital de día day health care service.

servicio interno environmental service.

servicio de salud maternoinfantil maternal and child (MCH) service.

servicio de toxicología detoxification service.

servicio de urgencias emergency department.

servicio de urgencias de psiquiatría psychiatric emergency service.

sesamoide *adj.* sesamoid.

sesamoideo, -a *adj.* sesamoid.

sesamoiditis *f.* sesamoiditis.

sesgo *m.* bias.

  sesgo de detección detection bias.

sesión *f.* round.

  sesión clínico-patológica clinical-pathologic conference.

  sesión docente teaching round.

seudoartrosis *f.* pseudarthrosis, pseudoarthrosis.

seudoembarazo *m.* pseudopregnancy.

sexo *m.* sex.

  sexo cromosómico chromosomal sex.

  sexo endocrinológico endocrinologic sex.

  sexo genético genetic sex.

  sexo gonadal gonadal sex.

  sexo morfológico morphological sex.

  sexo nuclear nuclear sex.

  sexo psicológico psychological sex.

  sexo seguro safe sex.

  sexo social social sex.

sexología *f.* sexology.

sexopatía *f.* sexopathy.

sextigrávida *f.* sextigravida.

sextillizo, -za *adj.* sextuplet.

sextípara *f.* sextipara.

sexto par craneal *m.* sixth cranial nerve.

sexual *adj.* sexual.

sexualidad *f.* sexuality.

  sexualidad infantil infantile sexuality.

shock *m.* shock.

shunt *m.* shunt.

sialorrea *f.* sialorrhea.

sibilancia *f.* sibilant rales, wheeze, whistling rales.

sibilante *adj.* sibilant.

sicosis *f.* sycosis.

  sicosis de la barba sycosis barbae.

sideremia *f.* blood iron.

sideroblasto *m.* sideroblast.

siderocito *m.* siderocyte.

siderosis *f.* siderosis.

sien *f.* temple.

sierra *f.* saw.

sífilis *f.* syphilis.

sifilítico, -ca *adj.* syphilitic.

sigmoide *m. y adj.* sigmoid.

sigmoidectomía *f.* sigmoidectomy.

sigmoideo, -a *adj.* sigmoid.

sigmoides *m.* sigmoid.

significación *f.* significance.

  significación estadística statistical significance.

signo *m.* sign.

  signo físico physical sign.

  signo meníngeo meningeal sign.

  signo neurológico leve soft neurologic sign.

  signo positivo de embarazo positive sign of pregnancy.

  signo de presunción presumptive sign.

  signo prodrómico prodromic sign.

  signo visual visual sign.

  signo vital vital sign.

silbido *m.* whistle.

silencio *m.* silence.

silencioso, -sa *adj.* silent.

silente *adj.* silent.

silicona *f.* silicone.

  silicona inyectable injectable silicone.

silicosis *f.* silicosis.

silla *f.* chair, sella.

  silla de parto birthing chair.

silla de ruedas wheelchair.

silueta *f.* silhouette.

silueta cardíaca cardiac silhouette.

simbiosis *f.* symbiosis.

símbolo *m.* symbol.

simetría *f.* symmetry.

simétrico, -ca *adj.* symmetrical, symmetric.

sí mismo *m.* self.

simpatectomía *f.* sympathectomy.

simpatía *f.* sympathy.

simpático *m. y adj.* sympathetic, sympathic.

simple *adj.* simple.

simulación *f.* simulation.

simulador *m.* simulator.

simulador, -ra *adj.* simulator.

simultáneo, -a *adj.* simultaneous.

sinapsis *f.* synapse, synapsis.

sináptico, -ca *adj.* synaptic.

sincopal *adj.* syncopal.

síncope *m.* syncope.

síncope anginoso syncope anginosa.

síncope cardíaco cardiac syncope.

sincrónico, -ca *adj.* synchronous.

sincronismo *m.* synchronism.

sindactilia *f.* syndactylia, syndactyly.

síndrome *m.* syndrome.

síndrome de abstinencia abstinence syndrome, withdrawal syndrome.

síndrome de abstinencia del alcohol withdrawal syndrome for alcohol.

síndrome de abstinencia de sedantes withdrawal syndrome for sedatives.

síndrome de abuso del niño abused-child syndrome.

síndrome de accidente vascular stroke syndrome.

síndrome alcohólico fetal, síndrome de alcoholismo fetal fetal alcohol syndrome.

síndrome anginoso anginal syndrome, anginose syndrome.

síndrome de ansiedad anxiety syndrome.

síndrome de apnea del sueño sleep apnea syndrome.

síndrome de aspiración fetal fetal aspiration syndrome.

síndrome compartimental compartmental syndrome.

síndrome de dificultad respiratoria del adulto (SDRA) adult respiratory distress syndrome (ARDS).

síndrome de distrés respiratorio del recién nacido respiratory distress syndrome of the newborn.

síndrome de distrés respiratorio del adulto (SDRA) adult respiratory distress syndrome (ARDS).

síndrome de Henoch-Schönlein Henoch-Schönlein syndrome.

síndrome de injerto contra huésped runting syndrome.

síndrome de inmunodeficiencia adquirida (SIDA) acquired immunodeficiency syndrome (AIDS).

síndrome de insuficiencia respiratoria del recién nacido respiratory distress syndrome of the newborn.

síndrome del intestino irritable irritable bowel syndrome.

síndrome de mala absorción, síndrome de malabsorción malabsorption syndrome.

síndrome de la muerte súbita del lactante (SMSL) sudden infant death syndrome (SIDS).

síndrome de la mujer maltratada (SMM) battered woman syndrome (BWS).

síndrome nefrítico nephritic syndrome.

síndrome nefrótico nephrotic syndrome.

síndrome del niño maltratado battered child syndrome.

síndrome del niño hiperactivo hyperactive child syndrome.

síndrome del ovario poliquístico polycystic ovary syndrome.

síndrome paleoestriado, síndrome paleoestriatal paleostriatal syndrome.

síndrome posconmoción, síndrome posconmocional postconcussion, postconcussional syndrome.

sindrómico, -ca *adj.* syndromic.

sinequia *f.* synechia.

sinergia *f.* synergy, synergia.

sinérgico, -ca *adj.* synergic.

sinergismo *m.* synergism.

sínfisis *f.* symphysis.

sinistralidad *f.* sinistrality.

sinósqueo *m.* synoscheos.

sinovitis *f.* synovitis.

síntesis *f.* synthesis.

síntoma *m.* symptom.

síntoma de abstinencia abstinence symptom.

síntoma concomitante concomitant symptom.

síntoma diana target symptom.

síntoma diferido delayed symptom.

síntoma de presentación presenting symptom.

síntoma prodrómico prodromal symptom.

sintomático, -ca *adj.* symptomatic.

sinuitis *f.* sinuitis.

sinusitis *f.* sinusitis.

sistema *m.* system.

sistema digestivo digestive system.

sistema endocrino endocrine system.

sistema esquelético skeletal system.

sistema fagocítico mononuclear (SFM) mononuclear phagocyte system (MPS).

sistema genital genital system.

sistema glandular glandular system.

sistema de grupos sanguíneos blood group system.

sistema de Havers, sistema haversiano Haversian system.

sistema hematopoyético, sistema hemopoyético hematopoietic system.

sistema inmunitario, sistema inmunológico immune system.

sistema internacional de unidades (SI) international system of units.

sistema linfático lymphatic system.

sistema locomotor locomotor system.

sistema mononuclear fagocítico mononuclear phagocyte system.

sistema muscular muscular system.

sistema nervioso nervous system.

sistema nervioso autónomo autonomic nervous system.

sistema nervioso central central nervous system.

sistema nervioso parasimpático parasympathetic nervous system.

sistema nervioso periférico systema nervosum periphericum.

sistema nervioso simpático, sistema nervioso del tronco simpático sympathetic nervous system.

sistema nervioso vegetativo vegetative nervous system.

sistema nervioso visceral visceral nervous system.

sistema neuromuscular neuromuscular system.

sistema reproductor reproductive system.

sistema respiratorio system respiratorium.

sistema urinario urinary system.

sistema urogenital urogenital system.

sistema vegetativo vegetative nervous system.

sistematizado, -da *adj.* systematized.

sistémico, -ca *adj.* systemic.

sístole *f.* systole.

situación *f.* situation.

sobrealimentación *f.* overfeeding, superalimentación.

sobrecarga *f.* overloading.

sobredosificación *f.* overdosage.

sobredosis *f.* overdose.

sodio *m.* sodium.

sofoco *m.* flush.

sol *m.* sol.

sólido, -da *m. y adj.* solid.

solitario, -ria *adj.* solitary.

solubilidad *f.* solubility.

soluble *adj.* soluble.

solución *f.* solution, solutio.

somático, -ca *adj.* somatic.

somatización *f.* somatization.

sombra *f.* shadow.

sombra acústica acoustic shadow.

somnífero, -ra *adj.* somniferous, somnific.

somnolencia *f.* somnolence, somnolency, somnolentia.

somnoliento, -ta *adj.* somnolent.

sonambulismo *m.* sleepwalking, somnambulance, somnambulism.

sonámbulo, -la *m., f.* sleepwalker, somnambulist.

sonda *f.* probe, sound, tube.

sonda de alimentación feeding tube.

sonda esofágica esophageal sound, esophageal tube, probang.

sonda gástrica stomach tube.

sonda nasogástrica nasogastric tube.

sonda nasotraqueal nasotracheal tube.

sonda de nefrostomía nephrostomy tube.

sondaje femenino *m.* female catheterization.

sondaje gástrico *m.* gastric intubation.

sondaje masculino *m.* male catheterization.

sondar *v.* probe, sound.

sonido *m.* sound, sonitus.

sonido auscultatorio auscultatory sound.

sonido cardíaco heart sound.

sonido respiratorio respiratory sound.

soplo *m.* murmur, souffle.

soplo cardíaco cardiac souffle, heart murmur.

sopor *m.* drowsiness, sopor.

soporífero, -ra *adj.* soporiferous.

soporte *m.* assistant, holder, rest, support, sustentaculum.

soporte vital life support.

sordera *f.* deafness.

sordo, -da *adj.* deaf.

sordomudez *f.* deaf-mutism, surdi-mutitas.

sordomudo, -da *adj.* deaf-mute, surdimute.

subagudo, -da *adj.* subacute.

subconsciencia *f.* subconsciousness.

subconsciente *m.* subconscious.

subcutáneo, -a *adj.* subcutaneous.

sublingual *adj.* sublingual.

subluxación *f.* subluxation.

succión *f.* suction.

succión del pulgar thumbsucking.

sucedáneo, -a *adj.* succedaneous.

sudar *v.* sweat.

sudor *m.* sweat, sudor.

sudoríparo, -ra *adj.* sudoriparous.

suelo *m.* floor, solum.

sueño¹ *m.* dream.

sueño² *m.* sleep.

sueño ligero, sueño liviano light sleep.

sueño de movimientos oculares rápidos (MOR) rapid eye movement sleep, REM sleep.

sueño NREM NREM sleep.

sueño profundo deep sleep.

sueño rápido fast sleep.

sueño REM REM sleep.

suero *m.* whey, serum.

suficiencia *f.* competence.

sufrimiento *m.* distress, suffering.

sufrimiento fetal fetal distress.

sugestión *f.* suggestion.

suicida¹ *m., f.* suicide.

suicida² *adj.* suicidal.

suicidio *m.* suicide.

sujeción *f.* restraint.

sujetar *v.* subject.

sujeto *m.* subject.

sulfamida *f.* sulfa drug, sulfonamide.

sumergido *m.* submerged.

superacidez *f.* superacidity.

superácido, -da *adj.* superacid.

superactividad *f.* superactivity.

superagudo, -da *adj.* superacute.

superalimentación *f.* superalimentation.

superficial *adj.* superficial, superficialis.

superficie *f.* surface.

superinfección *f.* superinfection.

superposición *f.* overlap, oversampling, superposition.

supersensibilidad *f.* supersensitivity.

supinación *f.* supination.

supinación del antebrazo supination of the forearm.

supinación del pie supination of the foot.

supinador *m.* supinator.

supinar *v.* supinate.

supino, -na *adj.* supine.

suplementario, -ria *adj.* supplemental.

suplente *m.* surrogate.

supraespinoso, -sa *adj.* supraspinous.

suprapúbico, -ca *adj.* suprapubic.

suprarrenal *adj.* adrenal, suprarenal.

supraspinoso, -sa *adj.* supraspinous.

supresión *f.* suppression.

supresor, -ra *m. y adj.* suppressant.

supuración *f.* suppuration.

supurar *v.* suppurate.

supurativo, -va *adj.* suppurative.

surco *m.* furrow, groove, sulcus.

susceptibilidad *f.* susceptibility.
  susceptibilidad genética genetic susceptibility.

susceptible *adj.* susceptible.

suspensión *f.* suspension.

suspiro *m.* sigh.

sustancia *f.* substance, substantia.

sustitución *f.* replacement, substitution.
  sustitución de cadera hip replacement.
  sustitución de rodilla knee replacement.
  sustitución total de la cadera total hip replacement.

sustitutivo, -va *m., f. y adj.* substitutive.

sustituto, -ta *m., f.* substitute.
  sustituto plasmático plasma substitute.
  sustituto de sangre blood substitute.
  sustituto de volumen volume substitute.

sustituyente *adj.* substituent.

susto *m.* fright.

sustrato *m.* substrate, substratum.

susurro *m.* susurrus.
  susurro auricular susurrus aurium.

sutura¹ *f.* suture, sutura.
  sutura anatómica anatomical suture.

sutura² *f.* suture.
  sutura absorbible absorbable suture, absorbable surgical suture.
  sutura no absorbible, sutura quirúrgica no absorbible non-absorbable surgical suture.

suturar *v.* stitch.

T

tabaco *m.* tobacco.

tabacosis *f.* tabacosis.

tábano *m.* gadfly, horsefly, warblefly.

tabaquera anatómica *f.* anatomic snuffbox, anatomical snuffbox, anatomist's snuffbox.

tabaquismo *m.* tabacism, tabagism.

tabes *f.* tabes.

tabique *m.* partition, septum.

tabla *f.* table, tabula.

tableta *f.* tablet.
  tableta bucal buccal tablet.
  tableta comprimida compressed tablet.
  tableta con cubierta entérica enteric coated tablet.
  tableta sublingual sublingual tablet.

tabular *adj.* tabular.

táctil *adj.* tactual, tactile.

tacto *m.* touch, tactus.

tacto rectal rectal touch.

tacto vaginal vaginal touch.

talalgia *f.* talalgia.

talámico, -ca *adj.* thalamic.

tálamo *m.* thalamus.

talasemia *f.* thalassemia.

talla *f.* height, stature.

talla baja short stature.

talle *m.* waist.

tallo *m.* stalk.

tallo corporal body stalk.

tallo óptico optic stalk.

talón *m.* heel, talus.

talón anterior anterior heel.

talón doloroso painful heel.

tampón *m.* sponge, tampon.

tampón menstrual menstrual sponge.

tánatos *m.* thanatos.

tapón *m.* plug.

tapón de cerumen cerumen plug.

taponamiento *m.* pack, packing, tamponade.

taponamiento cardíaco cardiac tamponade.

taponamiento nasal nasal packing.

taponamiento pericárdico pericardial tamponade.

taponar *v.* tampon.

taquiarritmia *f.* tachyarrhythmia.

taquicardia *f.* tachycardia.

taquicardia auricular atrial tachycardia.

taquicardia auriculoventricular atrioventricular tachycardia, auriculoventricular tachycardia.

taquicardia fetal fetal tachycardia.

taquicardia sinusal sinus tachycardia.

taquicardia supraventricular (TSV) supraventricular tachycardia (SVT).

taquicárdico, -ca *adj.* tachycardiac, tachycardic.

taquipnea *f.* tachypnea.

tara *f.* tare.

tardío, -a *adj.* late, tardive, tardy.

tarsal *adj.* tarsal.

tarsalgia *f.* tarsalgia.

tarso *m.* tarsus.

tartamudez *f.* stuttering.

tasa *f.* rate.

tasa de filtración glomerular (TFG) glomerular filtration rate (GFR).

tasa de morbididad morbidity rate.

tasa de mortalidad death rate.

tatuaje *m.* tattoo, tattooing.

taxonomía *f.* taxonomy.

teca[1] *f.* theca.

teca[2] *f.* theque.

técnica *f.* technique.

técnica de relajación relaxation technique.

técnica de reproducción asistida assisted reproduction technique.

tejido *m.* tissue, textus.

tejido adiposo adipose tissue.

tejido cartilaginoso cartilaginous tissue.

tejido cicatricial cicatricial tissue, scar tissue.

tejido conectivo connective tissue.

tejido conjuntivo connective tissue.

tejido conjuntivo laxo loose connective tissue.

tejido elástico, amarillo elastic tissue.

tejido embrionario embryonic tissue.

tejido esponjoso cancellous tissue.

tejido esquelético skeletal tissue.

tejido fibroelástico fibroelastic tissue.

tejido linfático lymphatic tissue.

tejido linfoide lymphoid tissue.

tejido muscular muscular tissue.

tejido nervioso nervous tissue.

tejido óseo bone tissue, osseous tissue.

tejido subcutáneo subcutaneous tissue.

telangiectasia *f.* telangiectasia.

telediastólico, -ca *adj.* telediastolic.

telepatía *f.* telepathy.

telofase *f.* telophase.

telómero *m.* telomere.

temblor *m.* tremor.

temblor esencial, temblor esencial benigno, temblor esencial hereditario benign essential tremor, essential tremor, hereditary essential tremor.

temblor familiar familial tremor.

temblor fisiológico physiologic tremor.

temblor postural postural tremor.

temblor de reposo rest tremor, resting tremor.

temblor senil senile tremor.

tembloroso, -sa *adj.* tremulous.

temor *m.* fear.

temperamento *m.* temperament.

temperamento bilioso choleric temperament.

temperamento colérico choleric temperament.

temperatura *f.* temperature.

temperatura ambiental ambient temperature, room temperature.

temperatura axilar axillary temperature.

temperatura basal basal temperature.

temperatura corporal body temperature.

temperatura del lactante temperature of infant.

templado *m.* template.

templado, -da *adj.* warm.

temporal[1] *adj.* temporal.

temporal[2] *adj.* temporalis.

tendencia *f.* trend.

tendinitis *f.* tendinitis, tendonitis.

tendinoso, -sa *adj.* tendinous.

tendón *m.* sinew, tendon, tendo.

tendón de Aquiles Achilles' tendon, tendo Achillis.

tendón desgarrado pulled tendon.

tendosinovitis *f.* tendosynovitis.

tenesmo *m.* straining, tenesmus.

tenesmo rectal rectal tenesmus.

tenesmo vesical vesical tenesmus.

tenia[1] *f.* tapeworm, taenia.

tenia[2] *f.* tenia, taenia.

teniasis *f.* taeniasis, teniasis.

tensiómetro *m.* tensiometer.

tensión[1] *f.* stress.

tensión[2] *f.* tension.

tensión arterial arterial tension, arterial pressure.

tensión emocional strain.

tensión de fatiga fatigue tension.

tensión intraocular intraocular pressure.

tensión muscular muscular tension.

tensión de oxígeno oxygen tension.

tenso, -sa *adj.* tense.

teñir *v.* stain.

teorema *m.* theorem.

teoría *f.* theory.

teoría de Baeyer Baeyer's theory.

teórico, -ca[1] *m., f.* theorist, theoretical.

terapia *f.* therapeutics, therapy, therapia.

terapia adyuvante adjuvant therapy.

terapia anticoagulante anticoagulant therapy.

terapia biológica biological therapy.

terapia combinada combined therapy.

terapia electroconvulsiva (TEC) electroconvulsive therapy.

terapia de inhalación inhalation therapy.

terapia de inmunización immunization therapy.

terapia inmunosupresora immunesuppresive therapy.

terapia intravenosa intravenous therapy.

terapia con oxígeno oxygen therapy.

terapia de relajación relaxation therapy.

terapia sexual sexual therapy.

terapia de shock shock therapy.

terapia con vacunas vaccine therapy.

terapeuta *m., f.* therapist.

terapeuta físico physical therapist.

terapeuta del lenguaje speech therapist.

terapeuta ocupacional occupation therapist.

terapeuta sexual sexual therapist.

terapéutico, -ca *adj.* therapeutic.

teratogénesis *f.* teratogenesis.

teratogenia *f.* teratogenesis.

teratógeno *m.* teratogen.

teratógeno, -na *adj.* teratogenous.

teratoma *m.* teratoma.

terciana *f.* tertian fever.

terciano, -na *adj.* tertian.

termal *adj.* thermal.

térmico, -ca *adj.* thermal, thermic.

terminación *f.* ending, termination, terminatio.

terminación nerviosa nerve ending.

terminal *m. y adj.* terminal.

término *m.* term, terminus.

terminología *f.* terminology.

termoestable *adj.* thermostabile, thermostable.

termolábil *adj.* heat labile, thermolabile.

termómetro *m.* thermometer.

termómetro de Celsius, termómetro centígrado Celsius thermometer.

termómetro electrónico electronic thermometer.

termómetro de Fahrenheit Fahrenheit thermometer.

termómetro para la fiebre fever thermometer.

termómetro de mercurio mercury thermometer.

termómetro rectal rectal thermometer.

termorreceptor, -ra *m., f. y adj.* thermoreceptor.

termorregulación *f.* thermoregulation.

termostato, termóstato *m.* thermostat.

  termostato hipotalámico hypothalamic thermostat.

terror *m.* terror.

  terror nocturno night terror.

test *m.* test.

  test de inteligencia intelligence test.

  test intracutáneo intradermal skin test.

  test de personalidad personality test.

testamento vital *m.* living will.

testicular *adj.* testicular.

testículo *m.* testicle, testis.

  testículo ectópico ectopic testicle.

  testículo no descendido undescended testicle.

testosterona *f.* testosterone.

tetania *f.* tetany.

  tetania hipocalcémica hypocalcemic tetany.

  tetania neonatal neonatal tetany.

  tetania posoperatoria postoperative.

  tetania del recién nacido neonatal tetany.

tetanización *adj.* tetanization.

tetanizar *v.* tetanize.

tétanos *m.* tetanus.

tetralogía *f.* tetralogy.

  tetralogía de Fallot Fallot's tetralogy, tetralogy of Fallot.

tetraplejía *f.* tetraplegia.

tetrapléjico, -ca *adj.* tetraplegic.

tetrasomía *f.* tetrasomy.

tiacida *f.* thiazide.

tibia *f.* tibia.

  tibia valga tibia valga.

  tibia vara tibia vara.

tibial *adj.* tibial, tibialis.

tibio, -bia *adj.* tepid.

tic *m.* tic.

  tic convulsivo convulsive tic.

  tic crónico chronic tic.

  tic diafragmático diaphragmatic tic.

  tic doloroso, tic doloroso de la cara tic douloureux.

  tic espasmódico spasmodic tic.

  tic facial tic facial.

  tic local local tic.

tiempo *m.* time.

  tiempo de coagulación clotting time.

  tiempo de protrombina prothrombin time.

  tiempo de reacción reaction time.

  tiempo de relajación relaxation time.

  tiempo de sedimentación sedimentation time.

  tiempo de trombina thrombin.

  tiempo de tromboplastina parcial (TTP) partial thromboplastin time (PTT).

  tiempo de trombloplastina parcial activada (TTPa) activated partial thromboplastin time (APTT).

tifus *m.* typhus.

tijeras *f.* scissors.

tiloma *m.* tyloma.

timbre *m.* timbre.

timo *m.* thymus.

tímpano *m.* eardrum, tympanum.

tinción *f.* tinction.

tinea *f.* ringworm, tinea.

tinnitus *m.* tinnitus.

tiña *f.* ringworm, tinea.

tiña del cuero cabelludo ringworm of the scalp.

tiña del cuerpo tinea corporis.

tioflavina *f.* thioflavine.

tipificación *f.* typing.

tipificación de los grupos sanguíneos blood typing.

tipificación de los HLA HLA typing.

tipo *m.* type.

tipo constitucional constitutional type.

tipología *f.* typology.

tira *f.* strip.

tira reactiva dipstrip.

tiro *m.* tugging.

tiroidectomía *f.* thyroidectomy.

tiroidectomizado, -da *adj.* thyroidectomize.

tiroideo, -a *adj.* thyroid.

tiroides *m.* thyroid.

tiroidismo *m.* thyroidism.

tiroiditis *f.* thyroiditis.

tirotoxicosis *f.* thyrotoxicosis, tyrotoxicosis.

tiroxina *f.* tyroxine.

tísico, -ca *adj.* phthisic.

tisis *f.* phthisis.

tisular *adj.* tissular.

titubeo *m.* titubation.

titulación *f.* titration.

titular *v.* titrate.

título *m.* titer.

tobillo *m.* ankle.

tocología *f.* tocology.

tocólogo, -ga *m., f.* obstetrician.

tofo *m.* tophus.

tolerancia *f.* tolerance.

tolerancia al dolor tolerance pain.

tolerancia al ejercicio exercise tolerance.

tolerancia farmacológica, tolerancia a los fármacos drug tolerance.

tolerancia inmunológica immunologic tolerance.

toma *f.* collection, sampling.

tomografía *f.* tomography.

tomografía axial computadorizada (TAC) computer axial tomography (CAT).

tomografía computadorizada (TC) computed tomography (CT).

tomografía computadorizada por emisión (TCE) emission computed tomography (ECT).

tomografía computadorizada por emisión de fotón único (SPECT) single-photon emission computed tomography (SPECT).

tomografía por emisión de positrones (PET) positron emission tomography (PET).

tonicidad *f.* tonicity, tonus.

tónico, -ca *m. y adj.* tonic.

tono *m.* tone, tonus.

tono afectivo affective tone.

tono cardíaco heart tone.

tono cardíaco fetal (TCF) fetal heart tone (FHT).

tono muscular muscular tone.

tono vagal vagal tone.

tonoclónico, -ca *adj.* tonoclonic.

tonsilar *adj.* tonsillar, tonsillary.

tonsilectomía *f.* tonsillectomy.

tonsilitis *f.* tonsillitis.

tópico *m.* topicum.

tópico, -ca *adj.* topical.

toracentesis *f.* thoracentesis.

torácico, -ca *adj.* thoracic.

tórax *m.* chest, thorax.

torcedura *f.* sprain.

torniquete *m.* tourniquet.

tórpido, -da *adj.* torpid.

torsión *f.* torsion.

   torsión testicular, torsión del testículo torsion of the testis.

torso *m.* torso.

tortícolis, torticolis *f.* torticollis.

tortuoso, -sa *adj.* tortuous.

tos *f.* cough, tussis.

   tos blanda wet cough.

   tos convulsa whooping cough.

   tos ferina whooping cough.

   tos espasmódica paroxysmal cough.

   tos húmeda wet cough.

   tos no productiva non-productive cough.

   tos productiva productive cough.

   tos seca dry cough, hacking cough.

tosferina *f.* whooping cough.

totipotencial *adj.* totipotential.

toxemia *f.* toxemia.

   toxemia del embarazo toxemia of pregnancy.

   toxemia gravídica toxemia of pregnancy.

toxicidad *f.* toxicity.

   toxicidad aguda acute toxicity.

tóxico *m.* toxin.

tóxico, -ca *adj.* toxic.

toxicología *f.* toxicolgy.

toxicológico, -ca *adj.* toxicologic.

toxicosis *f.* toxicosis.

toxina *f.* toxin.

toxoplasmosis *f.* toxoplasmosis.

trabajo *m.* work.

   trabajo del duelo work of mourning.

   trabajo de parto labor, travail.

   trabajo de parto espontáneo spontaneous labor.

trabécula *f.* trabecula.

trabeculado, -da *adj.* trabeculate.

trabecular *adj.* trabecular.

tracción *f.* traction.

tracoma *m.* trachoma.

tracto *m.* tract, tractus.

trance *m.* trance.

tranquilizante *m. y adj.* tranquilizer.

   tranquilizante mayor major tranquilizer.

   tranquilizante menor minor tranquilizer.

transaminasemia *f.* transaminasemia.

transcutáneo, -a *adj.* transcutaneous.

transdérmico, -ca *adj.* transdermal.

transducción *f.* transduction.

transexual *adj.* transsexual.

transexualismo *m.* transsexualism.

transferencia¹ *f.* transfer.

   transferencia intratubárica de gametos (TITG) gamete intrafallopian traction (GIFT).

transferencia² *f.* transference.

   transferencia negativa negative transference.

transferencia positiva positive transference.

transformación f. transformation.

transfundir v. transfuse.

transfusión f. transfusion.

transfusión arterial arterial transfusion.

transfusión fetomaterna fetomaternal transfusion.

transfusión gemelo-gemelar twin-to-twin transfusion.

transfusión por goteo drip transfusion.

transfusión de sangre blood transfusion.

transgénico, -ca adj. transgenic.

tránsito m. transit.

tránsito intestinal intestinal transit.

transitorio, -a adj. transient.

translocación f. translocation.

translocación balanceada balanced translocation.

translocación equilibrada balanced translocation.

transmembrana f. transmembrane.

transmigración f. transmigration.

transmisible adj. transmissible.

transmisión f. transmission.

transmisión sináptica synaptic transmission.

transmural adj. transmural.

transparente adj. transparent.

transpirable adj. transpirable.

transpiración f. transpiration.

transplacentario, -a adj. transplacental.

transporte m. transport.

trapecio m. trapezium.

tráquea f. trachea.

traqueal adj. tracheal.

traqueítis f. tracheitis, trachitis.

traqueostomía f. tracheostomy.

traqueostomizar v. tracheostomize.

traqueotomía f. tracheotomy.

trascendencia f. trascendence.

trascendental adj. trascendent.

traslación f. traslation.

traslado m. transfer.

traslocación f. translocation.

trasplantar¹ v. transplant.

trasplantar² adj. trasplantar.

trasplante m. transplant, transplantation.

trasplante cardiaco, trasplante de corazón heart transplant.

trasplante corneal, trasplante de córnea corneal transplant.

trasplante hepático liver transplant.

trasplante HLA idéntico HLA-identical transplant.

trasplante de médula ósea bone marrow transplant.

trasplante pancreático pancreatic transplant.

trasplante postmortem postmortem graft.

trasplante renal renal transplant.

trasplante de tejido fetal fetal tissue transplant.

trasplante tendinosos, trasplante del tendón tendon transplant.

trastorno m. disorder.

trastorno por abuso de sustancias substance abuse disorder.

trastorno adaptativo adjustment disorder.

trastorno afectivo affective disorder.

trastorno de ansiedad anxiety disorder.

trastorno antisocial de la personalidad antisocial personality disorder.

trastorno del aprendizaje learning disorder.

trastorno autista, trastorno autístico autistic disorder.

trastorno bipolar bipolar disorder.

trastorno ciclotímico cyclotimic disorder.

trastorno del comportamiento behavior disorder.

trastorno de la conducta alimentaria eating disorder.

trastorno por déficit de atención con hiperactividad attention-deficit hyperactive disorder.

trastorno del desarrollo developmental disorder.

trastorno depresivo mayor major depressive disorder.

trastorno por dolor pain disorder.

trastorno esquizoafectivo schizoaffective disorder.

trastorno esquizoide de la personalidad schizoid personality disorder.

trastorno del estado del ánimo mood disorder.

trastorno por estrés agudo acute stress disorder.

trastorno por estrés postraumático post-traumatic stress disorder.

trastorno funcional functional disorder.

trastorno hereditario inherited disorder.

trastorno hipocondriaco hypochondriac disorder.

trastorno de la identidad sexual sexual identity disorder.

trastorno por inmunodeficiencia immunodeficiency disorder.

trastorno maniacodepresivo maniac-depressive disorder.

trastorno de la marcha gait disorder.

trastorno mental mental disorder.

trastorno metabólico metabolic disorder.

trastorno multifactorial multifactorial disorder.

trastorno neurótico neurotic disorder.

trastorno de pánico panic disorder.

trastorno sexual sexual disorder.

trastorno del sueño sleep disorder.

trasudación *f.* transudation.

trasudado *m.* transudate.

tratamiento *m.* treatment.

tratamiento activo active treatment.

tratamiento adyuvante adjuvant treatment.

tratamiento causal causal treatment.

tratamiento coadyuvante coadjuvant treatment.

tratamiento combinado combined modality treatment.

tratamiento conservador conservative treatment.

tratamiento curativo curative treatment.

tratamiento de la diabetes diabetic treatment.

tratamiento dietético dietetic treatment.

tratamiento empírico empiric treatment.

tratamiento escalonado stepped treatment.

tratamiento específico specific treatment.

tratamiento higiénico hygienic treatment.

tratamiento inmunosupresor immunosuppressive treatment.

tratamiento orgánico organ treatment.

tratamiento paliativo palliative treatment.

tratamiento preventivo preventive treatment.

tratamiento profiláctico prophylactic treatment.

tratamiento quirúrgico surgical treatment.

tratamiento radical radical treatment.

tratamiento sintomático symptomatic treatment.

tratamiento sustitutivo substitutive treatment.

tratar *v.* treat.

trauma *m.* trauma.

trauma acústico acoustic trauma.

trauma craneoencefálico cranioencephalic trauma.

trauma por herida de bala missile wound trauma.

trauma del nacimiento birth trauma.

trauma psíquico psychic trauma.

traumático, -ca *adj.* traumatic.

traumatismo *m.* traumatism.

traumatología *f.* traumatology.

traumatólogo, -ga *m.* traumatologist.

travestido, -da *m., f.* transvestite.

travestismo *m.* transvestism.

trayecto *m.* path.

trazado *m.* plot, tracing.

trazador *m.* tracer.

trazar *v.* plot.

trazo *m.* tracing.

trémulo, -la *adj.* tremulous.

trepanación *f.* trepanation.

trepanador, -ra *m., f.* trepanner.

trepanar *v.* trephine.

trépano *m.* drill, trepan.

tríada *f.* triad.

triángulo *m.* triangle, triangulum.

triangulum triangulum.

tricíclico, -ca *adj.* tricyclic.

tricipital *adj.* tricipital.

tricosis *f.* trichosis.

tricúspide *adj.* tricuspid, tricuspidal, tricuspidate.

trifásico, -ca *adj.* triphasic.

trigémino *m.* trigeminus.

triglicérido *m.* triglyceride.

trigonitis *f.* trigonitis.

trígono *f.* trigone, trigonum.

trilaminar *adj.* trilaminar.

trilateral *adj.* trilateral.

trillizo, -za *adj.* triplets.

trilogía *f.* trilogy.

trimestral *adj.* trimensual.

trimestre *m.* trimester.

tripanosoma *m.* trypanosome.

tripanosomiasis *f.* trypanosomiasis

trípara f. tripara.

triple adj. triplex.

triplete m. triplet.

tripsinógeno m. trypsinogen.

tríptico, -ca adj. tryptic.

triquinosis f. trichinosis.

trisomía f. trisomy, trisomia.

tristeza f. sadness.

triturar v. triturate.

trocánter m. trochanter.

trócar m. trocar.

trófico, -ca adj. trophic.

trofismo m. trophism.

trofoblasto m. trophoblast.

trofología f. trophology.

trombectomía f. thrombectomy.

trombina f. thrombin.

trombo m. thrombus.

trombocitemia f. thrombocythemia.

trombocitemia esencial essential thrombocythemia.

trombocitosis f. thrombocytosis.

tromboembolia f. thromboembolism.

tromboembolismo m. thromboembolism.

trombofilia f. thrombophilia.

tromboflebitis f. thrombophlebitis.

trombolítico, -ca adj. thrombolytic.

trombopenia f. thrombopenia, thrombopeny.

trombosado, -da adj. thrombosed.

trombosis f. thrombosis.

trombosis venosa venous thrombosis.

trombótico, -ca adj. thrombotic.

trompa f. tube, tuba.

tronco m. trunk, truncus.

tropismo m. tropism.

troquíter m. trochiter.

truncado, -da adj. truncate, truncatus.

truncar v. truncate.

tubárico, -ca adj. tubal.

tuberculina f. tuberculin.

tuberculocida[1] m. tuberculocide.

tuberculocida[2] adj. tuberculocidal.

tuberculosis f. tuberculosis.

tuberculosis pulmonar pulmonar tuberculosis.

tuberculoso, -sa adj. tuberculous.

tuberculostático, -ca adj. tuberculostatic.

tuberosidad f. tuberosity, tuberositas.

tubo m. tube, tubus.

tubo de alimentación feeding tube.

tubo de drenaje drainage tube.

tubo de ensayo test tube.

tubo de rayos X X-ray tube.

tubular adj. tubular.

túbulo m. tubule, tubulus.

tuerto, -ta adj. one-eyed.

tularemia f. tularemia.

tumefacción f. tumefaction.

tumefaciente adj. tumefacient.

tumor m. tumor.

tumor benigno benign tumor.

tumor maligno malignant tumor.

tumoroso, -sa adj. tumorous.

túnel m. tunnel.

túnica f. tunic, tunica.

turbiedad f. turbidity.

turbio, -bia adj. turbid.

tusivo, -va adj. tussal, tussive.

tzetzé f. tzetze.

U

úlcera *f.* ulcer, sore, ulcus.

  úlcera aftosa aphthous ulcer.

  úlcera crónica chronic ulcer.

  úlcera curada healed ulcer.

  úlcera esofágica Barrett's ulcer.

  úlcera del estómago ulcer of the stomach.

  úlcera gástrica gastric ulcer.

  úlcera inflamada inflamed ulcer.

  úlcera péptica peptic ulcer.

  úlcera perforante perforating ulcer.

  úlcera venérea venereal sore, venereal ulcer.

ulceración *f.* ulceration.

ulcerado, -da *adj.* ulcerated.

ulcerar *v.* ulcerate.

ulcus *f.* ulcer, sore, ulcus.

ultrasónico, -ca *adj.* ultrasonic.

ultrasonografía *f.* ultrasonography.

ultravioleta *adj.* ultraviolet.

umbilicación *f.* umbilication.

umbilicado, -da¹ *adj.* umbilicate.

umbilicado, -da² *adj.* umbilicated.

umbilical *adj.* umbilical.

umbral *m.* threshold.

unción *f.* unction.

ungueal *adj.* ungual.

ungüento *m.* ointment, unguent.

  ungüento ocular, ungüento oftálmico eye ointment, ophthalmic ointment.

unicelular *adj.* unicellular.

unidad *f.* unit.

  unidad clínica clinical unit.

  unidad de cuidados intensivos

  (UCI) intensive care unit (ICU).

  unidad de cuidados intensivos neonatales (UCIN) neonatal intensive care unit (NICU).

  unidad internacional international unit.

unigrávida *adj.* unigravida.

unión¹ *f.* attachment.

unión² *f.* junction.

unión³ *f.* union.

unipotente *adj.* unipotent.

unir *v.* bind.

universal *adj.* universal.

univitelino, -na *adj.* univitelline.

uña *f.* fingernail, nail, toenail, unguis.

  uña encarnada, uña incardinada, uñero unguis aduncus.

  uña encarnada, uña incardinada, uñero unguis incarnatus.

  uña en cuchara spoon nail.

  uña encarnada ingrowing toenail, unguis aduncus, unguis incarnatus.

  uña incardinada ingrowing toenail, unguis aduncus, unguis incarnatus.

  uña con hoyuelos pitted nail.

uñero *m.* ingrown toenail , ingrowing toenail, unguis aduncus, unguis incarnatus.

urea *f.* urea.

uremia *f.* uremia.

urémico, -ca *adj.* uremic.

uréter *f.* ureter.

uretra *f.* urethra.

  uretra masculina urethra masculina.

  uretra membranosa membranous urethra.

uretra peneana penile urethra.

uretra prostática prostatic urethra.

uretral *adj.* urethral.

uretritis *f.* urethritis.

urgencia¹ *f.* emergency.

urgencia² *f.* urgency.

urgencia motora motor urgency.

urgencia sensorial sensory urgency.

uricemia *f.* uricemia.

úrico, -ca *adj.* uric.

uricosuria *f.* uricosuria.

urinario, -ria *adj.* urinary.

urogenital *adj.* urogenital.

urografía *f.* urography.

urología *f.* urology.

urológico, -ca *adj.* urologic.

urólogo, -ga *m., f.* urologist.

urotelio *m.* urothelium.

urticante *adj.* urticant.

urticaria *f.* urticaria.

uterino, -na *adj.* uterine.

útero *m.* uterus.

útero grávido gravid uterus.

utrículo *m.* utricle, utriculus.

úvea *f.* uvea, uveal tract.

uveítis *f.* uveitis.

úvula *f.* uvula.

uvulitis *f.* uvulitis.

V

vaciado *m.* casting.

vacío *m.* vacuum.

vacuna *f.* vaccine, vaccinum.

vacuna absorbida de toxoide diftérico y tetánico y de la tos ferina (DTP) adsorbed diphtheria and tetanus toxoids and pertussis vaccine (DTP).

vacuna antidiftérica diphtheria vaccine.

vacuna antigripal influenza virus vaccine.

vacuna antimeningocócica de polisacáridos meningococcal polysaccharide vaccine.

vacuna antineumocócica pneumococcal vaccine.

vacuna antiparotiditis, vacuna antiparotidítica mumps virus vaccine.

vacuna antipertussis pertussis vaccine.

vacuna antipoliomielitis, vacuna antipoliomielítica poliovirus vaccine.

vacuna antipoliomielítica inactivada (IPV) inactivated poliovirus vaccine (IPV).

vacuna antipoliomielítica oral (OPV) oral poliovirus vaccine (OPV).

vacuna antipoliomielítica de Sabin Sabin's oral vaccine.

vacuna antipoliomielítica de Salk Salk vaccine.

vacuna antirrábica antirabic vaccine.

vacuna antirrábica preparada de células diploides humanas, vacuna antirrábica preparada en células diploides humanas (HDRV) human diploid cell rabies vaccine (HDRV).

vacuna antirrubéola, vacuna antirrubeólica rubella virus vaccine.

vacuna antirrubeólica de virus vivos live rubella virus vaccine.

vacuna antisarampión, vacuna antisarampionosa measles vaccine, measles virus vaccine.

vacuna antitetánica tetanus vaccine.

vacuna antitosferinosa pertussis vaccine.

vacuna antituberculosa tuberculosis vaccine.

vacuna atenuada attenuated vaccine.

vacuna del bacilo de Calmette-Guérin (BCG) (bacillus) Calmette-Guérin vaccine (BCG).

vacuna bacteriana, vacuna bactérica bacterial vaccine.

vacuna de la difteria diphtheria vaccine.

vacuna estafilocócica, vacuna de estafilococo staphylococcus vaccine.

vacuna estreptocócica, vacuna de estreptococos streptococcic vaccine.

vacuna de la fiebre amarilla yellow fever vaccine.

vacuna de la hepatitis B, vacuna contra la hepatitis B hepatitis B vaccine.

vacuna inactivada inactivated vaccine.

vacuna de organismos muertos killed vaccine.

vacuna de la poliomielitis poliovirus vaccine.

vacuna polivalente combined vaccine, polyvalent vaccine.

vacuna de la rabia rabies vaccine.

vacuna recombinante de la hepatitis B recombinant hepatitis B vaccine.

vacuna de Salk Salk vaccine.

vacuna del sarampión measles vaccine, measles virus vaccine.

vacuna contra el sarampión, la parotiditis y la rubéola (MMR) measles, mumps and rubella vaccine (MMR).

vacuna de la tos ferina, vacuna contra la tos ferina pertussis vaccine, whooping cough vaccine.

vacuna de toxoide diftérico, tetánico y de la tos ferina (DTP) diphtheria and tetanus toxoids and pertussis vaccine (DTP).

vacuna de toxoide diftérico, tetánico y antipertussis (DTP) diphtheria, tetanus toxoids and pertussis vaccine (DTP).

vacuna triple, vacuna triple vírica triple vaccine, trivalent vaccine.

vacuna de la tuberculosis tuberculosis vaccine.

vacuna de la viruela smallpox vaccine.

vacuna de virus de influenza, vacuna de virus de la influenza influenza virus vaccine.

vacunación *f.* vaccination.

vacunal *adj.* vaccinal.

vacuola *f.* vacuole.

vagal *adj.* vagal.

vagina *f.* vagina.

  vagina septada septate vagina.

  vagina tabicada septate vagina.

vaginal *adj.* vaginal.

vaginismo *m.* vaginismus.

vaginosis *f.* vaginosis.

vago *m.* vagus.

vagotomía *f.* vagotomy.

vahído *m.* giddiness, swoon.

vaina *f.* sheath, vagina.

valgo, -ga *adj.* valgus.

validación *f.* validation.

validez *f.* validity.

válido, -da *adj.* valid.

valle *m.* valley.

valor *m.* value.

  valor medio mean value.

  valor normal normal value.

  valor umbral threshold value.

valoración¹ *f.* assay.

valoración² *f.* assessment, measurement, testing.

  valoración del dolor pain assessment.

  valoración física physical assessment.

  valoración gestacional gestational assessment.

  valoración neurológica neurologic assessment.

valoración³ *f.* analysis, titration.

  valoración química titration.

valvotomía *f.* valvotomy.

válvula *f.* valve, valvule, valva.

  válvula cardíaca protésica prosthetic heart valve.

valvular *adj.* valvular.

valvulitis *f.* valvulitis.

valvulopatía cardíaca *f.* valvular heart disease.

vapor *m.* vapor.

vaporización *f.* vaporization.

vaporizador *m.* vaporizer.

variabilidad *f.* variability.

  variabilidad basal de la frecuen-

  cia cardíaca fetal baseline variability of fetal heart rate.

variable *f. y adj.* variable.

variación *f.* variation.

variante *f. y adj.* variant.

varianza *f.* variance.

varicela *f.* chickenpox, varicella.

varicocele *m.* varicocele.

varicosidad *f.* varicosity.

varicoso, -sa *adj.* varicose.

variedad *f.* variety.

varo, -ra *adj.* varus.

varón *m.* male.

vascular *adj.* vascular.

vascularidad *f.* vascularity.

vascularizado, -da *adj.* vascularized.

vascularización *f.* vascularization.

vasculitis *f.* vasculitis.

vasculopatía *f.* vasculopathy.

vasectomía *f.* vasectomy.

vasectomizado, -da *adj.* vasectomized.

vaselina *f.* petrolatum.

vaso *m.* vessel, vas.

vasoconstricción *f.* vasoconstriction.

vasoconstrictivo, -va *adj.* vasoconstrictive.

vasoconstrictor, -ra *adj.* vasoconstrictive, vasoconstrictor.

vasodilatación *f.* vasodilatation.

vasodilatador, -ra *adj.* vasodilative, vasodilator.

vasomotor, -ra *adj.* vasomotive.

vasopresina (VP) *f.* vasopressin (VP).

vasospasmo *m.* vasospasm.

vasovagal *adj.* vasovagal.

vector *m.* vector.

vector biológico biological vector.

veganismo *m.* veganism.

vegetación *f.* vegetation.

vegetación adenoide adenoid vegetation.

vegetación bacteriana bacterial vegetation.

vegetarianismo *m.* vegetarianism.

vegetariano, -na *m., f.* vegetarian.

vegetativo, -va *adj.* vegetative.

vejez *f.* old age.

vejiga *f.* bladder, vesica.

vejiga biliar vesica biliaris.

vejiga urinaria, vesica urinalis, vesica urinaria urinary bladder, cystis urinaria, vesica urinaria.

vello *m.* hair, vellus.

vello pubiano, vello púbico pubic hair.

vellosidad *f.* villus.

vellosidad amniotica amniotic villus.

vellosidad intestinales intestinal villi, villi intestinale.

velloso, -sa *adj.* villose, villous.

velo *m.* veil, velum.

velocidad *f.* rate, speed, velocity.

velocidad de sedimentación sedimentation rate, sedimentation velocity.

vena *f.* vein, vena.

venda *f.* bandage.

venda elástica elastic bandage.

vendaje *m.* bandage, dressing, strapping.

vendaje adhesivo adhesive bandage, strap.

vendaje de inmovilización immobilizing bandage.

vendar *v.* bandage, bind, strap.

veneno *m.* poison, venom.

veneno de las serpientes snake venom.

veneno de víbora viper venom.

venepuntura *f.* venipuncture.

venéreo, -a *adj.* venereal.

venereología *f.* venereology.

venipuntura *f.* venipuncture.

venografía *f.* venography.

venopunción *f.* venepuncture.

venoso, -sa *adj.* venous, venose.

ventana *f.* window, fenestra.

ventilación *f.* ventilation.

ventilación artificial artificial ventilation.

ventilación asistida assisted ventilation.

ventilador *m.* ventilator.

ventilar *v.* ventilate.

ventosa *f.* cup, cupping glass.

ventral *adj.* ventral, ventralis.

ventricular *adj.* ventricular.

ventrículo *m.* ventricle, ventriculus.

vénula *f.* venule, venula.

venular *adj.* venula.

verborrea *f.* verbiage.

verde *adj.* green.

verga *f.* penis.

vermis vermis.

verruga *f.* wart, verruga, verruca.

verruga vulgar verruca vulgaris.

versión *f.* version.

vértebra *f.* vertebra.

vertebrado, -da *adj.* vertebrated.

vertebral *adj.* vertebral.

vertex vertex.

vertical[1] *adj.* vertical.

vertical[2] *adj.* vertical, verticalis.

vértice *m.* vertex.

vertiginoso, -sa *adj.* vertiginous.

vértigo *m.* vertigo.

  vértigo de altura height vertigo.

  vértigo central central vertigo.

  vértigo laberíntico labyrinthine vertigo.

  vértigo periférico peripheral vertigo.

  vértigo posicional, vértigo de posición positional vertigo.

  vértigo posicional incapacitante disabling positional vertigo.

  vértigo postural postural vertigo.

  vértigo rotatorio rotary vertigo, rotatory vertigo.

vesical *adj.* vesical.

vesícula *f.* blister, vesicle, vesicula.

  vesícula biliar gallbladder, vesicula bilis, vesicula fellea.

  vesícula seminal seminal vesicle, vesicula seminalis.

vesicular *adj.* vesicular.

vestibular *adj.* vestibular.

vestíbulo *m.* vestibule, vestibulum.

vestigio *m.* vestige, vestigium.

vía *f.* path, pathway, route, way, via.

  vía accesoria accessory pathway.

  vía de administración route of administration.

  vía aérea superior upper airway.

  vía alternativa alternative pathway.

  vía arterial arterial line.

  vía central central line.

  vía natural via naturale.

  vía respiratorias respiratory tract.

  vía urinarias urinary tract.

viabilidad *f.* viability.

viable *adj.* viable.

vial *m.* vial.

vibración *f.* vibration.

vibrador *m.* vibrator.

vibrante *adj.* vibrative.

vibrión *m.* vibrio.

vicio *m.* vice, vitium.

vicioso, -sa *adj.* vicious.

vida *f.* life.

  vida antenatal prenatal life.

  vida artificial artificial life.

  vida intrauterina prenatal life.

  vida media average life, mean lifetime.

  vida media plasmática plasma half life.

  vida posnatal postnatal life.

  vida prenatal prenatal life.

  vida sedentaria sedentary living.

  vida sexual sexual life.

  vida uterina prenatal life.

  vida vegetativa vegetative life.

vidrio *m.* glass.

vientre *m.* belly, venter.

  vientre en tabla wooden belly.

vigilancia *f.* surveillance, survey.

  vigilancia inmune, vigilancia inmunológica inmune surveillance, inmunological surveillance.

  vigilancia metastática metastatic survey.

vigilia *f.* vigilance, wakefulness.

vigor *m.* vigor.

vinculación *f.* bonding.

  vinculación afectiva f. bonding.

  vinculación maternoinfantil f. maternal-infant bonding.

vínculo *m.* vinculum.

violáceo, -a *adj.* violaceous.

violación *f.* rape, violation.

violación marital marital rape.

violación de menores statutory rape.

violación por conocido date rape, acquaintaince rape.

violar *v.* rape.

violeta *adj.* violet.

viral *adj.* viral.

viremia *f.* viremia.

virgen *adj.* virgin.

virginidad *f.* virginity.

viriasis *f.* viral infection.

viricida *adj.* viricidal.

vírico, -ca *adj.* viral.

viril *adj.* virile.

virilidad *f.* virility.

virilización *f.* virilization.

virilizante *adj.* virilizing.

virión *m.* virion.

virosis *f.* virosis.

　virosis hemorrágica del noroeste bonaerense Argentine hemorrhagic fever.

virtual *adj.* virtual.

virucida *adj.* viricidal.

viruela *f.* smallpox, variola.

virulento, -ta *adj.* virulent.

virus *m.* virus.

virustático, -ca *adj.* virustatic.

víscera *f.* viscera, viscus.

visceral *adj.* visceral.

visceralgia *f.* visceralgia.

viscoelasticidad *f.* viscoelasticity.

viscosidad *f.* viscosity.

visibilidad *f.* visibility.

visible *adj.* visible.

visión *f.* sight, vision.

　visión central central vision.

　visión de cerca near sight.

visión de color color vision.

visión corta short sight.

visión diurna day sight.

visión doble double vision.

visión escotópica scotopic vision.

visión estereoscópica stereoscopic vision.

visión de lejos long sight, far sight.

visión monocular monocular vision.

visión nocturna night vision.

visita *f.* visit.

vista *f.* sight, view.

　vista cansada presbyopia.

　vista cercana short sight.

　vista corta short sight.

　vista diurna day sight.

　vista doble double vision.

　vista larga, vista lejana long sight.

　vista nocturna night sight.

visual *adj.* visual.

visualización *f.* visualization.

visualizar *v.* visualize.

vital *adj.* vital.

vitalidad *f.* vitality.

vitalizar *v.* vitalize.

vitamina *f.* vitamin.

vitaminoterapia *f.* vitamin therapy.

vitelino, -na *adj.* vitelline.

vitíligo *m.* vitiligo.

vitrectomía *f.* vitrectomy.

vítreo *m.* vitreous body, corpus vitreum.

　vítreo desprendido detached vitreous body.

vivencia *f.* internal experience.

vivíparo, -ra *adj.* viviparous.

vivisección *f.* vivisection.

vivo, -va *adj.* alive.

vocal *adj.* vocal.

volátil *adj.* volatile.

volemia *f.* blood volume.

volumen *m.* volume .

   volumen corpuscular medio (VCM) mean corpuscular volume (MCV).

   volumen sanguíneo blood volume .

voluntad *f.* will.

voluntario, -ria *adj.* voluntary.

vólvulo *m.* volvulus.

vómer *m.* vomer.

vomitar *v.* vomit.

vomitivo *m.* vomitory.

vomitivo, -va *adj.* vomitive.

vómito[1] *m.* vomit.

   vómito bilioso bilious vomit.

   vómito hiperácido gastroxynsis.

   vómito negro black vomit, vomitus niger.

   vómito en posos de café coffee-ground vomit.

   vómito de sangre hematemesis.

vómito[2] *m.* vomiting.

   vómito del embarazo vomiting of pregnancy.

   vómito incoercible incoercible vomiting.

   vómito matinal morning vomiting.

   vómito periódico periodic vomiting.

   vómito en escopetazo projectile vomiting.

   vómito recurrente recurrent vomiting.

vómito[3] *m.* vomitus.

   vómito negro vomitus niger.

vortex vortex.

voyeurismo *m.* voyeurism, scopophilia.

voz *f.* voice, voix, vox.

   voz cavernosa cavernous voice.

   voz de falsete eunuchoid voice.

   voz susurrada whispered voice.

vuelta *f.* tour.

vulgar *adj.* vulgaris.

vulnerabilidad *f.* vulnerability.

vulnerable *adj.* vulnerable.

vulva *f.* vulva.

vulvar *adj.* vulval, vulvar.

vulvitis *f.* vulvitis.

X

xantelasma *m.* xanthelasma.

xantelasmatosis *f.* xanthelasmatosis.

xantina *f.* xanthin, xanthine.

xantogranuloma *m.* xanthogranuloma.

xantogranulomatosis *f.* xanthogranulomatosis.

xantoma *m.* xanthoma.

xantomatosis *f.* xanthomatosis.

xantosis *f.* xanthosis.

xenofobia *f.* xenophobia.

xenofonía *f.* xenophonia.

xenoinjerto *m.* xenograft.

xerodermia *f.* xeroderma

xerosis *f.* xerosis.

xerostomía *f.* xerostomia.

xifoide *adj.* xiphoid.

xifoides *adj.* xiphoid.

xifoiditis *f.* xiphoiditis.

xilosa *f.* xylose.

Y-Z

yatrogénesis *f.* iatrogenesis.
yatrogenia *f.* iatrogeny.
yatrogénico, -ca *adj.* iatrogenic.
yatrógeno, -na *adj.* iatrogenic.
yeso[1] *m.* cast.
yeso[2] *m.* gypsum, plaster.
yeyunal *adj.* jejunal.
yeyunectomía *f.* jejunectomy.
yeyunitis *f.* jejunitis.
yeyuno *m.* jejunum.
yo *m.* ego.
yodado, -da *adj.* iodinated, iodized.
yodar *v.* iodinate, iodize.
yódico, -ca *adj.* iodic.
yodo *m.* iodine.
yodopsina *f.* iodopsin.
yodoterapia *f.* iodotherapy.
yoduro *m.* iodide.
yugular *adj.* jugular.
yunque *m.* anvil, incus.
yuxtaarticular *adj.* juxta-articular.
zambo, -ba *adj.* knock-kneed.
zapato *m.* shoe.
  zapato para escayola cast shoe.

zapato de horma normal normal last shoe.
  zapato ortopédico de tacón bajo orthopedic Oxford shoe.
zigoma *m.* zygoma.
zimógeno, -na *adj.* zymogenic, zymogenous, zymogic.
zona *f.* area, site, zone, zona.
  zona de apoyo rest area.
  zona de descarga relief area.
  zona epileptógena epileptogenic zone, epileptogenous zone.
  zona erógena, zona erotógena erogenous zone, erotogenic zone.
  zona gatillo trigger zone.
  zona visual visual zone.
zoofilia *f.* zoophilia.
zoología *f.* zoology.
zoom *m.* zoom.
zoonosis *f.* zoonosis.
zoospermia *f.* zoospermia.
zoster *m.* zoster.
  zoster oftálmico ophthalmic zoster, zoster ophthalmicus.
zumbido *m.* hum, bourdonnement, tinnitus.
  zumbido vibratorio vibratory tinnitus.
zurdo, -da *m. y adj.* left-handed.

Medical Spanish Phrasebook

Greetings and Basics

Hello.	Hola.
My name is…	Me llamo…
I am your nurse. (male)	Soy su enfermero.
I am your nurse. (female)	Soy su enfermera.
I am your doctor. (male)	Soy su doctor.
I am your doctor. (female)	Soy su doctora.
Good morning.	Buenos días.
Good afternoon.	Buenas tardes.
Good evening.	Buenas noches.
How are you?	¿Cómo está?
Very well.	Muy bien.
Nice to meet you.	Mucho gusto.
Thank you.	Gracias.
You're welcome.	De nada.
Please.	Por favor.
Do you speak English?	¿Habla inglés?
Do you understand?	¿Entiende?
I don't understand.	No entiendo.
Speak slower, please.	Hable más despacio, por favor.
Repeat, please.	Repita, por favor.
Do you have any questions?	¿Tiene preguntas?

Patient Admission

What is your name?	¿Cómo se llama?
What is your address?	¿Cuál es su dirección?

What is your phone number?	¿Cuál es su número de teléfono?
What is your Social Security number?	¿Cuál es su número de seguro social?
What medical insurance do you have?	¿Cuál seguro médico tiene?
Do you have your medical insurance card?	¿Tiene su tarjeta de seguro médico?
Do you take any medication?	¿Toma medicina?
How old are you?	¿Cuántos años tiene?
What is your date of birth?	¿Cuál es su fecha de nacimiento?
Where are you from?	¿De dónde es?
Are you married? (to a male)	¿Es casado?
Are you married? (to a female)	¿Es casada?
Are you single? (to a male)	¿Es soltero?
Are you single? (to a female)	¿Es soltera?
Are you widowed? (to a male)	¿Es viudo?
Are you widowed? (to a female)	¿Es viuda?
Do you have any children?	¿Tiene hijos?
Do you have a relative with you?	¿Tiene un pariente con usted?
Sign here to give your consent.	Firme aquí para dar su consentimiento.

Medical History

Have you or anyone in your family had . . .	¿Ha tenido o tiene alguien en su familia…
. . . allergies?	… alergias?
. . . asthma?	… asma?
. . . bleeding problems?	… problemas de hemorragia?
. . . breast disease?	… enfermedad de los senos?
. . . bronchitis?	… bronquitis?

. . . cancer? What type?	. . . cáncer? ¿Qué tipo?
. . . convulsions?	. . . convulsiones?
. . . diabetes?	. . . diabetes?
. . . emotional problems or depression?	. . . problemas emocionales o depresión?
. . . frequent headaches?	. . . dolores frecuentes de cabeza?
. . . glaucoma?	. . . glaucoma?
. . . heart attack?	. . . ataque del corazón?
. . . heart disease?	. . . enfermedad del corazón?
. . . high blood pressure?	. . . presión alta?
. . . high cholesterol?	. . . colesterol alto?
. . . kidney disease?	. . . enfermedad de los riñones?
. . . liver disease?	. . . enfermedad del hígado?
. . . obesity?	. . . obesidad?
. . . osteoporosis?	. . . osteoporosis?
. . . pneumonia?	. . . neumonía?
. . . rheumatic fever?	. . . fiebre reumática?
. . . strokes or blood clots?	. . . derrames cerebrales o coágulos de sangre?
. . . surgeries? What type?	. . . operaciones? ¿Qué tipo?
. . . thyroid disease?	. . . enfermedad de la tiroides?
. . . tuberculosis?	. . . tuberculosis?
. . . venereal diseases?	. . . enfermedades venéreas?
Is your mother living or deceased?	¿Está su madre viva o muerta?
Is your father living or deceased?	¿Está su padre vivo o muerto?
Do you smoke?	¿Fuma?
How many cigarettes do you smoke in a day?	¿Cuántos cigarrillos fuma en un día?

Do you drink alcohol?	¿Toma alcohol?
How many beers do you drink in a day?	¿Cuántas cervezas toma en un día?
What drugs do you use for fun?	¿Cuáles drogas usa para divertirse?
How often?	¿Con qué frecuencia?
Would you say that you . . .	**¿Diría que…**
. . . are healthy?	… es saludable?
. . . are sickly?	… es enfermizo?
. . . sometimes get sick?	… a veces se enferma?
. . . never get sick?	… nunca se enferma?
Would you say that your weight . . .	**¿Diría que su peso…**
. . . has gone down?	… ha bajado?
. . . has gone up?	… ha subido?
. . . is the same as always?	… es igual que siempre?
Do you feel less hungry than usual?	¿Siente menos hambre que de costumbre?

Chief Complaint

What's going on?	¿Qué pasa?
What's wrong, sir?	¿Qué tiene, señor?
What's wrong, ma'am?	¿Qué tiene, señora?
Why did you come to the hospital?	¿Por qué vino al hospital?
Do you have pain?	¿Tiene dolor?
When did this problem start?	¿Cuándo comenzó este problema?
Does this stop you from working?	¿Le impide este problema trabajar?
Has this problem affected . . .	**¿Este problema ha afectado…**
. . . your life at home?	… su casa?
. . . your work?	… su trabajo?
. . . your social activities?	… sus actividades sociales?

Have you had this problem before?	¿Ha tenido este problema antes?
Did it start suddenly?	¿Comenzó de repente?
Did it start little by little?	¿Comenzó poco a poco?
Do you have this problem constantly?	¿Tiene este problema constantemente?
How many times a day?	¿Cuántas veces al día?
When do you feel worse . . .	**¿Cuándo se siente peor…**
. . . in the morning?	… en la mañana?
. . . in the afternoon?	… en la tarde?
. . . at night?	… en la noche?
Do you have any additional symptoms?	¿Tiene síntomas adicionales?
Have you seen the doctor lately?	¿Ha visto al doctor recientemente?
Is there anything that helps relieve this problem?	¿Hay algo que le ayude a aliviar este problema?
Are you taking medicine you brought from your country?	¿Toma medicina traída de su país?
What is the worst thing that is happening?	¿Qué es lo peor que está pasando?

Pain

Do you have pain?	¿Tiene dolor?
Did it develop slowly?	¿Le apareció lentamente?
Did it develop suddenly?	¿Le apareció de repente?
Is there anything that alleviates the pain?	¿Hay algo que alivie el dolor?
When did the pain begin?	¿Cuándo comenzó el dolor?
Where does it hurt?	¿Dónde le duele?
Does it hurt when I apply pressure?	¿Le duele cuando pongo presión?
Does it hurt when I remove pressure?	¿Le duele cuando quito presión?

Do you have the pain . . .	¿Tiene el dolor…
. . . all the time?	… todo el tiempo?
. . . in the morning?	… por la mañana?
. . . at night?	… por la noche?
. . . before eating?	… antes de comer?
. . . after eating?	… después de comer?

What kind of pain is it?	¿Qué tipo de dolor es?
A little?	¿Un poco?
A lot?	¿Mucho?
Dull?	¿Sordo?
Severe?	¿Severo?
Mild?	¿Leve?
Sharp?	¿Agudo?
Stabbing?	¿Punzante?
Throbbing?	¿Pulsativo?
Shooting? Like a knife?	¿Fulgurante? ¿Como un cuchillo?
Burning?	¿Quemante?
Constant?	¿Constante?
Intermittent?	¿Intermitente?
Cramping?	¿Como un calambre?

Physical Exam

I am going to examine you. (to a male)	Lo voy a examinar.
I am going to examine you. (to a female)	La voy a examinar.
I am going to tap here.	Voy a dar un golpecito aquí.
I am going to listen to your heart.	Voy a escuchar su corazón.

I am going to take . . .	**Voy a tomar…**
. . . a sample.	… una muestra.
. . . your pulse.	… su pulso.
. . . your blood pressure.	… su presión de sangre.
. . . your temperature.	… su temperatura.
I am going to examine your . . .	**Voy a examinar su…**
. . . abdomen.	… abdomen.
. . . throat.	… garganta.
. . . ear.	… oído.
. . . rectum.	… recto.
. . . vagina.	… vagina.
I am going to palpate your abdomen.	Voy a palpar el abdomen.
Tell me if it hurts.	Dígame si le duele.
Does it hurt when I press down?	¿Le duele cuando presiono?
Does it hurt when I let go?	¿Le duele cuando retiro la mano?
Raise your head.	Levante la cabeza.
Turn on your side.	Dése la vuelta a su lado.
Take a deep breath.	Respire profundo.
Exhale.	Exhale.

Medication Instructions

Take . . .	**Tome…**
. . . a drop.	… una gota.
. . . a teaspoon.	… una cucharadita.
. . . a tablespoon.	… una cucharada.
. . . a glass.	… un vaso.
. . . two inhalations.	… dos inhalaciones.
Apply it . . .	**Aplíquelo…**
. . . one time a day.	… una vez al día.

. . . two times a day.	. . . dos veces al dia.
. . . three . . .	. . . tres. . .
. . . four . . .	. . . cuatro. . .
. . . five . . .	. . . cinco. . .
. . . six . . .	. . . seis. . .

This medicine is taken . . .	**Esta medicina se toma. . .**
. . . by mouth.	. . . por la boca.
. . . by rectum.	. . . por el recto.
. . . intravenously.	. . . por las venas.
. . . under the tongue.	. . . por debajo de la lengua.
. . . by patch.	. . . en parche.
. . . under the skin.	. . . por debajo de la piel.
. . . orally.	. . . por la boca.
. . . nasally.	. . . por la nariz.

Avoid sunlight.	Evite la luz del sol.
Don't drive while taking this medicine.	No maneje cuando tome esta medicina.
Don't take medicine from any healer.	No tome otra medicina de ningún sanador.

Take this medicine . . .	**Tome esta medicina. . .**
. . . a half hour before every meal.	. . . media hora antes de cada comida.
. . . one hour after every meal.	. . . una hora después de cada comida.
. . . before bedtime.	. . . antes de acostarse.
. . . with food.	. . . con la comida.
. . . on an empty stomach.	. . . con el estómago vacío.

This medicine will . . .	**Esta medicina. . .**
. . . give you diarrhea.	. . . le dará diarrea.
. . . lower your blood sugar.	. . . le bajará el nivel de su azúcar en la sangre.

. . . lower your blood pressure.	. . . le bajará su presión de sangre.
. . . relieve fever and inflammation.	. . . le aliviará la fiebre y la inflamación.
. . . relieve your pain.	. . . le aliviará el dolor.

Emergencies and Injuries

Did you have . . .	¿Tuvo...
. . . an accident?	. . . un accidente?
. . . an allergic reaction?	. . . una reacción alérgica ?
. . . an anxiety attack?	. . . un ataque de ansiedad?
. . . bleeding?	. . . hemorragia?
. . . a bee sting?	. . . una picadura de abeja ?
. . . a blow to the head?	. . . un golpe a la cabeza?
. . . a bruise?	. . . un moretón?
. . . a burn?	. . . una quemadura?
. . . chest pain?	. . . dolor del pecho?
. . . a cut?	. . . una cortada?
. . . dizziness?	. . . mareos?
. . . a dog bite?	. . . una mordida de perro?
. . . domestic abuse?	. . . abuso doméstico?
. . . a fall?	. . . una caída?
. . . a fight?	. . . una pelea?
. . . a fracture?	. . . una fractura?
. . . frostbite?	. . . congelamiento?
. . . heat stroke?	. . . insolación?
. . . an overdose?	. . . una sobredosis?
. . . pain?	. . . dolor?
. . . a spasm?	. . . un espasmo?
. . . a stabbing?	. . . una puñalada?

. . . a stroke?	. . . un derrame cerebral?
Can you tell me what happened?	¿Puede decirme lo que pasó?
Do you know where you are?	¿Sabe dónde está?
Where does it hurt?	¿Dónde le duele?
Show me.	Enséñeme.
What happened to your . . .	**¿Qué le pasa a su . . .**
. . . abdomen?	. . . abdomen?
. . . ankle?	. . . tobillo?
. . . arm?	. . . brazo?
. . . back?	. . . espalda?
. . . chest?	. . . pecho?
. . . ear?	. . . oído?
. . . eye?	. . . ojo?
. . . face?	. . . cara?
. . . finger?	. . . dedo?
. . . foot?	. . . pie?
. . . hand?	. . . mano?
. . . head?	. . . cabeza?
. . . knee?	. . . rodilla?
. . . leg?	. . . pierna?
. . . mouth?	. . . boca?
. . . neck?	. . . cuello?
. . . nose?	. . . nariz?
. . . shoulder?	. . . hombro?
. . . skin?	. . . piel?
. . . stomach?	. . . estómago?
. . . teeth?	. . . dientes?
Was it burned?	¿Fue quemado?

Was it cut?	¿Fue cortado?
Was it fractured?	¿Fue fracturado?
Was it infected?	¿Fue infectado?
Was it swollen?	¿Fue hinchado?

Diagnostic Tests and Treatments

You need to have . . .	Usted necesita tener...
. . . a blood test.	... un examen de sangre.
. . . a neurological exam.	... un examen neurológico.
. . . a pregnancy test.	... una prueba de embarazo.
. . . a scan.	... un escán.
. . . an echocardiogram.	... un ecocardiograma.
. . . an EKG.	... un electrocardiograma.
. . . an ultrasound.	... un examen de ultrasonido.
. . . an x-ray.	... una radiografía.

You need . . .	Usted necesita...
. . . an antibiotic.	... un antibiótico.
. . . a bandage.	... un vendaje.
. . . a blood transfusion.	... una transfusión de sangre.
. . . a cast.	... un yeso.
. . . first aid.	... los primeros auxilios.
. . . an IV.	... un suero.
. . . medicine.	... medicina.
. . . an operation.	... una operación.
. . . oxygen.	... oxígeno.
. . . physical therapy.	... terapia física.
. . . a shot.	... una inyección.
. . . a sling.	... un cabestrillo.

| . . . stitches. | . . . los puntos. |
| . . . urgery. | . . . la cirugía. |

Specialties

You need to see a specialist in . . .	Necesita ver un especialista en...
. . . ENT.	. . . los oídos, la nariz y la garganta.
. . . ophthalmology.	. . . oftalmología.
. . . cardiology.	. . . cardiología.
. . . gastroenterology.	. . . gastroenterología.
. . . OB-GYN.	. . . ginecología.
. . . endocrinology.	. . . endocrinología.
. . . orthopedics.	. . . ortopedia.
. . . pediatrics.	. . . pediatría.
. . . neurology.	. . . neurología.
. . . dermatology.	. . . dermatología.
. . . obstetrics.	. . . obstetricia.
. . . oncology.	. . . oncología.
. . . psychiatry.	. . . psiquiatría.
. . . surgery.	. . . cirugía.

Pregnancy

It is important to take care of yourself during pregnancy.	Es importante cuidar su salud durante su embarazo.
How many times have you been pregnant?	¿Cuántas veces ha estado embarazada?
How many children do you have?	¿Cuántos hijos tiene?
Do you breast-feed them?	¿Les da pecho?
Have you ever been pregnant?	¿Ha estado alguna vez embarazada?

How many . . .	¿Cuántos…
. . . pregnancies?	… embarazos?
. . . children?	… hijos?
. . . miscarriages?	… abortos espontáneos?
. . . abortions?	… abortos?

What is the date of your last period? ¿Cuándo fue su última regla?

You are . . . weeks pregnant. **Tiene… semanas de embarazo.**

. . . six . . . … seis…

. . . ten . . . … diez…

Have you had any bleeding? ¿Ha sangrado?

Birth Control

Are you using birth control now? ¿Usa algún método para evitar el embarazo?

Do you use . . .	¿Usa…
. . . the pill?	… la píldora anticonceptiva?
. . . the diaphragm?	… el diafragma?
. . . an IUD?	… el dispositivo intrauterino?
. . . condoms?	… preservativos?
. . . the rhythm method?	… el método del ritmo?
. . . abstinence?	… abstinencia?

How long have you used this method? ¿Cuánto tiempo ha usado este método?

Have you experienced any of the following taking the pill? **¿Ha sentido alguna de estas molestias tomando la píldora?**

Headaches? ¿Dolores de cabeza ?

Vision changes? ¿Cambios de la visión?

Pain or swelling in the legs? ¿Dolor o hinchazón en las piernas?

Chest pain? ¿Dolor en el pecho?

| Shortness of breath? | ¿Falta de aire? |
| Weight loss or gain? | ¿Pérdida o aumento de peso? |

Diabetic Patients

Are you a diabetic? (to a male)	¿Es diabético?
Are you a diabetic? (to a female)	¿Es diabética?
Do you take insulin?	¿Toma insulina?
What type of insulin?	¿Qué tipo de insulina?
Oral or by injection?	¿Oral o inyectada?
When was the last time you took insulin?	¿Cuándo fue la última vez que tomó insulina?
When did you last eat?	¿Cuándo fue la última vez que comió?
Are you measuring your sugar?	¿Mide su azúcar?
Before and after meals?	¿Antes y después de las comidas?
Are you keeping a record of your sugar levels?	¿Toma notas de los niveles de su azúcar?
Are you taking your insulin?	¿Toma su insulina?
Are you exercising?	¿Hace ejercicio?
Have you had your vision checked?	¿Ha tenido su visión chequeada?
Have you had your feet checked?	¿Ha tenido sus pies chequeados?
You need to have . . .	**Necesita tener…**
. . . blood sugar records.	… notas del nivel del azúcar.
. . . better control of your blood sugar.	… mejor control de los niveles de su azúcar.
. . . a dilated eye exam.	… un examen con los ojos dilatados.
. . . a finger stick test.	… un examen pinchando el dedo.
. . . a foot exam.	… un examen del pie.
. . . a urine protein test.	… un examen de la proteína en la orina.

Pay attention to . . .	**Preste más atención a...**
. . . not smoking.	… evitar fumar.
. . . blood sugar count before and after meals.	… contar el nivel del azúcar antes y después de las comidas.
. . . changes in vision.	… los cambios de la visión.
. . . changes in your skin.	… los cambios de la piel.
. . . decreased sense of touch.	… la disminución del sentido del tacto.
. . . difficulty picking up small objects.	… las dificultades para recoger objetos pequeños.
. . . lack of sensation in any part of the body.	… la falta de sensación en alguna parte del cuerpo.
. . . swelling in your legs or hands.	… la hinchazón en las piernas y las manos.

Eat your meals at the same time each day.

Coma sus comidas a la misma hora cada día.

Take your medicine at the same time each day.

Tomar su medicina a la misma hora cada día.

Monitor your cholesterol level.

Controle el nivel de su colesterol.

Check your blood pressure regularly.

Chequee regularmente su presión de la sangre.

Are you eating measured portions?

¿Come porciones medidas?

You need to have a diet . . .	**Necesita tener una dieta...**
. . . low in cholesterol.	… baja en colesterol.
. . . low in sodium.	… baja en sodio.
. . . low in sugar.	… baja en azúcar.
. . . high in fiber.	… alta en fibra.
. . . low in carbohydrates.	… baja en carbohidratos.

Cardiovascular System

Do you have . . .	**¿Tiene…**
Have you had . . .	**¿Ha tenido…**
. . . cardiovascular disease?	… enfermedad cardiovascular?
. . . chest pain?	… dolor de pecho?
. . . embolism?	… embolismo?
. . . fainting?	… desmayos?
. . . high blood pressure?	… presión alta?
. . . infarction?	… infarto?
. . . irregular heartbeat?	… latidos irregulares del corazón?
. . . low blood pressure?	… presión baja?
. . . mitral valve prolapse?	… prolapso de la válvula mitral?
. . . obesity?	… obesidad?
. . . palpitations?	… palpitaciones?
. . . poor circulation?	… mala circulación de la sangre?
. . . shortness of breath?	… falta de aire?
. . . stroke?	… derrame cerebral?
. . . thrombosis?	… trombosis?
Have you ever had a heart attack?	¿Ha tenido alguna vez un ataque de corazón?
Has this ever happened before?	¿Ha ocurrido esto antes?
Do you have a history of heart problems?	¿Tiene un historial de problemas del corazón?
Have you had . . .	**¿Ha tenido…**
. . . chest pain?	… dolor en el pecho?
. . . headaches?	… dolores de cabeza?
. . . pressure in your chest?	… presión en el pecho?
. . . shortness of breath?	… falta de aire?

. . . swollen ankles?	. . . los tobillos hinchados?
. . . dizziness?	. . . mareos?
. . . irregular heartbeat?	. . . latidos irregulares del corazón?
Do you have shortness of breath when . . .	**¿Tiene la falta de aire cuando...**
. . . at rest?	. . . descansa?
. . . walking?	. . . camina?
. . . climbing stairs?	. . . sube las escaleras?
. . . exercising?	. . . hace ejercicio?
Is there anyone in your family who has . . .	**¿Hay alguien en su familia que haya...**
. . . suffered from heart problems?	. . . sufrido de problemas del corazón?
. . . suffered from high blood pressure?	. . . sufrido de presión alta?
. . . had a stroke?	. . . tenido un derrame cerebral?
Where does it hurt?	¿Dónde le duele?
Does the pain radiate to the arms?	¿Corre el dolor a los brazos?
Does it hurt when you breathe?	¿Le duele cuando respira?
You need to have . . .	**Usted necesita tener...**
. . . an angiogram.	. . . un angiograma.
. . . an angioplasty.	. . . una angioplastia.
. . . blood tests.	. . . pruebas de sangre.
. . . a breathing test.	. . . una prueba de la respiración.
. . . catheterization.	. . . cateterismo.
. . . a chest x-ray.	. . . una radiografía del pecho.
. . . an echocardiogram.	. . . un ecocardiograma.
. . . an EKG.	. . . un electrocardiograma.
. . . heart surgery.	. . . cirugía del corazón.
. . . a Holter monitor.	. . . un monitor de Holter.

. . . an MRI.	. . . una imagen de resonancia magnética.
. . . a pacemaker.	. . . un marcapaso.
. . . a stress test.	. . . un examen del estrés.
. . . a triple bypass.	. . . un bypass triple.
. . . a quadruple bypass.	. . . un bypass cuádruple.

Gastrointestinal System

Do you have problems with . . .	**¿Tiene problemas con...**
. . . abdominal tenderness?	. . . dolor tocando el abdomen?
. . . constipation?	. . . estreñimiento?
. . . diarrhea?	. . . diarrea?
. . . indigestion?	. . . indigestión?
. . . cramps?	. . . calambres?
. . . vomiting?	. . . vómitos?
. . . dizziness?	. . . mareos?
Does it hurt when I press here?	¿Le duele cuando presiono aquí?
Are you moving your bowels normally?	¿Es su excremento regular?
Any blood in the urine or stools?	¿Hay sangre en la orina o el excremento?
Have you ever had . . .	**Ha tenido alguna vez...**
. . . a stomach ulcer?	. . . una úlcera en el estómago?
. . . inflammatory bowel disease?	. . . enfermedad inflamatoria del intestino?
. . . history of GI disease or bleeding?	. . . un historial de enfermedad o sangrado gastrointestinal?
Do you have . . .	**¿Tiene...**
. . . stomach acid in your throat?	. . . ácido del estómago en la garganta?

. . . stomach pain?	. . . dolor en el estómago?
. . . gas?	. . . gas?
. . . a metallic taste in your mouth?	. . . un sabor metálico en la boca?

Do you eat or drink . . . **¿Toma...**

. . . more than one cup of coffee a day?	. . . más de una taza de café al día?
. . . carbonated drinks?	. . . bebidas gaseosas?
. . . spicy food?	. . . la comida picante?

You need to . . . **Necesita...**

. . . lower alcohol use.	. . . bajar el uso del alcohol.
. . . stop smoking.	. . . no fumar.
. . . stop overeating.	. . . dejar de comer demasiado.
. . . eliminate coffee.	. . . eliminar el café.
. . . eliminate carbonated drinks.	. . . eliminar las bebidas gaseosas.
. . . eliminate spicy food.	. . . eliminar la comida picante.
. . . sleep with your head elevated.	. . . dormir con la cabeza elevada.

Neurological Exam

Have you had . . . **¿Ha tenido...**

. . . changes or vision problems?	. . . cambios o problemas con la visión?
. . . fainting?	. . . desmayos?
. . . dizzy spells?	. . . mareos?
. . . difficulty moving part of your body?	. . . dificultad para mover una parte del cuerpo?
. . . problems remembering things?	. . . problemas recordando cosas?
. . . a recent head injury?	. . . una herida en la cabeza recientemente?
Are you taking any medications?	¿Toma medicamentos?

What were you doing before you had the seizure?	¿Qué estaba haciendo antes del ataque?
Has it happened before?	¿Ha pasado antes?
Can you describe what happened before the seizure?	¿Puede describir qué pasó justo antes del ataque?
Were you unconscious?	¿Estuvo inconsciente?
For how long?	¿Por cuánto tiempo?
Is there any part of your body that feels . . .	**¿Hay alguna parte de su cuerpo que sienta…**
. . . numb?	… dormida?
. . . like pins and needles?	… como hormigueo?
. . . weak?	… débil sin fuerzas?
. . . painful?	… con dolores?
. . . heavy?	… pesada?
I'm going to check your eyes.	Voy a revisarle los ojos.
Follow my fingers with your eyes without moving your head.	Siga mis dedos con los ojos sin mover la cabeza.
Open your mouth and say "ahhh."	Abra la boca y diga "aaaah".
Shrug your shoulders.	Levante los hombros.
Smile.	Sonría.
Close your eyes.	Cierre los ojos.
Open your eyes.	Abra los ojos.
Touch the tip of your nose with your finger.	Toque la punta de su nariz con el dedo.
I'm going to check your strength.	Voy a chequear su fuerza.
Pull.	Jale.
Push.	Empuje.
Squeeze my fingers.	Apriete mis dedos.
Stand and close your eyes.	Párese y cierre los ojos.

Walk on your toes.	Camine de puntillas.
Walk on your heels.	Camine con los talones.

Mental Health

Do you feel . . .	**¿Siente…**
. . . sadness?	… tristeza?
. . . anxiety?	… ansiedad?
. . . emptiness?	… vacío?
. . . hopelessness?	… desesperanza?
. . . guilt?	… culpabilidad?
. . . worthlessness?	… inutilidad?
. . . irritability?	… irritabilidad?
How long have you felt this way?	¿Hace cuánto tiempo que se ha sentido así?
Do you have interest in activities?	¿Tiene interés en actividades?
Do you have difficulty concentrating?	¿Tiene dificultad para concentrarse?
Do you feel . . .	**¿Siente…**
. . . decreased energy?	… falta de energía?
. . . difficulty concentrating?	… dificultad para concentrarse?
. . . difficulty remembering?	… dificultad para recordar?
. . . insomnia?	… insomnio?
. . . lack of appetite?	… que le falta el apetito?
. . . you eat too much?	… que come demasiado?
. . . you have digestive disorders?	… que tiene trastornos de digestión?
. . . chronic pain?	… dolor crónico?
Do you wake up earlier than normal?	¿Siente que se despierta más temprano que lo normal?
Do you oversleep?	¿Siente que duerme demasiado?

Do you think about dying?	¿Piensa en la muerte?
Do you think about suicide?	¿Piensa en el suicidio?
Do you feel . . .	**¿Siente…**
. . . mania?	… manía?
. . . excessive elation?	… un estado excesivo de elación?
. . . racing thoughts?	… pensamientos acelerados?
. . . irritable?	… irritable?
Do you have more energy than usual?	¿Tiene más energía que lo normal?
Do you have less need for sleep?	¿Necesita dormir menos?
How long have you felt this way?	¿Hace cuánto tiempo que se ha sentido así?